Neurological Disorders and Imaging Physics, Volume 2

Engineering and clinical perspectives of multiple sclerosis

Neurological Disorders and Imaging Physics, Volume 2

Engineering and clinical perspectives of multiple sclerosis

Ayman El-Baz
University of Lousiville, USA

Jasjit S Suri
AtheroPoint, CA, USA

IOP Publishing, Bristol, UK

ISBN 978-0-7503-1762-7 (ebook)
ISBN 978-0-7503-1760-3 (print)
ISBN 978-0-7503-1763-4 (mobi)

DOI 10.1088/978-0-7503-1762-7

Version: 20191101

IOP ebooks

British Library Cataloguing-in-Publication Data: A catalogue record for this book is available from the British Library.

Published by IOP Publishing, wholly owned by The Institute of Physics, London

IOP Publishing, Temple Circus, Temple Way, Bristol, BS1 6HG, UK

US Office: IOP Publishing, Inc., 190 North Independence Mall West, Suite 601, Philadelphia, PA 19106, USA

With love and affection to my mother and father, whose loving spirit sustains me still.
Ayman El-Baz
To my late loving parents, immediate family, and children.
Jasjit S Suri

Contents

Preface

This volume of the book discusses the state-of-the-art topics that investigate multiple sclerosis (MS), which is the most common immune-mediated disorder affecting the central nervous system. In 2015, about 2.3 million people were affected globally with rates varying widely in different regions and among different populations. That year about 18 900 people died from MS, up from 12 000 in 1990. Multiple sclerosis is a demyelinating disease in which the insulating covers of nerve cells in the brain and spinal cord are damaged. This damage disrupts the ability of parts of the nervous system to communicate, resulting in a range of signs and symptoms, including physical, mental, and sometimes psychiatric problems. Specific symptoms can include double vision, blindness in one eye, muscle weakness, trouble with sensation, or trouble with coordination. The symptons of MS will be covered in this book, in addition to several related active research topics, such as exoskeleton-assisted rehabilitation training, combinational drug therapies, characterization of balance disorders, hope, transcranial direct current stmiulation, oxidative stress, auditory neuroprosthetics, neuropsychological assessment, imaging disconnection, gait analysis, brain–computer interfaces, and dysarthria.

In summary, the main aim of this book is to help advance scientific research within the broad field of MS. This book focuses on major trends and challenges in this area, and it presents work aimed to identify new techniques and their use in biomedical image analysis.

Ayman El-Baz
Jasjit S Suri

Acknowledgements

The completion of this book could not have been possible without the participation and assistance of so many people whose names may not all be enumerated. Their contributions are sincerely appreciated and gratefully acknowledged. However, the editors would like to express their deep appreciation and indebtedness particularly to Dr Ali H Mahmoud and Heba Kandil for their endless support.

Ayman El-Baz
Jasjit S Suri

Editor biographies

Ayman El-Baz

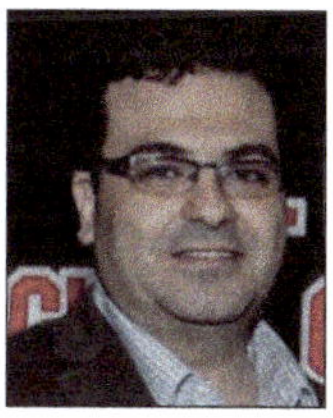

Ayman El-Baz is a Professor, University Scholar, and Chair of the Bioengineering Department at the University of Louisville, Kentucky. Dr El-Baz earned his BSc and MSc degrees in electrical engineering in 1997 and 2001, respectively. He earned his PhD in electrical engineering from the University of Louisville in 2006. In 2009, Dr El-Baz was named a Coulter Fellow for his contributions to the field of biomedical translational research. Dr El-Baz has 17 years of hands-on experience in the fields of bio-imaging modeling and non-invasive computer-assisted diagnosis systems. He has authored or coauthored more than 500 technical articles (133 journals, 25 books, 57 book chapters, 212 refereed conference papers, 143 abstracts, and 27 US patents and Disclosures).

Jasjit S Suri

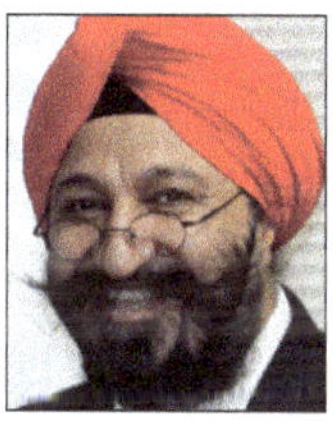

Jasjit S Suri is an innovator, scientist, visionary, industrialist and an internationally known world leader in biomedical engineering. Dr Suri has spent over 25 years in the field of biomedical engineering/devices and its management. He received his PhD from the University of Washington, Seattle and his Business Management Sciences degree from Weatherhead, Case Western Reserve University, Cleveland, Ohio. Dr Suri was crowned with President's Gold medal in 1980 and made Fellow of the American Institute of Medical and Biological Engineering for his outstanding contributions. In 2018, he was awarded the Marquis Life Time Achievement Award for his outstanding contributions and dedication to medical imaging and its management.

List of contributors

Marika Berchicci
Department of Movement, Human and Health Sciences, University of Rome 'Foro Italico', Rome—Italy

Giuliana Lucci
Department of Human Science University G. Marconi

Sabrina Pitzalis
Department of Movement, Human and Health Sciences, University of Rome 'Foro Italico', Rome—Italy and Santa Lucia Foundation (IRCCS Fondazione Santa Lucia)

Valentina Sulpizio
Santa Lucia Foundation (IRCCS Fondazione Santa Lucia) and Department of Biomedical and Neuromotor Sciences, University of Bologna, Bologna—Italy

Maria Grazia Grasso
Santa Lucia Foundation (IRCCS Fondazione Santa Lucia)

Maurizio Ripani
Department of Movement, Human and Health Sciences, University of Rome 'Foro Italico', Rome—Italy

Stefano Paolucci
Santa Lucia Foundation (IRCCS Fondazione Santa Lucia)

Marco Iosa
Santa Lucia Foundation (IRCCS Fondazione Santa Lucia)

Gaspare Galati
Department of Psychology University of Rome 'La Sapienza' and Santa Lucia Foundation (IRCCS Fondazione Santa Lucia)

Francesco Di Russo
Department of Movement, Human and Health Sciences, University of Rome 'Foro Italico', Rome—Italy

Ian Cock
Griffith University

Matthew Cheesman
Griffith University

Hua CAO
HEI—Yncrea Hauts-de-France

Laurent Peyrodie
HEI—Yncrea Hauts-de-France

Olivier Agnani
Groupe Hospitalier de l'Institut Catholique de Lille (GHICL)

Andrew Soundy
University of Birmingham

Khadije Janalipour
Urmia University

Michael Shaw
New York University Langone Health

Giuseppina Pilloni
University of Cagliari/New York University Langone Health

Leigh Charvet
New York University Langone Health

Necat Yilmaz
SBU-AEAH

Esin Eren
SBU-AEAH

Shashank Ghai
Institute of Sports Science, Leibniz University Hannover, Germany

Ishan Ghai
RSGBIOGEN, New Delhi, India

Ornella Argento
IRCCS 'Santa Lucia' Foundation, Rome

Ugo Nocentini
IRCCS 'Santa Lucia' Foundation, Rome

Riccardo Manca
University of Sheffield

Basil Sharrack
Sheffield Teaching Hospital

Annalena Venneri
University of Sheffield

Hilal Keklicek
Trakya University

Sezer Ulukaya
Trakya University

Víctor Martínez-Cagigal
University of Valladolid

Eduardo Santamaría-Vázquez
University of Valladolid

Javier Gomez-Pilar
University of Valladolid

Roberto Hornero
University of Valladolid

Kostas Konstantopoulos
European University Cyprus

Dimitrios Karangioules
European University Cyprus

Heba Kandil
University of Louisville

Ahmed Soliman
University of Louisville

Ali Mahmoud
University of Louisville

Ahmed Shalaby
University of Louisville

Fatma Taher
Zayed University

Mohammed Ghazal
Abu Dhabi University

Adel Elmagraby
University of Louisville

Ayman El-Baz
University of Louisville

IOP Publishing

Neurological Disorders and Imaging Physics, Volume 2
Engineering and clinical perspectives of multiple sclerosis
Ayman El-Baz and Jasjit S Suri

Chapter 1

Exoskeleton-assisted rehabilitation training improves cognitive and motor functions in multiple sclerosis patients

M Berchicci, G Lucci, S Pitzalis, V Sulpizio, MG Grasso, M Ripani, S Paolucci, M Iosa, G Galati and F Di Russo

Background: As previously found, a single exoskeleton application did improve mobility in multiple sclerosis (MS) patients, with effects also at brain level.

Objective: To evaluate the use of the same exoskeleton, the 'Human Body Posturizer' (HBP), to assist rehabilitation processes in MS patients during a 6-week intervention using a pilot randomized controlled trial.

Methods: Twelve patients were evaluated using multiple neurological, motor, functional and cognitive testing before and after 6-week multidisciplinary rehabilitation training performed wearing normal clothes (control group) or wearing the HBP (experimental group). Participants were randomly assigned to control or experimental group. Event-related potentials were recorded to measure temporal brain dynamics during cognitive testing.

Results: Both groups improved performance as shown by neurologic, motor and functional testing, but only the experimental group showed positive treatment effects in cognitive tasks, disability status and fatigue severity. In cognitive tasks, the experimental group showed significant benefits in terms of processing speed and response accuracy, and, at brain level, they showed enhancement in proactive preparatory activity in frontal and prefrontal cortices, and stronger post-stimulus reactive activity in the anterior insula related to a more efficient stimulus-response decision making. No effects were reported for visual information processing.

Conclusion: Both rehabilitation protocols are supported by objective neurophysiological and mobility improvements, but the HBP intervention was more effective especially reducing disability status and fatigue, likely stimulating cognitive processing in prefrontal cortex.

doi:10.1088/978-0-7503-1762-7ch1

1.1 Introduction

Multiple sclerosis (MS) is a neurological disease characterized by a multi-focal inflammation in the central nervous system, leading to the demyelination of axons. Its aetiology is still unknown and both environmental and genetic factors seem to increase the risk of developing the disease [52]. People with MS experience several symptoms, such as fatigue, weakness, spasticity, walking difficulties, visual, bladder and bowel problems, sexual dysfunction, pain, numbness and tingling [46]; less common symptoms are headache and tremor. The first intervention is the pharmacological treatment (e.g. beta interferon and glatiramer acetate) that modifies the disease progression [28]. Medicines diminish the relapse rates in relapsing remitting MS types, which is the most common form of MS; thus, drugs reduce and delay the development of disability [28]. Several researches have investigated different therapies for treating MS symptoms to improve the quality of life, such as nutritional, cognitive, speech-language therapies, and multidisciplinary rehabilitation, with this latter being considered one of the most effective [29].

Walking is considered as an outcome in clinical research and practice involving MS patients [36]. Many MS patients face increasing difficulties with walking, which interfere with the ability to adequately exercise. Physical exercise has proven to have many benefits for people with MS, preventing secondary disorders, such as weight gain, cardiovascular disease, metabolic syndrome and osteoporosis [37], but also influencing fatigue, cardiovascular fitness, muscle strength, walking and gait ability, and even depression. It has been proposed that walking performance could be used as a measure of physical activity [48].

Another common symptom in MS is the cognitive impairment (experienced by approximately 50% of MS patients), especially when assessed by neuropsychological tests that focus on mental processing speed, episodic memory, and some aspects of executive function, since these cannot be clearly recognizable in routine neurological examination [3, 45]. There has been increasing interest in cognitive benefits of physical exercise in neurological population. Indeed, one of the worst MS effects at the brain level is the hippocampal atrophy, which leads to memory deficits. Since both animal and human findings [22, 53] agree on the positive effects played by physical exercise on hippocampal neurogenesis, the benefits of aerobic exercise on memory impairments assessed in MS patients has been supported [14, 33, 38, 48]. There is further evidence of coupling between walking performance and cognitive processing speed in MS [4, 21]. However, when the mobility and ambulation deficits are more severe, it is quite difficult to walk and, thus, to exercise. Technological devices, such as lower extremity gait trainer, may provide further improvements in MS patients' neurorehabilitation, supporting adequate stability needed for successful walking and improving the ability to perform frequent and repetitive movements, which would, in turn, also allow changes in the brain. In an earlier study [19], we observed that one application of a passive and fully articulated exoskeleton, called Human Body Posturizer (HBP), improved mobility, response accuracy and ambulation in MS patients. Notably, these effects were associated with changes at the brain level, particularly in the prefrontal cortex, as revealed by electrophysiological measures. The HBP, transmitting proprioceptive signals on correct posture to supra-axial nerves, facilitates the central nervous system in integrating and interpreting body signals of postural dynamics [19]. The HBP may increase the degree of symmetry in trunk and lumbar regions of the spinal column and also reduce the risk of falling in the elderly [16, 17]. Here, we evaluate the use of the HBP to assist the rehabilitation process in individuals with MS during a 6-week intervention using a pilot randomized controlled trial. Figure 1.1 displays the HBP worn by a model.

The primary goal of this study is to compare the effects of a 6-week multi-disciplinary rehabilitation intervention on cognitive functions of MS patients following the intervention alone, and patients following the same intervention and also wearing the HBP during physical exercise. Cognitive functions were objectively recorded during a complex visuo-motor discriminative response task (DRT) at both brain level, measuring the electroencephalographic (EEG)-based event-related potentials (ERP), and behavioural level, measuring response speed and accuracy.

The second aim is to compare the two rehabilitation trainings in terms of improvements on neurological and functional problems frequently experienced by MS patients, such as fatigue, gait deficits, and balance disturbance, quantified using

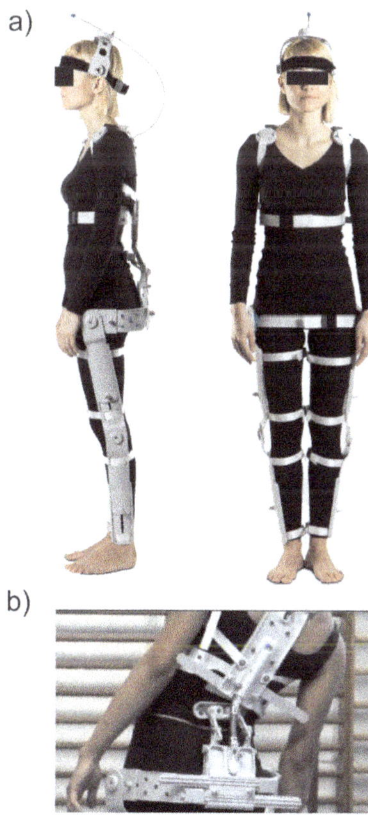

Figure 1.1. a) Lateral and front view of the HBP exoskeleton. b) Rear view showing the articulation capacities (The subject of the photograph has given written informed consent).

the most common neurological scales. Our hypothesis is that rehabilitation reinforced by the HBP could improve cognitive brain functions (especially executive functions) and mobility, and could mitigate fatigue perception during rehabilitation training.

1.2 Methods

1.2.1 Participants

Twelve MS patients were initially recruited for the study; they were randomly divided into a control and an experimental group. However, two control patients and one experimental patient did not complete the experiments and were excluded from further analysis. The two groups were age- and gender-matched (univariate tests showed lack of significant differences $p > 0.8$), as follows: control group: $N = 4$, 2 females, mean age 50.3 ± 7.3 years; experimental group: $N = 5$, 2 females, mean age 49.0 ± 7.3 years. The MS patients were selected based on the absence of other neurological disorders and gross visual pathologies, and with Expanded Disability Status Scale (EDSS) between 5 and 7. All participants were right handed (Edinburgh handedness inventory). The participants' written consent was obtained according to the Declaration of Helsinki after approval by the ethical committee of the IRCCS Santa Lucia Foundation.

1.2.2 Intervention

All patients participated in a multidisciplinary rehabilitation intervention program consisting in twice-daily exercise sessions, each 45 min long, performed 5 days a week, and lasting about 6 weeks. The program, which focused on Activities of Daily Living (ADL), was devised and coordinated by the treating physicians, and administered by qualified physiotherapists from Santa Lucia Foundation. The intervention consisted of muscle stretching, postural alignment especially at the height of the axial segments, active-assisted mobilizations and neuromuscular facilitations to improve motor recruitment. Balance training was performed during standing and dynamic tasks using exercises with progressive restrictions of support base and the use of unstable surfaces like wobble boards, balance pads or stability balls in different positions (bridge, sitting, quadrupedal, half-kneeling, kneeling, standing, one leg standing; Brichetto *et al* [13]). In the dynamic condition, dual task exercises were introduced by using a ball to create open tasks [15]. The exercises were carried out both in eyes-closed and eyes-open conditions. The control group executed these exercises wearing normal clothes, while the experimental group wore the HBP over their clothes. The HBP was calibrated for each patient regulating the subclavian and lumbosacral thrusts in order to improve the rachis straightening reactions and the stability between shoulder and pelvic girdles. Patients were instructed to perceive the proprioceptive adjustments and stimulations offered by the exoskeleton.

1.2.3 Functional and neurological assessment

The following functional measures were performed before and after the treatment:

1. 2 min Walk Test (2-WT): measurement of endurance by assessing walking distance over two minutes [24];
2. Timed 25 Foot Walk Test (T25-FW): quantitative mobility and leg function performance test based on timing walking for a distance of 25 feet [36];
3. Fatigue Severity Scale: self-report questionnaire designed to assess disabling fatigue [31];
4. Tinetti test: gait and balance test [51];
5. Berg Balance Scale (BBS): balance function assessing the performance of a functional task [10].

The following neurological measures were administered before and after the treatment:

1. Barthel scale: measurement of activities of daily living [34];
2. Expanded Disability Status Scale (EDSS): the scale quantifies disability in eight functional systems (i.e. pyramidal, cerebellar, brainstem, sensory, bowel and bladder, visual, cerebral, other), allowing neurologists to assign a functional system score in each domain [32];
3. Rivermead Mobility Index (RMI) test: mobility test [18].

Statistical analysis was performed using a 2 (Group: control versus experimental) × 2 (Treatment: pre versus post) ANOVA separately for each measure. Bonferroni post hoc comparisons were used, and the alpha level was set at 0.05.

1.2.4 Cognitive testing

1.2.4.1 Experimental task

Participants were individually tested during the discriminative response task (DRT) in a dimly lit room after mounting the EEG cap on their scalp. They were seated in front of a monitor (distance: 114 cm) with a pushbutton under the right hand. Four visual stimuli (i.e. squared configurations made by vertical and horizontal bars) were randomly displayed for 250 ms with equal probability ($p = 0.25$), and their stimulus-onset asynchrony varied from 1 to 2 s. Participants were required to press a button with their right index finger as fast and accurately as possible when the target appeared (Go stimuli; $p = 0.5$), and to withhold the response when the non-target appeared (No-Go stimuli; $p = 0.5$). The order of presentation was randomized within blocks and across participants. A total of 640 trials (320 targets and 320 non-targets) was collected during a session of about 30 min (including breaks across the 8 blocks of trials). The task was performed before and after 6 weeks in both groups following the same procedure.

1.2.4.2 Behavioral recording and analysis

Behavioral performance during the DRT was assessed measuring response time (RT) for correct trials and accuracy measured as omission errors (OM%, i.e. missed responses to targets) and commission errors (CE%, i.e. responses to non-targets). Performance consistency was also calculated as the intra-individual coefficient of variation (standard deviation of RT/mean RT). Each measure was submitted to a 2 (Group: control versus experimental) × 2 (Treatment: pre versus post) analysis of variance (ANOVA) using Bonferroni correction for multiple comparisons. Alpha level was 0.05.

1.2.4.3 Electrophysiological recording and analysis

During the DRT, EEG was recorded using two BrainAmp™ amplifiers (BrainProducts, Germany) system with 64 electrodes referenced to the left mastoid. Horizontal and vertical electrooculogram (EOG) was recorded in bipolar modality. The EEG was digitized at 250 Hz, amplified (bandpass of 0.01–60 Hz including a 50 Hz notch filter) and stored for offline averaging. The continuous signal was band-pass filtered (0.1–30 Hz) to remove movement artifacts before performing the independent component analysis (ICA; Jung *et al* [27]) that was used to correct eye-movement artifacts. Artifact rejection was performed prior to signal averaging in a semi-automatic way to discard epochs contaminated by blinks, eye movements or other signals exceeding the amplitude threshold of ±50 μV. The signal was segmented in epochs lasting 2 s: from 1100 ms before to 900 ms after stimulus onset. Pre-stimulus ERP components were measured with respect to a −1100/−900 ms baseline and target and non-target conditions were averaged. Post-stimulus ERP components were calculated with respect to the typical −200/0 ms baseline and the epochs were separately averaged for each condition (target and non-target).

Selection of time windows and sites for statistical analyses was based on both topographical distribution and previous studies (e.g. Di Russo *et al* [20]). The pre-stimulus components were measured as the mean amplitude in the −500/0 ms time windows on the following sites: the pN on Fp2 and the BP on Cz. Since no condition effects were expected in the pre-stimulus phase (i.e. the stimuli were randomly presented), the pN and the BP were calculated by averaging target and non-target trials. Both pN and BP were submitted to a 2 (Group: control versus experimental) × 2 (Treatment: pre versus post) ANOVA.

Post-stimulus ERP components were calculated as the peak amplitude and latency in the following time windows and electrodes: the P1 and the pN1 (80–150 ms) components at PO8 and AFz, respectively, and the N1 and the pP1 (130–200 ms) components at PO8 and Fp2, respectively. The pP2 and the P3 were calculated as the mean amplitude on the following time windows and sites, respectively: 200–500 ms at Fp2; 400–600 ms at Pz. Each post-stimulus ERP component was submitted to a 2 (Group: control versus experimental) × 2 (Treatment: pre versus post) × 2 (Task: target versus non-target) ANOVA separately for peak amplitude and latency.

According to the approach adopted in previous papers [11, 12, 39], an additional 2 (Group: control veresus experimental) × 2 (Treatment: pre versus post) ANOVA was performed on the peak amplitude and latency of the differential pP2 wave target minus non-target; hereafter referred to as dpP2) on Fp2 site, where the amplitude reached the maximum. Bonferroni post-hoc comparisons were used, and the alpha level was set at 0.05.

1.3 Results

1.3.1 Functional and neurological testing

Table 1.1 shows rehabilitation and neurological data obtained by each group before and after 6 week treatment for both groups. For the 2-WT, ANOVA showed a significant effect of Treatment ($F_{1,7} = 10.18$, $p < 0.02$, ${}_{\mathrm{p}}\eta^2 = 0.592$), with lower scores in pre- than post-treatment test. The T25-FW showed a marginally significant effect of Treatment ($F_{1,7} = 5.54$, $p = 0.0508$, ${}_{\mathrm{p}}\eta^2 = 0.441$), with higher scores in post-than pre-test. The FSS showed a significant effect of Group ($F_{1,7} = 6.46$, $p < 0.04$, ${}_{\mathrm{p}}\eta^2 = 0.479$), but also a significant interaction Treatment by Group ($F_{1,7} = 5.72$, $p < 0.05$, ${}_{\mathrm{p}}\eta^2 = 0.433$); post-hoc showed a significant fatigue reduction from pre- to post-treatment for the experimental group only ($p < 0.05$). The Tinetti test showed a significant effect of Treatment ($F_{1,7} = 10.68$, $p < 0.02$, ${}_{\mathrm{p}}\eta^2 = 0.604$), with lower scores in pre- than post-treatment. The BBS showed significant effect of Treatment ($F_{1,7} = 8.31$, $p < 0.025$, ${}_{\mathrm{p}}\eta^2 = 0.543$), with lower scores in pre- than post-treatment. The Barthel scale indicated significant effect of Treatment ($F_{1,7} = 16.53$, $p = 0.005$, ${}_{\mathrm{p}}\eta^2 = 0.703$), with lower scores in pre- than post-treatment. The EDSS showed a marginally significant effect of Treatment ($F_{1,7} = 5.22$, $p = 0.058$, ${}_{\mathrm{p}}\eta^2 = 0.476$), with higher scores in pre- than post-treatment. The RNMT-3 indicated a significant effect of Treatment ($F_{1,7} = 10.68$, $p < 0.02$, ${}_{\mathrm{p}}\eta^2 = 0.606$), with lower scores in pre- than post-treatment.

1.3.2 Cognitive testing

1.3.2.1 Behavioral results

ANOVA on RT displayed a significant Group by Treatment interaction ($F_{1,7} = 19.7$, $p < 0.009$, ${}_{\mathrm{p}}\eta^2 = 0.649$), with post-hoc showing a significant RT reduction ($p > 0.004$) in the experimental group from pre- to post-treatment and faster RT in the experimental group in the post-test ($p > 0.02$). With respect to the accuracy,

Table 1.1. Rehabilitation and neurological parameters.

	Control group		Experimental group	
	Pre Mean ± SD	Post Mean ± SD	Pre Mean ± SD	Post Mean ± SD
2-WT (m)	54.7 ± 12.4	69.7 ± 20.5	57.4 ± 16.4	66.0 ± 14.6
T25-FW (s)	16.3 ± 6.1	14.1 ± 7.6	15.5 ± 4.6	12.1 ± 3.8
FSS	6.2 ± 0.6	6.1 ± 0.3	4.2 ± 0.2	3.6 ± 0.5
Tinetti	22.5 ± 4.3	24.3 ± 4.2	15.4 ± 4.6	23.8 ± 4.9
BBS	39.3 ± 7.3	44.3 ± 7.6	37.0 ± 7.5	44.6 ± 6.6
Barthel	84.5 ± 4.6	91.0 ± 5.7	73.2 ± 16.2	88.4 ± 6.1
EDSS	6.4 ± 0.4	6.1 ± 0.4	6.3 ± 0.5	6.2 ± 0.5
RMI	7.8 ± 1.9	9.3 ± 1.8	6.2 ± 1.3	7.8 ± 1.3

Table 1.2. Behavioral data. RT: response time (ms); CE: commission error (%); OM: omission (%); ICV: intra-individual coefficient of variation.

	Control group		Experimental group	
	Pre Mean ± SD	Post Mean ± SD	Pre Mean ± SD	Post Mean ± SD
RT (ms)	607 ± 41.4	629 ± 38.3	621 ± 18.4	547 ± 31.5
CE%	29.2 ± 10	31.2 ± 8.8	28.8 ± 6.3	13.5 ± 9.7
OM%	4.9 ± 3.6	8.4 ± 5.6	6.4 ± 5.3	5.7 ± 3.9
ICV	0.20 ± 0.04	0.29 ± 0.07	0.23 ± 0.06	0.21 ± 0.05

ANOVA on CE% revealed a significant Group by Treatment interaction ($F_{1,7} = 15.49$, $p < 0.006$, ${}_{p}\eta^2 = 0.688$); post-hoc revealed that the CE% at the post-treatment of the experimental group was significantly lower than the others ($p < 0.01$). The analysis of the OM% showed a significant Group by Treatment interaction ($F_{1,7} = 5.81$, $p > 0.05$, ${}_{p}\eta^2 = 0.427$); post-hoc indicated OM% increasing in the post-treatment for the control group compared to the pre-test ($p < 0.01$). The analysis of the ICV did not show statistical effects. Table 1.2 shows the mean ± SD of the behavioral data.

1.3.2.2 Electrophysiological results

Grand-averaged pre-stimulus ERP waveforms (target and non-target are collapsed) for the experimental (solid lines) and control (dashed lines) groups before and after the intervention are reported in figure 1.2(a). Before stimulus onset, the typical slow rising negativity (the BP component) over the central–parietal site is visible, with larger amplitude after the treatment in the experimental group. A similar pattern of activity is detectable for the prefrontal negativity (pN) component over Fp2. Statistical analysis of the pN on Fp2 site revealed significant Group ($F_{1,7} = 6.44$, $p = 0.029$, ${}_{p}\eta^2 = 0.63$) and Treatment ($F_{1,7} = 5.19$, $p = 0.045$, ${}_{p}\eta^2 = 0.62$) effects, and an interaction Group by Treatment ($F_{1,7} = 12.35$, $p = 0.001$, ${}_{p}\eta^2 = 0.74$). ANOVA on the BP component over CPz revealed a significant effect of Group ($F_{1,7} = 7.15$, $p = 0.023$, ${}_{p}\eta^2 = 0.61$), and an interaction Group by Treatment ($F_{1,7} = 12.35$, $p = 0.001$, ${}_{p}\eta^2 = 0.74$). Post-hoc comparisons showed that in the experimental group only, both pN and BP were larger in the post- than in the pre-treatment phase ($p < 0.005$), while in the control group these two components did not differ from each other. See table 1.3 for the components' amplitude values. The topographic distribution of the BP and the pN is reported in figure 1.2(b): the BP focused on medial central–parietal sites and the pN focused on bilateral prefrontal sites. These scalp distributions were quite similar between groups and conditions.

Figure 1.3 shows the grand-average post-stimulus ERP waveforms superimposed for the two groups before and after the treatment, for the Go condition, on the most relevant sites. Major ERP components (P1, N1, pN1, pP1, pP2 and P3) were clearly visible in both groups and conditions. Statistical analysis showed a Treatment effect

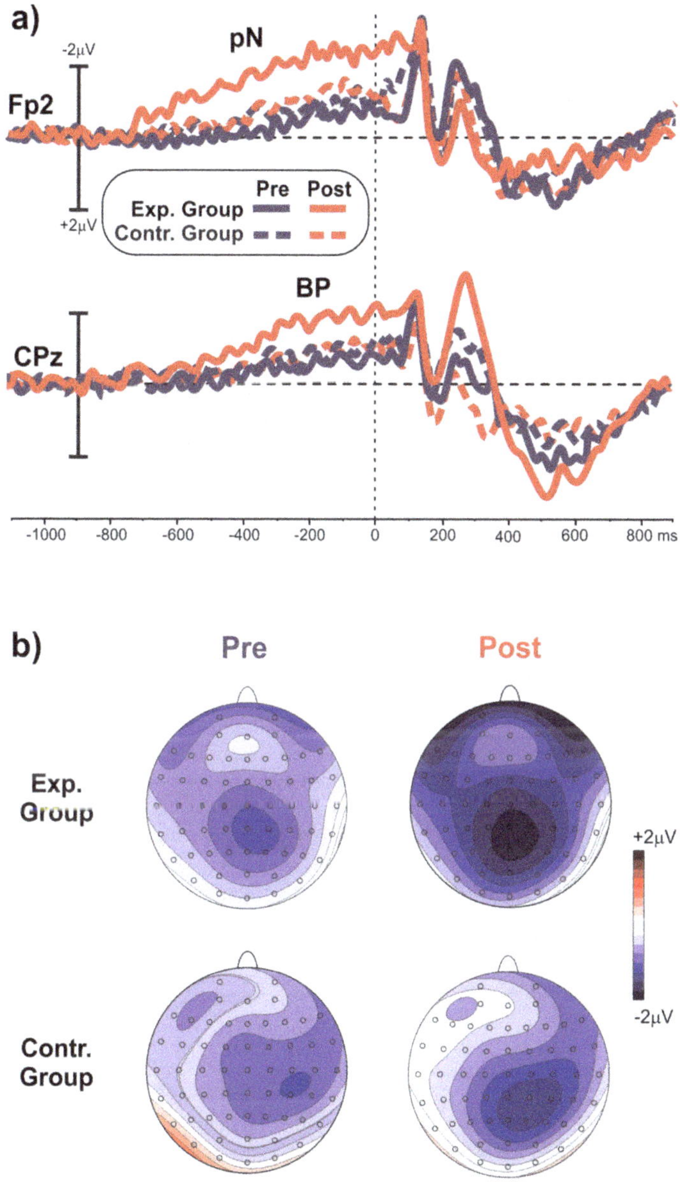

Figure 1.2. (a) Grand-averaged pre-stimulus ERP waveforms from the experimental (solid lines) and the control (dotted lines) groups before (blue lines) and after (red lines) the treatment. Two representative electrodes are shown: left frontopolar (Fp2) and medial central–parietal (CPz) electrodes. The main components are labelled in the figure: the Bereitschaftspotential (BP) and the prefrontal negativity (pN). (b) Scalp topography of the grand-averaged data from the experimental and the control groups before and after the treatment. Top-flat view maps report the mean activity in the last 500 ms before stimulus onset.

Table 1.3. Mean amplitude (μV) of the pre-stimulus ERP components. BP: Bereitschaftspotential; pN: prefrontal negativity.

	Control group		Experimental group	
	Pre Mean ± SD	Post Mean ± SD	Pre Mean ± SD	Post Mean ± SD
BP	−0.67 ± 0.26	−0.66 ± 0.19	−0.62 ± 0.16	−2.12 ± 0.55
pN	−0.62 ± 0.21	−0.55 ± 0.08	−0.51 ± 0.18	−1.88 ± 0.41

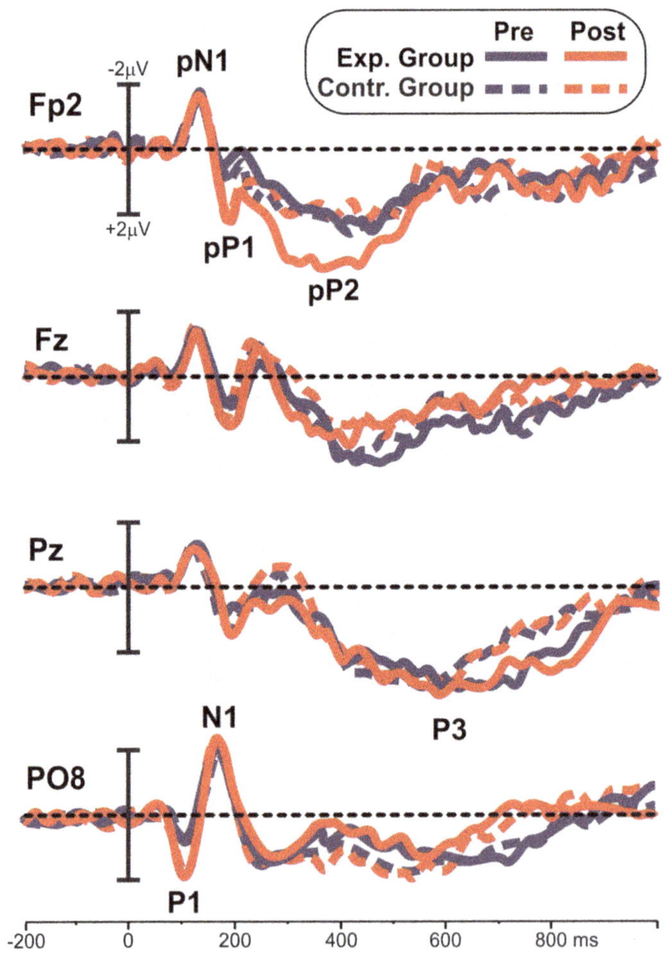

Figure 1.3. Grand-averaged post-stimulus ERP waveforms from the experimental (solid lines) and the control (dotted lines) groups before (blue lines) and after (red lines) the treatment only for Target trials. The most representative electrodes are shown: left frontopolar (Fp2), medial frontal (Fz), medial parietal (Pz), and left parietal–occipital (PO8) electrodes. The main components are labelled in the figure.

for the P1 amplitude ($F_{1,7} = 9.12$, $p = 0.012$, ${}_{p}\eta^2 = 0.80$) that was larger in the post-treatment conditions, whereas no effect of Group, Task and interactions were observed. No significant effects were found for the P1 latency, the N1 amplitude and latency (all ps > 0.05). With respect to the prefrontal components, both peak latency and amplitude of the pN1 were not significant, as well as the pP1 latency. A Treatment effect was reported for the pP1 amplitude ($F_{1,7} = 7.65$, $p = 0.01$, ${}_{p}\eta^2 = 0.71$), indicating larger amplitude in the post-treatment conditions, whereas the other factors were not significant. ANOVA was performed on the mean amplitude of the pP2 component, which showed a significant effect for Task ($F_{1,7} = 19.56$, $p = 0.0013$, ${}_{p}\eta^2 = 0.82$), being larger for target trials. The Group by Treatment interaction was also significant ($F_{1,7} = 8.68$, $p = 0.015$, ${}_{p}\eta^2 = 0.73$). Post-hoc comparisons showed that in the post-treatment condition the pP2 amplitude of the experimental group was larger than the control group. The last analyzed component, the P3, showed a significant Task effect ($F_{1,7} = 9.14$, $p = 0.013$, ${}_{p}\eta^2 = 0.73$) with larger amplitude for Target stimuli.

Figure 1.4 shows the differential waves (target minus non-target) for the two groups and conditions at Fp2 site where the dpP2 was maximum. Statistical analysis performed on the dpP2 peak amplitude revealed a Group effect ($F_{1,7} = 8.65$, $p = 0.014$, ${}_{p}\eta^2 = 0.70$), a Treatment effect ($F_{1,7} = 8.02$, $p = 0.017$, ${}_{p}\eta^2 = 0.68$), and an interaction Group by Treatment ($F_{1,7} = 9.89$, $p = 0.010$, ${}_{p}\eta^2 = 0.72$), indicating that after the intervention the experimental group, compared to the control group, had larger pP2. No effects were observed for the peak latency. Table 1.4 shows the peak amplitudes for all considered post-stimulus ERP components, whereas table 1.5 shows the peak latencies of the same ERP components.

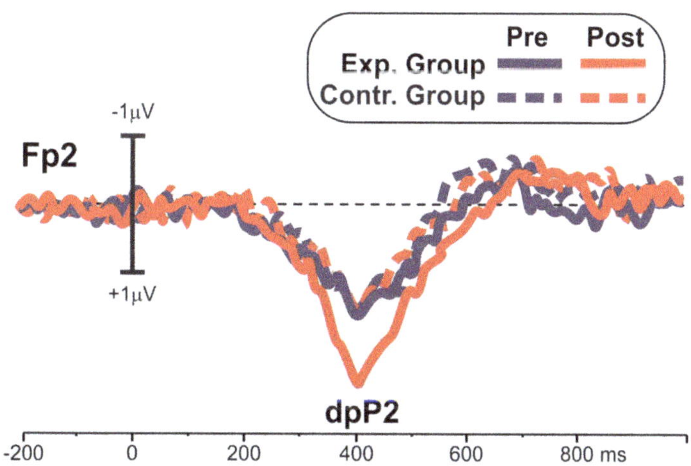

Figure 1.4. Target minus non-target differential pP2 (dpP2) waves from the experimental (solid lines) and the control (dotted lines) groups before (blue lines) and after (red lines) the treatment over prefrontal site (Fp2).

Table 1.4. Peak amplitude (μV) of the post-stimulus ERP components for both target (Go) and non-target (No-Go).

	Control group		Experimental group	
	Pre Mean ± SD	Post Mean ± SD	Pre Mean ± SD	Post Mean ± SD
P1 Go	0.87 ± 0.23	1.98 ± 0.46	0.98 ± 0.29	2.02 ± 0.54
P1 No-Go	0.86 ± 0.21	2.09 ± 0.49	0.92 ± 0.35	2.15 ± 0.62
N1 Go	−2.57 ± 0.78	−2.56 ± 0.56	−2.64 ± 0.82	−2.62 ± 0.62
N1 No-Go	−2.81 ± 0.62	−2.83 ± 0.55	−2.85 ± 0.65	−2.80 ± 0.63
pN1 Go	−1.77 ± 0.38	−1.71 ± 0.35	−1.95 ± 0.42	−1.88 ± 0.44
pN1 No-Go	−1.82 ± 0.37	−1.79 ± 0.39	−2.04 ± 0.48	−2.01 ± 0.46
pP1 Go	1.26 ± 0.29	2.24 ± 0.38	1.17 ± 0.38	2.28 ± 0.47
Ppl No-Go	0.98 ± 0.21	2.21 ± 0.49	1.08 ± 0.35	2.28 ± 0.47
pP2 Go	1.98 ± 0.51	1.89 ± 0.57	1.94 ± 0.56	3.25 ± 0.74
pP2 No-Go	0.23 ± 0.12	0.17 ± 0.08	0.19 ± 0.1	0.39 ± 0.11
dpP2	1.75 ± 0.28	1.72 ± 0.35	1.76 ± 0.31	2.86 ± 0.63
P3 Go	3.83 ± 0.82	3.80 ± 0.75	3.72 ± 0.78	3.75 ± 0.59
P3 No-Go	2.84 ± 0.66	2.75 ± 0.51	2.77 ± 0.58	2.72 ± 0.62

Table 1.5. Peak latency (ms) of the post-stimulus ERP components for both target (Go) and non-target (No-Go).

	Control group		Experimental group	
	Pre Mean ± SD	Post Mean ± SD	Pre Mean ± SD	Post Mean ± SD
P1 Go	108 ± 26	108 ± 28	107 ± 25	108 ± 24
P1 No-Go	108 ± 29	108 ± 25	108 ± 22	109 ± 30
N1 Go	168 ± 38	168 ± 36	169 ± 40	169 ± 44
N1 No-Go	168 ± 41	168 ± 40	169 ± 38	169 ± 37
pN1 Go	130 ± 25	130 ± 22	130 ± 26	129 ± 24
pN1 No-Go	130 ± 23	130 ± 26	130 ± 24	130 ± 22
pP1 Go	191 ± 39	190 ± 38	189 ± 40	190 ± 37
Ppl No-Go	190 ± 40	190 ± 39	189 ± 42	190 ± 40
dpP2	398 ± 58	400 ± 60	400 ± 64	399 ± 62

1.4 Discussion

To our knowledge, this is the first study implementing exoskeleton in multidisciplinary rehabilitation training for MS patients measuring neural, behavioural, functional, and clinical data. With respect to the first aim of this study, we confirm cognitive and behavioural improvement in the discriminative response task, especially in the group that underwent the rehabilitation in conjunction with the HBP intervention. While response times of the control group increased, the experimental group was faster and more accurate (reduction of omission and commission errors) during the post-treatment session. This result is extremely interesting, because both processing speed and executive functions are mostly affected during MS, as confirmed by the control group results, whose performance worsen over time. The paradigm proposed in this study, also known as Go/No-Go task, involves many cognitive processes, such as proactive and reactive inhibition [1], decision-making [26], motor preparation [5], speed processing and behavioral execution. Most of these cognitive processing falls under the name of executive functions, which are particularly affected by MS. The processing speed, which is deteriorated in MS patients, is required to correctly perform the task (respond as fast as possible to target stimuli). Present findings indicate that the use of HBP during rehabilitation intervention improves both executive functions and processing speed, mitigating the cognitive decline associated to MS.

Moving to the typical neurological and rehabilitation measures, we observed an improved performance in both groups after the treatments and in all tests. This is of great importance, because it means that rehabilitation processes did properly work in mitigating the MS symptoms. However, the HBP played its main effects at two important levels: overall disability (EDSS) and fatigue perception (FSS). Indeed, the experimental group performance on these latter scales was much better than before.

The EDSS is the main scale used by neurologists to quantify the MS disability in eight functional systems; observing effects on this scale is of massive importance. The use of more complex systems, such as the exoskeleton and robotic devices, allows the reduction of the disability as measured by the EDSS; furthermore, the exoskeleton can have an easier application, although it is not included in standard rehabilitation treatments.

With respect to the FSS, we have already showed a correlation between prefrontal activities and fatigue perception [7, 35]; in this case, we observe an increased prefrontal activity together with a reduction of self-report fatigue, in line with previous interpretation on conscious perception of fatigue. Further, since the HBP should exert its effect throughout proprioceptive mechanisms, it might be responsible for perception modification. Besides the interpretation of this finding, which needs to be further supported, the decreased perception of fatigue is very important, because it is one of the most debilitation symptoms in MS.

At brain level, we analyzed ERP activities preceding stimulus presentation, contrary to previous study [19] where we analyzed the pre-movement phase (i.e. movement-related cortical potential; MRCP). We focused on two slow negative components: the well-known Bereitschaftspotential (BP), associated with motor preparation in premotor areas, and the prefrontal negativity (pN), reflecting cognitive preparation and proactive inhibition [5] with source in the inferior frontal gyrus [20, 50]. Present data highlight the importance of the HBP treatment in increasing the amplitude of both components, partially confirming previous findings. Indeed, in the previous study we showed an enhancement of activity over prefrontal regions in MS patients after only one session of HBP. In the present study, the HBP treatment was incorporated in the typical rehabilitation session for 6 weeks, leading to similar results: indeed, the increased amplitude of the pN component is detectable only in the experimental group and, further, this result is accompanied by the same amplitude trend over motor-related regions. The pN amplitude has been associated with the proactive inhibitory control, basically the core of the executive functions; thus, the larger the pN, the stronger the inhibitory control. An increased pN amplitude, for example, has been shown in the elderly during a discriminative and simple response task [5], wherein young participants did not need to recruit these high-order brain regions to accomplish the task. Indeed, the elderly hyperactivated the PFC to fulfill task requirements, because it requires higher cognitive effort to quickly perform the task without errors. The results of the present study are in line with previous data in the elderly [5, 6, 8]. We have also proposed that the prefrontal negative activity is responsible for a proactive response inhibition as far as the movement is not needed; basically, if the need to perform an action is approaching, but it is not yet the time to execute it, the prefrontal cortex works like a brake to freeze the action until the right time [20]. Present findings confirm this interpretation, showing also an increased BP amplitude over motor-related regions after the HBP intervention in the experimental group only. The BP amplitude has also been associated with the RT during the Go/No-Go task (the larger the BP, the faster the RT), whereas the pN has been associated with the accuracy (the larger the pN, the better the accuracy) [40]; these data also support this interpretation, because in the experimental group RT are faster and performance accuracy greater, together with increased amplitude of the BP and the pN components. Thus, the use of the HBP induces proactive modification in the brain during the preparation to the stimulus presentation on premotor and prefrontal regions; these modifications might support improvements at both cognitive and behavioral level, as explained before.

With respect to the post-stimulus component, both treatments increased the P1 component, but we did not observe specific changes induced by the HBP during early sensory processing. We did not expect to observe any amplitude or latency change at sensory processing level, because the intervention was not aimed at improving either processing of visual stimuli or the spatial attention [55], but it is important to note that both treatments positively affected early visual processing in extrastriate areas, despite the progressive visual degeneration affecting MS patients (for a review see Balcer *et al* [2]). However, in several studies in which the same paradigm has been employed, we have introduced the existence of activities at prefrontal sites concomitant to the well-known occipital components: the earliest negative component concomitant to the occipital P1, named prefrontal N1 (pN1), the second positive component concomitant to the occipital N1, named prefrontal P1 (pP1), and a third prefrontal positivity component, named prefrontal P2 (pP2), with amplitude peak at around 350 ms after stimulus onset (e.g. Berchicci *et al* [9]); these components were localized in the anterior Insula using fMRI recordings [20, 50]. The first two components were associated with sensory and sensory-motor awareness [42, 43, 47], while the pP2 has been associated with stimulus-response mapping in visual-motor tasks [41]. This latter component has been described in previous studies with different labels [23, 25, 49], even by our group. We have introduced this component in the previous study with HBP [19], showing larger amplitude after the single exoskeleton session. In the present study, while the pN1 was not affected by treatments, the pP1was larger after both types of treatment, indicating rehabilitation-related improvements in sensory-motor awareness, intended as sensory awareness for events requiring motor intervention (e.g. Di Russo *et al* [20]). In addition, the experimental treatment specifically increased the pP2 for target stimuli and the differential pP2, suggesting that the experimental intervention improves stimulus-response mapping in the Insular cortex, which has been associated with processing speed [12]. Regarding the P3, it is usually related to stimulus categorizations, working memory and movement execution [9]. Previous studies showed P3 alterations in MS patients compared to controls [44, 54], and changes after cognitive interventions [30], whereas we did not observe any modification. This result is not in line with our previous study [19], in which an increased amplitude of the P3 was reported, in both patients and controls. However, note that the non-specific P3 effect observed in Di Russo *et al* [19] might have been biased by the learning process involved during the second recording session (made only one hour after the previous one), because amplitude modification was present in both groups. In the present case, this interpretation cannot be applied because both groups did not show any P3 changes, whereas the behavioural effect (shorter RT) was present in the experimental group only.

In conclusion, we found here that the HBP intervention was very effective, especially in reducing the disability status and fatigue, likely stimulating cognitive processing in prefrontal cortex. Of course, we recognize as the main limitation of this study the low number of subjects and we are aware that a larger sample is needed to confirm present results. Nonetheless, the timing of this study is particularly fruitful because exoskeletons may be available for home use. A demonstration of successful exoskeleton intervention on different systems level in MS may translate into a new rehabilitation treatment, and, within a few years, into a means of independent home exercise and/or independent ambulation for individuals with MS.

References

[1] Aron A R 2011 From reactive to proactive and selective control: developing a richer model for stopping inappropriate responses *Biol. Psychiatry* **69** e55–68

[2] Balcer L J, Miller D H, Reingold S C and Cohen J A 2014 Vision and vision-related outcome measures in multiple sclerosis *Brain* **138** 11–27

[3] Benedict R H B and Zivadinov R 2011a Risk factors for and management of cognitive dysfunction in multiple sclerosis *Nat. Rev. Neurosci.* **7** 332–42

[4] Benedict R H B, Holtzer R, Motl R W, Foley F W, Kaur S, Hojnacki D and Weinstock-Guttman B 2011b Upper and lower extremity motor function and cognitive impairment in multiple sclerosis *J. Int. Neuropsychol. Soc.* **17** 643–53

[5] Berchicci M, Lucci G, Pesce C, Spinelli D and Di Russo F 2012 Prefrontal hyperactivity in older people during motor planning *Neuroimage* **62** 1750–60

[6] Berchicci M, Lucci G and Di Russo F 2013b The benefits of physical exercise on the aging brain: The role of the prefrontal cortex *J. Gerontol. A Biol. Sci. Med. Sci.* **68** 1337–41
[7] Berchicci M, Menotti F, Macaluso A and Di Russo F 2013a The neurophysiology of central and peripheral fatigue during sub-maximal lower limb isometric contractions *Front. Hum. Neurosci.* **7** 135
[8] Berchicci M, Lucci G, Perri R L, Spinelli D and Di Russo F 2014 Benefits of physical exercise on basic visuo-motor functions across age *Front. Aging Neurosci.* **6** 48
[9] Berchicci M, Spinelli D and Russo F 2016 New insights into old waves. Matching stimulus- and response-locked ERPs on the same time-window *Biol. Psychol.* **117** 202–15
[10] Berg K, Wood-Dauphinée S, Williams J I and Gayton D 1989 Measuring balance in the elderly: preliminary development of an instrument *Physiother. Can.* **41** 304–11
[11] Bianco V, Perri R L, Di Russo F and Berchicci M 2016 Different proactive action control in fencers' and boxers' brains *Neuroscience* **343** 260–8
[12] Bianco V, Berchicci M, Perri R L, Quinzi F and Di Russo F 2017 Exercise-related cognitive effects on sensory-motor control in athletes and drummers compared to non-athletes and other musicians *Neuroscience* **360** 39–47
[13] Brichetto G, Piccardo E and Pedullà L *et al* 2015 Tailored balance exercises on people with multiple sclerosis: A pilot randomized, controlled study *Mult. Scler.* **21** 1055–63
[14] Briken S, Gold S M and Patra S *et al* 2014 Effects of exercise on fitness and cognition in progressive MS: a randomized, controlled pilot trial *Mult. Scler.* **20** 382–90
[15] Cattaneo D, Jonsdottir J and Zocchi M *et al* 2007 Effects of balance exercises on people with multiple sclerosis: A pilot study *Clin. Rehabil.* **21** 771–81
[16] Colaiacomo B, Mantini S, Ciccarelli A and Ripani M 2011 Human Body Posturizer (HBP): new orthosis for improving postural dynamics *Ital. J. Anat. Embryol.* **116** 46
[17] Ciccarelli A, Mantini S and Ripani M 2012 Evaluation of the Human Body Posturizer in postural diseases and its impact on of the fall risk in the elderly *Ital. J. Anat. Embryol.* **117** 41
[18] Collen F M, Wade D T, Robb G F and Bradshaw C M 1991 The Rivermead Mobility Index: a further development of the Rivermead Motor Assessment *Int. Disabil. Stud.* **13** 50–4
[19] Di Russo F, Berchicci M, Perri R L, Ripani F R and Ripani M 2013 A passive exoskeleton can push your life up: application on multiple sclerosis patients *PLoS One* **8** e77348
[20] Di Russo F, Lucci G, Sulpizio V, Berchicci M, Spinelli D, Pitzalis S and Galati G 2016 Spatiotemporal brain mapping of the preparation, perception and action phases *NeuroImage* **126** 1–14
[21] D'Orio V L, Foley F W, Armentano F, Picone M A, Kim S and Holtzer R 2012 Cognitive and motor functioning in patients with multiple sclerosis: neuropsychological predictors of walking speed and falls *J. Neurol. Sci.* **316** 42–6
[22] Erickson K I, Voss M W and Prakash R S *et al* 2011 Exercise training increases size of hippocampus and improves memory *Proc. Natl Acad. Sci.* **108** 3017–22
[23] Gajewski P D and Falkenstein M 2015 Lifelong physical activity and executive functions in older age assessed by memory based task switching *Neuropsychologia* **73** 195–207
[24] Gijbels D, Eijnde B O and Feys P 2011 Comparison of the 2- and 6-minute walk test in multiple sclerosis *Mult. Scler.* **17** 1269–72
[25] Gonzalez-Rosa J J, Inuggi A, Blasi V, Cursi M, Annavazzi P, Comi G, Falini A and Leocani L 2013 Response competition and response inhibition during different choice-discrimination tasks: Evidence from ERP measured inside MRI scanner *Int. J. Psychophysiol.* **89** 37–47

[26] Heekeren H R, Marrett S and Ungerleider L G 2008 The neural systems that mediate human perceptual decision making *Nat. Rev. Neurosci.* **9** 467–79
[27] Jung T P, Makeig S, Westerfield M, Townsend J, Courchesne E and Sejnowski T J 2000 Removal of eye activity artifacts from visual event-related potentials in normal and clinical subjects *Clin. Neurophysiol.* **111** 1745–58
[28] Katrych O, Simone T M, Azad S and Mousa S A 2009 Disease-modifying agents in the treatment of multiple sclerosis: a review of long term outcomes *CNS Neurol. Disord. Drug Targets.* **8** 512–9
[29] Khan F, Turner-Stokes L, Ng L and Kilpatrick T 2007 Multidisciplinary rehabilitation for adults with multiple sclerosis *Cochrane Database Syst. Rev.* **18** CD006036
[30] Kiiski H, Reilly R B, Lonergan R, Kelly S, O'Brien M and Kinsella K *et al* 2011 Change in PASAT performance correlates with change in P3 ERP amplitude over a 12-month period in multiple sclerosis patients *J. Neurological. Sci.* **305** 45–52
[31] Krupp L B, La Rocca N G, Muir-Nash J and Steinberg A D 1989 The Fatigue Severity Scale. Application to patients with multiple sclerosis and systemic lupus erythematosus *Arch. Neurol.* **46** 1121–3
[32] Kurtzke J F 1983 Rating neurological impairment in multiple sclerosis: an expanded disability status scale *Neurology* **33** 1444–52
[33] Leavitt V M, Cirnigliaro C and Cohen A *et al* 2014 Aerobic exercise increases hippocampal volume and improves memory in multiple sclerosis: preliminary findings *Neurocase* **20** 695–7
[34] Mahoney F and Barthel D 1965 Functional evaluation: the Barthel Index *Md. State Med. J.* **14** 61–5
[35] Menotti F, Berchicci M, Di Russo F, Damiani A, Vitulli S and Macaluso A 2014 The role of the prefrontal cortex in the development of muscle fatigue in Charcot–Marie–Tooth 1A patients *Neuromuscul. Disord.* **24** 516–23
[36] Motl R W, Cohen J A, Benedict R, Phillips G, LaRocca N and Hudson L D *et al* 2017 Validity of the timed 25-foot walk as an ambulatory performance outcome measure for multiple sclerosis *Mult. Scler.* **23** 704–10
[37] Motl R W and Sandroff B M 2015 Benefits of exercise training in multiple sclerosis *Curr. Neurol. Neurosci. Rep.* **15** 62
[38] Motl R W, Sandroff B M and Benedict R H B 2011 Cognitive dysfunction and multiple sclerosis: developing a rationale for considering the efficacy of exercise training *Mult. Scler.* **17** 1034–40
[39] Perri R L, Berchicci M, Lucci G, Spinelli D and Di Russo F 2014a The premotor role of the prefrontal cortex in response consistency *Neuropsychology* **29** 767–75
[40] Perri R L, Berchicci M, Lucci G, Spinelli D and Di Russo F 2014b Individual differences in response speed and accuracy are associated to specific brain activities of two interacting systems *Front. Behav. Neurosci.* **8** 251
[41] Perri R L, Berchicci M, Lucci G, Spinelli D and Di Russo F 2015 Why do we make mistakes? Neurocognitive processes during the preparation-perception-action cycle and error-detection *NeuroImage* **113** 320–8
[42] Perri R L, Berchicci M, Bianco V, Spinelli D and Di Russo F 2017 Brain waves from an 'isolated' cortex: Contribution of the anterior insula to cognitive functions *Brain Struct. Funct.* **223** 1343–55

[43] Perri R L, Berchicci M, Bianco V, Quinzi F, Spinelli D and Di Russo F 2018 Awareness of perception and sensory-motor integration: ERPs from the anterior insula *Brain Struct. Funct.* **223** 3577–92

[44] Pokryszko-Dragan A, Zagrajek M, Slotwinski K, Gruszka E, Bilinska M and Podemski R 2009 Neuropsychological testing and event-related potentials in the assessment of cognitive performance in the patients with multiple sclerosis—a pilot study *Clin. Neurol. Neurosurg.* **111** 503–6

[45] Prakash R S, Snook E M and Lewis J L *et al* 2008 Cognitive impairments in relapsing-remitting multiple sclerosis: a meta-analysis *Mult. Scler.* **14** 1250–61

[46] Samkoff L M and Goodman A D 2011 Symptomatic management in multiple sclerosis *Neurol. Clin.* **29** 449–63

[47] Sanchez-Lopez J, Pedersini C A, Di Russo F, Cardobi N, Fonte C, Varalta V, Prior M, Smania N, Savazzi S and Marzi C A 2017 Visually evoked responses from the blind field of hemianopic patients *Neuropsychologia* **128** 127–39

[48] Sandroff B M, Klaren R E and Pilutti L A *et al* 2014 Randomized controlled trial of physical activity, cognition, and walking in multiple sclerosis *J. Neurol.* **261** 363–72

[49] Schapkin S A, Gajewski P D and Freude G 2014 Age differences in memory-based task switching with and without cues: An ERP study *J. Psychophysiol.* **28** 187–201

[50] Sulpizio V, Lucci G, Berchicci M, Galati G, Pitzalis S and Di Russo F 2017 Hemispheric asymmetries in the transition from action preparation to execution *NeuroImage* **1** 390–402

[51] Tinetti M E, Williams T F and Mayewski R 1986 Fall Risk Index for elderly patients based on number of chronic disabilities *Am. J. Med.* **80** 429–34

[52] Trapp B D and Nave K A 2008 Multiple sclerosis: an immune or neurodegenerative disorder? *Annu. Rev. Neurosci.* **31** 247–69

[53] van Praag H, Christie B R, Sejnowski T J and Gage F H 1999 Running enhances neurogenesis, learning, and long-term potentiation in mice *Proc. Natl Acad. Sci.* **96** 13427–31

[54] Whelan R, Lonergan R, Kiiski H, Nolan H, Kinsella K and Hutchinson M *et al* 2010 Impaired information processing speed and attention allocation in multiple sclerosis patients versus controls: a high-density EEG study *J. Neurol. Sci.* **293** 45–50

[55] Woodman G F 2010 A brief introduction to the use of event-related potentials (ERPs) in studies of perception and attention *Atten. Percept. Psychophys.* **72** 2031–46

IOP Publishing

Neurological Disorders and Imaging Physics, Volume 2
Engineering and clinical perspectives of multiple sclerosis
Ayman El-Baz and Jasjit S Suri

Chapter 2

The early stages of multiple sclerosis: new targets for the development of combinational drug therapies

I E Cock and M J Cheesman

The current methods of treating multiple sclerosis (MS) do not address the early phases of the disease progression and instead merely treat the later phase symptoms. Whilst this approach may help to alleviate many of the symptoms and much of the discomfort associated with MS, it does not stop the disease progression and the destruction of neuronal tissue still occurs. Furthermore, a number of serious side effects are associated with the current treatment modalities. A better strategy may be to eradicate the cause of the disease, thereby bypassing the later phase events. Until recently, this has not been possible due to a lack of understanding of the etiology of MS. However, recent advances have identified *Acinetobacter baylyi* and *Pseudomonas aeruginosa* as bacterial triggers of the disease in genetically susceptible people, and have provided some understanding of the disease progression. An understanding of the early phases of the disease has identified a variety of new targets for anti-MS drug development which may allow for the development of new treatment regimens with increased efficacy and/or less serious side effects. This chapter examines the bacterial triggers of rheumatoid arthritis (RA) and how they may induce self-reactive antibody production. In so doing, this report highlights some targets for drug treatments aimed at blocking the early phases of MS before the more serious later phase events occur. Whilst it is unlikely that any single drug will be able to treat all aspects of this disease, resveratrol and other stilbenes are highlighted as a class of compounds which may have beneficial effects on several phases of MS disease progression. Similarly, several natural therapeutics with activities against several phases of MS progression are discussed.

doi:10.1088/978-0-7503-1762-7ch2

2.1 Introduction

Multiple sclerosis (MS) is a debilitating disease that afflicts approximately 0.03% of the world's population [1]. Interestingly, MS has a latitudinal correlation, with higher prevalences in far northern regions of the Northern Hemisphere and the far south regions of the Southern Hemisphere as compared with tropical regions. It is particularly prevalent in populations of Northern European descent (especially in Scandinavian populations), where the incidence has been estimated to be as high as 0.2% of the overall population [2]. It was originally believed that the increased incidence in the Scandinavian population might be entirely due to genetic susceptibilities. However, environmental conditions may be a major contributor to the increased prevalence of MS in Scandinavian populations and it has been proposed that the latitudinal correlation may be linked to the increased incidence of respiratory infections at these latitudes. The higher incidence of MS in Scandinavian populations may be due to people spending greater periods indoors because of climatic conditions, thus increasing the likelihood of spreading pathogens [2]. The disease onset is also predominant in young adults in their 20s and 30s, and its onset is rare in childhood or in people over 50 [3]. In common with several other autoimmune disorders including RA, MS occurs substantially more frequently in women than in men [3]. Indeed, a recent study by the World Health Organisation (WHO) estimated that women are twice as likely as men to develop MS [4].

MS is an autoimmune inflammatory disease in which the immune system of afflicted individuals recognizes and establishes an immune response against self-tissue, resulting in demyelination of central nervous system cells. Pathologically, MS results in the formation of central nervous system (CNS) lesions (also called plaques), inflammation and widespread areas of demyelinated neurons [2]. As this demyelination can affect a variety of neurons associated with a myriad of autonomic, sensatory and motor functions, MS may result in a wide array of different symptoms, dependent on the nature of the affected neurons [5]. Specific symptoms appear to be determined by the location of the lesions in the CNS of the afflicted individual and frequently include loss of tactile sensitivity, a 'tingling' sensation (paresthesia, numbness), muscle weakness, spasms, uncoordinated movement, pronounced reflexes, vocal and speech problems, difficulty swallowing, visual disturbances, chronic fatigue, sexual dysfunction, pain and heat intolerance [2]. Cogitative impairment and emotional issues (e.g. depression, unstable moods) are also relatively common for individuals suffering from MS [5]. The rate and pathway of MS progression is also highly variable. Most MS patients initially present with isolated (relapsing) attacks, which are generally followed by periods of complete or partial recovery, with no apparent symptoms [6]. However, these periods of symptom regression are transient and afflicted individuals will generally suffer relapses. The time between relapses and their severity also varies widely between afflicted individuals. For individuals presenting with the relapse-remitting form of the disease (RRMS), each new attack may be characterized by new symptoms, or may be a recurrence of the previously expressed symptoms. In contrast, 10%–15% of

MS patients accumulate neurological disabilities continuously from the disease etiology, without periods of remission. For these individuals, the number and severity of their symptoms increase continually throughout the remainder of their life without any remission.

There is no known cure for MS. Instead, current treatment strategies aim to alleviate the later phase symptoms of MS, thereby increasing the quality of life of the afflicted individuals. Few current therapies aim at blocking the etiology of MS or managing the early events of MS disease progression, and research is desperately required in this field. Most commonly, anti-inflammatory drugs are administered to MS sufferers to alleviate the late phase events and slow the disease progression. Non-steroidal anti-inflammatory drugs (NSAIDs) are frequently used for this purpose. However, NSAIDs merely target the symptoms of MS and do not affect the course of the disease. Thus, whilst NSAID use may alleviate suffering, MS-associated neuronal myelin degradation persists. Furthermore, NSAIDs should be used cautiously for individuals with gastrointestinal, cardiovascular or kidney problems [7]. For example, cyclooxygenase-2 (COX-2) inhibitors are a class of NSAIDs that directly target the COX-2 enzyme which is responsible for inflammation and pain. However, treatment with COX-2 inhibitors is often associated with an increase in myocardial infarction [1]. Treatment with steroidal anti-inflammatory drugs, such as high doses of corticosteroids (e.g. methylprednisolone), is often more effective for short term therapies, although they do not have a significant impact on long term recovery [8]. Furthermore, prolonged usage of corticosteroid therapy may be accompanied by significant side effects and toxicities [9]. Due to the inability to cure the disease or effectively halt its progression, sufferers are continually seeking better, more effective therapeutic options. The symptoms of MS may also be controlled through complementary and alternative therapies including diet, yoga, acupuncture, hyperbaric oxygen therapy, reflexology [10] and herbal medicines (including cannabis) [10, 11], with varied success.

Other treatment modalities aim to halt or modify MS disease progression through the usage of disease modifying treatments (DMTs). These are a diverse grouping of drugs with no common mechanism of action, and are grouped together based on their common usage to improve the symptoms of MS, decrease neuronal damage and improve patient function and quality of life. These drugs are generally only used when more conventional treatments are ineffective due to their prohibitively high costs and their adverse effects (lymphoma, serious infections including tuberculosis, heart failure etc). DMTs include the following:

- Interferons, which are a class of cytokine that reduces the rate of MS relapses. Interferon β1α (IB1A) and interferon β1b (IB1b) reduce relapses by approximately 30% and are relatively safe, making them ideal first line treatments [12]. However, only approximately 70% of MS patients are responsive to IB1A therapy [13] and the therapy is expensive.
- The cancer chemotherapeutic drug mitoxantrone, which is often used to treat secondary-progressive MS, and is effective at slowing the progression of the disease and extending the period between relapses [14].

- A number of monoclonal antibody drugs that target specific cellular components. Natalizumab targets the cell adhesion molecule α4-integrin, thereby inhibiting the passage of T-lymphocytes through the blood brain barrier. Natalizumab therapy reduces relapses in MS sufferers by 68% and slows the progression of the disease [15]. The monoclonal antibody alemtuzumab binds the glycoprotein CD52 on mature lymphocytes, targeting them for destruction [16]. Indeed, the authors of that study have suggested that alemtuzumab may not only block MS relapses, but may even reverse the effects. Similarly, ocrelizumab targets the CD20 glycoprotein on B cells with similar efficacy [17].
- Several immunomodulators also commonly used to treat MS, such as glatiramer acetate administration which decreases the incidence of MS relapse events [18]. Whilst its mechanism of action has not been fully elucidated, it has been suggested that it induces pro-inflammatory Th1 T cells to convert to regulatory Th2 T cells, thereby suppressing the inflammatory response [19]. Fingolimod is a sphingosine-1-phosphate receptor modulator which sequesters lymphocytes in lymph nodes, preventing them from contributing to the neuronal myelin damage in MS patients [20]. Teriflunomide inhibits pyrimidine synthesis, decreasing the numbers of activated T cells, thus decreasing MS associated neuronal damage [21].

There remains a need to develop safer, more effective drugs for the treatment of MS which will not only alleviate symptoms, but prevent the progression of the disease. Targeting earlier events prior to the induction of the immune response would not only reduce the symptoms and discomfort associated with MS, but would also lessen/prevent the neuronal damage and the formation of CNS lesions that are predominant features of the chronic stages of the disease. Targeting the trigger(s) of MS is an attractive option for safer, more effective treatments. Greater understanding of the etiology and progression of the disease should allow more relevant drug discovery and development. Based on the evidence linking specific bacterial infections with MS pathogenesis (outlined in later sections of this chapter), a mechanism of disease progression has been proposed (figure 2.1). From this proposed mechanism, several broad phases of MS disease progression can be recognised as targets for drug design and/or discovery:

1. *Acinetobacter* spp. And *Pseudomonas aeruginosa* acts as triggers for MS [22–24]. Thus, limiting *Acinetobacter* spp. And *P. aeruginosa* infections may prevent MS initiation and minimize its downstream effects.
2. *Acinetobacter* spp. And *P. aeruginosa* will not initiate the autoimmune events associated with MS unless they are able to interact with the immune system. Interaction via the gastrointestinal lumen is a common pathway to establish an immune response. This may occur when epithelial lesions (or other epithelial interruptions) elicit the production of anti-*Acinetobacter* spp. and *anti-P. aeruginosa* antibodies [25, 26]. Inhibition of the causes of gut lesions (e.g. Crohn's disease, giardiasis) would also be expected to decrease MS initiation events.

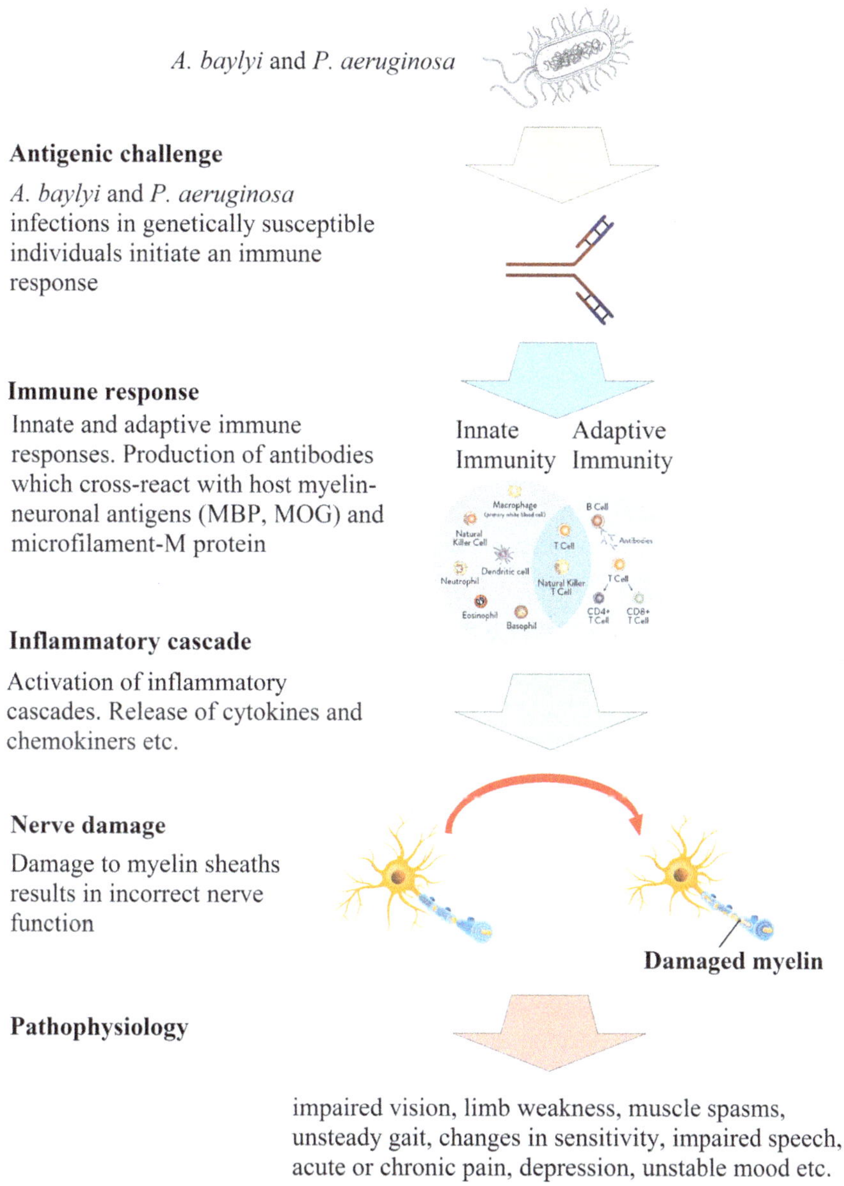

Figure 2.1. A schematic representation of the main events in MS disease etiology and progression. The main phases are the bacterial infection/antigenic challenge phase, the immune phase, inflammatory phase, and myelin damage and downstream symptoms. Only the major events are shown. It is the later phases (inflammation and pathophysiology) which are most frequently targeted by conventional MS therapies.

3. The prevention and early detection of *Acinetobacter* spp. And *P. aeruginosa* infections and/or the colonization at other sites (e.g. lungs) may block the onset of MS and lessen its downstream effects.
4. Blocking the immune response by blocking the interaction of *Acinetobacter* spp. And *P. aeruginosa* with immunological cells or by immunomodulation also prevents the production of self-reactive antibodies or the cross-reactivity with self-tissue, thereby diminishing the later phase events of MS and preventing the disease symptoms. However, immunomodulatory therapy should be used with caution as suppressing a patient's immunity would subsequently expose them to a variety of other infections.
5. Most current MS therapies target the later phase events by blocking the inflammatory cascades or by decreasing the symptoms of MS (e.g. loss of sensitivity, paresthesia, numbness, muscle weakness and uncoordinated movement, vocal and speech problems, difficulty swallowing, visual disturbances, chronic fatigue, pain). Whilst drugs targeting the late events are effective in easing patient discomfort, they still allow myelin tissue damage to occur in the neuronal tissue (which is associated with the self-reactive antibodies).

2.2 Evidence for the involvement of microbial triggers of MS

A greater understanding of the etiology of MS may highlight more relevant targets for drug discovery. This may facilitate the development of more effective chemotherapy options that both treat and prevent these diseases. Therapies that block the onset of MS may be particularly effective as they would not only block the downstream symptoms, but would also inhibit the early disease events, thus preventing the resultant damage to neuronal myelin. Furthermore, targeting the early phase events of MS would lessen the later phase events and alleviate the symptoms of MS. Whilst the etiological events of MS are still not completely understood, it is generally accepted that MS is triggered in susceptible individuals by specific antigens.

The causes of many autoimmune diseases are not fully understood. However, it is generally accepted that autoimmune diseases (including MS) are triggered in susceptible individuals by specific antigens. For many of these diseases the major triggers are bacterial and the responsible organisms are known [27]. Indeed, approximately 80 autoimmune diseases are recognised as being triggered by foreign antibodies, with bacterial pathogens being one of the most common triggers [28]. Bacteria may use several strategies to stimulate autoimmunity, including molecular mimicry, epitope spreading, bystander activation and polyclonal activation [29, 30]. Molecular mimicry is particularly relevant to the development of autoimmune diseases and results from similarities between bacterial and self-antigens (figure 2.2). When there is sufficient similarity between foreign and self-antigens, autoreactive T and/or B cells may be induced. A sub-population of antibodies are produced which not only recognise and react with the bacterial antigens, but may also cross-react with self-epitopes, resulting in tissue pathology (damage to neuronal myelin sheaths in the case of MS). Thus, the bacterial pathogens prompt the immune system to attack itself in genetically susceptible individuals.

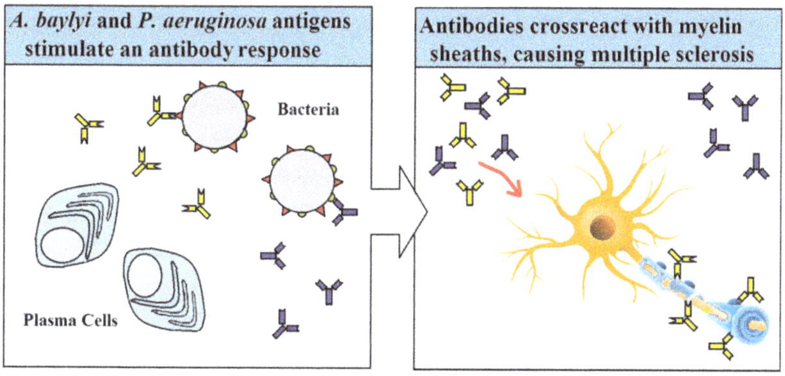

Figure 2.2. Molecular mimicry. Following pathogenic challenge (in this case, with *Acinetobacter* spp. And *P. aeruginosa*), the host produces antibodies against the bacterial antigens. When the host has antigens similar to the bacterial antigens, a subset of the antibodies (shown in yellow) will not only bind to the bacterial antigens, but will also cross-react with self-antigens, causing tissue damage.

Bacterial molecular mimicry is implicated in the etiology of several autoimmune inflammatory diseases. Rheumatoid arthritis (RA) is triggered in genetically susceptible individuals (with MHC class 2 allele HLA-DR4) by *Proteus* spp. infections [31–33]. Similarly, ankylosing spondylitis (AS) may be triggered in genetically susceptible individuals (with MHC class 1 allele HLA-B27) and *Klebsiella pneumoniae* has been identified as a bacterial trigger of that disease [34–39]. *Streptococcus pyogenes* infection may induce acute rheumatic fever (RF) in some individuals [40, 41]. There is a similarity between an MHC in genetically susceptible people and the *S. pyogenes* M-protein (cross reactive antigen), which results in breakdown of self-tolerance in immunocompromised individuals [27]. *Borrelia burgdorferi* is a trigger of Lyme disease [42]. Members of the Enterobacteriaceae family are associated with Graves' disease and Kawasaki syndrome [43, 44]. *Mycoplasma pneumoniae* triggers several demyelinating auto-immune diseases [45–47]. For all the autoimmune inflammatory diseases triggered by bacterial pathogens, treatments aimed at destroying the pathogen and inhibiting infection effectively block the trigger mechanisms of these diseases, thereby blocking the downstream symptoms. Whilst the causes of MS are not comprehensively understood, *Acinitobacter* spp. And *P. aeruginosa* have been linked to the disease's etiology [22–24, 48].

2.2.1 *Acinetobacter* spp. as a trigger of MS

Acinetobacter spp. infections have been confirmed as triggers of MS based on several lines of evidence:

- Increased IgA, IgM and IgG antibody levels are generally detected in MS patients [49].
- Many of these antibodies cross-react with myelin [23].
- *Acinetobacter* spp. specific cross-reactive antibodies are significantly elevated in the sera of individuals suffering from MS [23, 48, 49].

Table 2.1. The bacterial triggers of multiple sclerosis as the bacterial antigen and host susceptibility antigen sequences.

Bacterial trigger	Bacterial antigen	Bacterial sequence	Host antigen	Host sequence	References
Pseudomonas aeruginosa	ϒ-CMLD	TRHAYG	Myelin–neuronal antigen MBP	SRFSYG	[22, 48]
Acinetobacter spp.	4-CMLD	SRFAYG	Myelin–neuronal antigen MBP	SRFSYG	[22–24, 48]
	3-OACT-A	LTRAGK	Myelin–neuronal antigen MOG	LYRDGK	[22–24, 48]
	Acinetobacter regulatory protein	*KKVEEI	Neurofilament-M protein	*KKVEEI	[22–24, 48]

MOG = myelin oligodendrocyte glycoprotein; MBP = myelin basic protein; 4-CMLD = 4-carboxy-muconolactone decarboxylase; 3-OACT-A = 3-oxoadipate CoA-transferase; ϒ-CMLD = ϒ-carboxy-muconolactone decarboxylase. * indicates the sequence likely to be responsible for cross-reactivity although this is yet to be confirmed.

- Amino acid sequence homologies have been identified between the 'SRFSYG' motif present in the host's myelin basic protein (MBP) and the 'SRFAYG' amino acid sequence present in *Acinetobacter* spp. 4-carboxy-muconolactone decarboxylase (4-CMLD) antigen (table 2.1) [23, 48].
- Similarly, there is homology between the 'LYRDGK' of the host myelin oligodendrocyte glycoprotein antigen (MOG) and the 'LTRAGK' sequence 3-oxo-adipate-CoA-transferase subunit A (3-OACT-A) of *Acinetobacter* spp. [23, 48].
- A further sequence homology exists between the 'KKVEEI' sequence of human neurofilament M protein and the 'KKVEEI' motif present in *Acinetobacter* spp. regulatory protein [23, 48].

2.2.2 *Pseudomonas aeruginosa* as a trigger of MS

P. aeruginosa infections have also been confirmed as triggers of MS based on several lines of evidence:

- *P. aeruginosa* specific cross-reactive antibodies are significantly elevated in individuals suffering from MS [48, 49].
- An amino acid sequence homology has been identified between the 'TRHAYG' motif present in the host's myelin basic protein (MBP) and the 'SRFSYG' amino acid sequence present in *Acinetobacter* spp. ϒ-carboxy-muconolactone decarboxylase (ϒ-CMLD) antigen (table 2.1) [48, 49].

While both *P. aeruginosa* and *Acinetobacter* spp. have been linked with the induction of MS, they are a normal part of the microbial flora of soil and water, and are present within the normal flora of the human gastrointestinal tract. Gastrointestinal infections of these bacteria are generally not pathogenic in most individuals. However, both *P. aeruginosa* and *Acinetobacter* spp. frequently infect other tissues, with respiratory tract infections being relatively prevalent. Furthermore, *P. aeruginosa* and *Acinetobacter* spp. infections of the respiratory tract may result in other disease pathologies. Interestingly, an extensive study from the UK reported that 70% of individuals with recurrent MS had concurrent sinusitis [50]. *P. aeruginosa* infections may also stimulate other serious disease pathologies, particularly in immunocompromised individuals. Indeed, chronic *P. aeruginosa* respiratory infections are common in people with cystic fibrosis [51]. However, it is only when *P. aeruginosa* and *Acinetobacter* spp. interact with the bloodstream that they may stimulate an immune response, which may result in MS in genetically susceptible people [48, 49]. It has been postulated that *Acinetobacter* spp. and/or *P. aeruginosa* infections (most commonly as either gastrointestinal or lung infections) induce the production of antibodies that are cross-reactive with MBP, MOG and neurofilament M protein [22–24, 48] (table 2.1). Binding of these antibodies to self-antigens activates a number of downstream processes including inflammatory cascades involving acute phase proteins, components of the complement cascade, vasoactive amines, as well as cytokines, tumour necrosis factor-α (TNF-α) and various other cytotoxic components [48, 49]. The cross-reactivity also activates further cellular processes, which result in the development of *Acinetobacter* spp. (and *P. aeruginosa*) reactive MS. Initial infections often result in relatively mild symptoms. Recurrent infections result in enhanced production of cross-reactive antibodies and intensification of the immunological reactions, with further resulting neurological myelin damage.

2.3 Blocking the bacterial triggers of MS

Many antibiotics are already known to inhibit the growth and replication of *Acinetobacter* spp. and *P. aeruginosa* growth (e.g. amino glycosides, fluoroquinolones, tetracyclines, chloramphenicol). However, their use as an ongoing prophylactic therapy is not recommended as long term exposure of an antibiotic monotherapy to the microbiome is certain to induce the development of antibiotic resistant strains, rendering that antibiotic of reduced efficacy. Indeed, the development of super-resistant bacterial strains has already rendered many antibiotics of low efficacy for the treatment of many bacterial infections and care is required with future antibiotic usage to minimise reductions in our antibiotic repertoire. Combinational drug therapies may be a more sustainable therapeutic mode. Indeed, it has long been recognised that the development of antibiotic resistance occurs substantially less frequently when antibiotic combinations are used rather than for single drug therapies [52]. This is particularly true if the combination contains drugs which act via different mechanisms. A bacterium may evade the actions of a single antibiotic monotherapy, although it is substantially less likely to evade several antibiotics with different cytotoxic mechanisms, coadministered as a combinational therapy. There has also been a recent increase in interest in using plant-based antibiotic therapies, with thousands of studies published annually reporting the antibiotic properties of plant formulations. The antiseptic qualities and complex nature of medicinal plant extracts and essential oils make them attractive candidates for natural combinational therapies for promoting increases in treatment efficacy while reducing the risk of resistant bacterial strain development [53].

2.3.1 Targeting *A. baylyi* and *P. aeruginosa* to block the onset of MS using plant-derived therapeutics

Bacterial triggers of MS could be blocked in the GI and/or respiratory tracts before they interact with the immune system, preventing the downstream inflammatory phase of the disease. Thus, any plant extract that could target these bacteria (*A. baylyi* and *P. aeruginosa*) would be effective at preventing the disease onset and symptoms, or lessening the symptoms once the disease has been established. While a number of conventional antibiotics that target bacterial triggers of GI and/or respiratory diseases are available, the use of the pure antibiotics in prophylaxis leads to the development of resistant strains [54]. The use of these agents concomitantly with plant extracts or plant extract components would be preferable as it would arrest the development of resistant microorganisms while potentially reducing the adverse effects associated with use of the allopathic medicines. Specific targeting of two known bacterial triggers of MS, *A. baylyi* and *P. aeruginosa*, could play a vital role in arresting the onset and progression of MS.

A number of plant extracts have been reported to possess activity against these bacterial triggers of MS. Australian plants have featured prominently in this regard. For example, various extracts of *Terminalia ferdinandiana* Exell. (Kakadu plum) leaves [31] and fruit [55] potently inhibit the growth of *A. baylyi* and *P. aeruginosa* on agar, possibly as a result of the oxidative stress associated with high ascorbic acid content of the plant [56]. Multiple extracts of the *Tasmannia lanceolata* (Poir) A.C. Sm. (Tasmanian pepper) fruit, leaf and peppercorn also have strong antimicrobial activity towards both bacterial strains [57], with milder antimicrobial activities observed for *Tasmannia stipitata* (Vick.) A.C.Smith (Dorrigo pepper) extracts [58]. *Scaevola spinescens* R.Br. (currant bush) leaf extracts prepared with solvents of varying polarity (aqueous, methanol, ethyl acetate and chloroform) are also effective at inhibiting the growth of both *A. baylyi* and *P. aeruginosa* [59].

A number of other plant species have been found to exert antimicrobial effects against one or both of these two strains. Ethyl acetate extracts of *Glycyrrhiza glabra* L. (licorice) root potently inhibits *A. baylyi*, while *Plantago squarrosa* Murray and *Embelica officinalis* L. (Indian gooseberry) extracts inhibit the growth of both *A. baylyi* and *P. aeruginosa* [60–62]. A mild-moderate inhibition of both strains is also caused by frankincense (*Boswellia* spp.) resin extracted with water or methanol [63] as well as methanolic myrrh (*Commiphora molmol* (Engl.) Engl. Ex Tschirch) extracts [64]. A spectrum of Syzygium species are known to inhibit the growth of *P. aeruginosa* [65, 66]. Similarly, chamomile (*Chamaemelum nobile* L. All.) flower [67], *Rheum palmatum* L. (Chinese rhubarb) root [68] extracts, as well as the aqueous extracts of a panel of Kenyan and South African medicinal plants [69, 70] are all good inhibitors of these trigger bacterial species and would therefore be likely to be good inhibitors of the onset of MS.

2.3.2 Targeting the interaction between the bacterial triggers of MS and the immune system

A major pathway for the immune system to interact directly with *Acinitobacter* spp. and *P. aeruginosa* is via gastrointestinal interruptions [71]. Therefore, eradication/control of the causative agents of lesion forming conditions (e.g. Crohn's disease) would also be expected to inhibit MS initiation by blocking the interaction of the pathogens with the immune system. However, treatment of acute Crohn's disease is quite harsh and often involves the use of multiple classes of drugs. Antibiotics may be employed to eradicate the pathogenic causes of Crohn's disease [27, 72, 73]. Additionally, salicylates (e.g. 5-aminosalicylic acid) and corticosteroids (e.g. prednisone) may be used to reduce inflammation associated with Crohn's disease. Immunosuppressive drugs (e.g. azathioprine) may also be useful in severe cases. Some of these therapeutics may also directly assist with the symptoms and maintenance of inflammation and thus may have pluripotent effects in the treatment of MS.

Similarly, *Helicobacter pylori* infections also affect the integrity of the gastrointestinal epithelium, allowing interaction between the gut microflora and the host immune system. To avoid the highly acidic environment of the stomach, *H. pylori* burrow through the mucous lining of the stomach to inhabit the substantially less acidic environment of the epithelial cell layer [74]. Once it has colonized the epithelial layer, *H. pylori* further modifies its pH environment via the action of a urease enzyme which releases ammonia from urea. The ammonia neutralizes the gastric acids and increases the pH of *H. pylori* colony's local environment. These localized pH changes cause damage to the stomach epithelial cells, thereby disrupting the tight junctions between individual cells, allowing interaction between the immune system and gastric microflora (including *Acinitobacter* spp. and *P. aeruginosa*). The inflammation associated with the *H. pylori* infection may overwhelm the protective mechanisms of the stomach and duodenum, resulting in gastric ulcer formation. Even less severe *H. pylori* infections that fail to produce ulcers may still allow interaction between gut bacteria and the immune system due to a disruption of the tight junctions between gastric epithelial cells. Therefore, control of *H. pylori* (even when gastritis is not apparent) may be effective in inhibiting the triggering events of MS, and thus the later phase symptoms. Several treatments are already available for *H. pylori* induced gastric ulcers. These usually consist of proton pump inhibitors (e.g. omeprazole) in combination with the antibiotics clarithromycin and amoxicillin (or metronidazole) [75]. However, these treatments are not are very effective in the prevention of *H. pylori* infections and are best considered short term treatments (usually no more than 1 week). Furthermore, prolonged antibiotic administration is not advisable due to the likely formation of antibiotic resistant bacterial pathogens, rendering further similar therapy ineffective [54, 76]. Substantial research is directed towards *H. pylori* vaccination and this may become a useful approach to help decrease the incidence and severity of a number of diseases associated with *H. pylori* infections (e.g. MS, rheumatoid arthritis, stomach cancers, asthma, inflammatory bowel disease, gastroesophageal reflux disease).

Infection of other regions of the gastrointestinal tract may also allow interaction between the immune system and the gastrointestinal microflora. The gastrointestinal protozoal parasite *Giardia duodenalis* may infect the upper and middle regions of the small intestine (duodenum and jejunum). The parasite attaches to the brush border of the epithelial cells via a ventral attachment disc, which flattens the villi of the epithelial cells and forces open the tight junctions between the cells [77]. The disrupted tight junctions increase the permeability across the epithelial layer of the small intestine, allowing increased interaction between the immune system and the gut microflora [78]. Metronidazole is effective at treating acute infections of most strains of *G. duodenalis*, although prevention through hygienic food handling practices and the consumption of sterilized water is generally considered a better option.

2.4 Immunomodulation and immunosuppressants in controlling MS

Blocking the immune response by blocking the interaction of *Acinitobacter* spp. and *P. aeruginosa* with immunological cells (as outlined above), or by immunomodulation may prevent the production of self-reactive antibodies and thus would diminish neuronal myelin damage. Blocking the immune response may also prevent the production of self-reactive antibodies and thus would diminish neuronal myelin damage and the later phase disease symptoms. However, immune-modulatory therapy should be used with caution as inhibiting the patient's immune capability would also expose the patient to a variety of other infections. Cortisone was the first immuno-suppressant with widespread clinical usage. However, its usage has remained limited due to its wide (and often serious) range of side effects. Currently, cyclosporine, which suppresses the immune system by inhibiting the proliferation and function of T cells, has gained much wider acceptance due to its less serious side effects.

2.4.1 Chemotherapeutic approaches to immunomodulation

The predominant approach to immunomodulatory therapy via the use of conventional medicines involves the use of single chemicals or biologicals. Often these compounds have undergone synthetic modifications to increase their potency or bioavailability. What these drugs have in common is that they generally interact with a single specific component of the inflammatory pathway. Corticosteroids (e.g. methylprednisolone) lower the expression of cytokines and prevent leukocyte migration [79] while calcineurin inhibitors such as cyclosporin and tacrolimus lower cytokine production and subsequent T cell proliferation [80]. Immunosuppressant antibodies (also known as biologicals) reduce circulating levels of cytokines or lymphocytes by binding to specific targets [81]. The mTOR inhibitors block mTOR kinase and halt the cytokine-induced T and B cell cycle progression [82]. Other immunosuppressant drugs such as azathioprine and mycophenolate impair purine synthesis required for lymphocyte proliferation [83].

2.5 Targeting inflammatory processes to treat MS

Inflammation is a complex process involving multiple mechanisms which exist to amplify the response to a relatively small signal. However, the presence of multiple steps also allows for a multifactorial approach to MS chemotherapy. Currently, most MS therapies are monotherapies that target one specific process. These therapeutic approaches are generally tailored towards decreasing the late phase symptoms rather than inhibiting the intermediary phases of MS. A representation of the complexity of the inflammatory response is shown in figure 2.3. Although plant-derived compounds have been well documented in their ability to stimulate the immune system [84], there is also considerable evidence for the inhibition of several key steps in the inflammation pathway.

In order for inflammation to occur, migration of T cells from the bloodstream to the nervous system tissue is required, facilitating interaction with antigen-presenting cells (APCs). Disruptions to this process using plant compounds/extracts may occur in several ways:

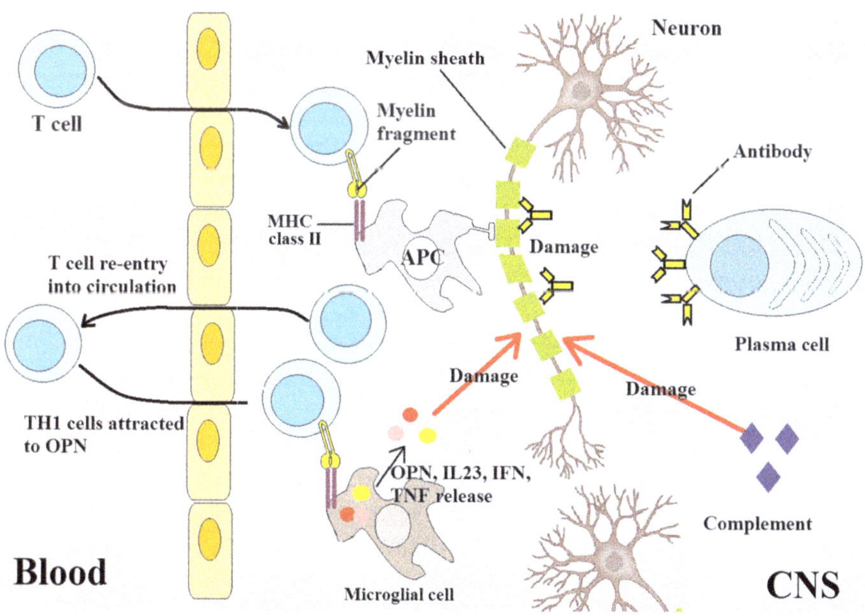

Figure 2.3. The inflammatory phase of multiple sclerosis. T cells, B cells and antigen presenting cells (APCs) enter the central nervous system (CNS) from the blood stream. They are stimulated to secrete cytokines and chemokines including osteopontin (OPN), interleukin-23 (IL23), IFN-ϒ and tumour necrosis factor (TNF), which directly damage neuronal myelin sheaths (and myelin producing cells). The released OPN also attracts T helper cells (TH1). At the same time, B cells (plasma cells) produce myelin specific antibodies, which (in combination with complement) induce further damage to the myelin sheath. The damaged myelin inhibits normal neuronal transduction, resulting in a myriad of symptoms, dependent on the degree of damage and which neurons are affected.

- The abundance of T lymphocytes can be reduced by inhibiting their proliferation. Treatment with several plant-derived alkaloids, including berberine and gelselegine, have been reported to cause substantial decreases in T lymphocyte proliferation [85, 86]. However, examination of plant extracts and purified compounds for the ability to inhibit T lymphocyte proliferation is relatively under-studied and far greater work is needed in developing novel plant-derived inhibitors.
- T cell maturation and activation may also be inhibited by phytophenols [87–89]. These compounds act by lowering the expression of major histocompatibility complex II (MHC-II) and costimulatory (e.g. CD40, CD80) cell surface molecules, thereby preventing T cell interaction with APCs such as dendritic cells. This interaction may be further suppressed by using oenothein B to induce dendritic cell apoptosis [90], or curcumin to stimulate antigen capture [91]. In the latter case, the specific capture of myelin fragments by plant compounds would be an especially key intervention in the pathway of inflammation occurring in the progression of multiple sclerosis. Compounds such as β-sitosterol, a common component in many plant-based foods, have also been reported to suppress IL-2 production from Jurkat T cells [92].
- Direct effects on the microglia, providing another avenue for the interaction of plant compounds in the inflammation pathway. Isoflavones such as daidzein, genistein and glycitein, predominantly found in soybeans, have anti-inflammatory and neuroprotective effects on microglial cells [93]. Phenolic compounds extracted from blueberries prevent the release of IL-1β, NO, PGE2 and TNF-α from activated microglia [94]. Curcumin possesses similar properties, whilst also reducing COX-2 induction in microglia by inhibiting NF-κB [95, 96] and suppressing IL-23 release from dendritic cells [97].
- Plant compounds which slow the progression of MS via neuronal protection. Anthocyanins such as those present in berries and blackcurrant, protect neuronal cells by reducing oxidative stress and reducing levels of pro-inflammatory cytokines [98]. Similar effects have been noted for flavanols [99] and olive oil phenolic compounds [100].

The inflammatory phases are currently the most extensively targeted processes in MS (and other autoimmune diseases) as they rapidly decrease the symptoms and make the patient more comfortable. As already summarised, several effective drug options are already available to target these processes. However, many plant-based therapies remain to be rigorously examined and further evaluation may yield more potent treatments with fewer side effects and toxicities. Whilst targeting the earlier disease events would inhibit MS progressing to the inflammatory stages, therapies targeting these later phase events should not be ignored and further study is urgently required.

2.6 Natural products and herbal medicines as anti-inflammatory agents

Several classes of phytochemicals have good anti-inflammatory activity and some target several aspects of the inflammatory process. A complete examination of phytochemicals with anti-inflammatory activities is beyond the scope of this chapter and has been adequately reviewed elsewhere [101, 102]. Instead, we have selected several classes of phytochemicals here for discussion.

2.6.1 Stilbenes

The stilbenes are particularly useful in treating autoimmune inflammatory diseases (including MS) due to their array of anti-inflammatory, immune-suppressive and antibacterial activities (figure 2.4). Resveratrol (figure 2.5(a)) is perhaps the most widely known and used stilbene for therapeutic purposes. It can directly inhibit the growth of several bacterial species via bacteriostatic mechanisms [103]. Resveratrol can also inhibit the conversion of some bacteria to a swarming form, which allows them to undergo biofilm formation. It also has direct effects in reducing the immune response to bacterial pathogens. Resveratrol inhibits the production of the

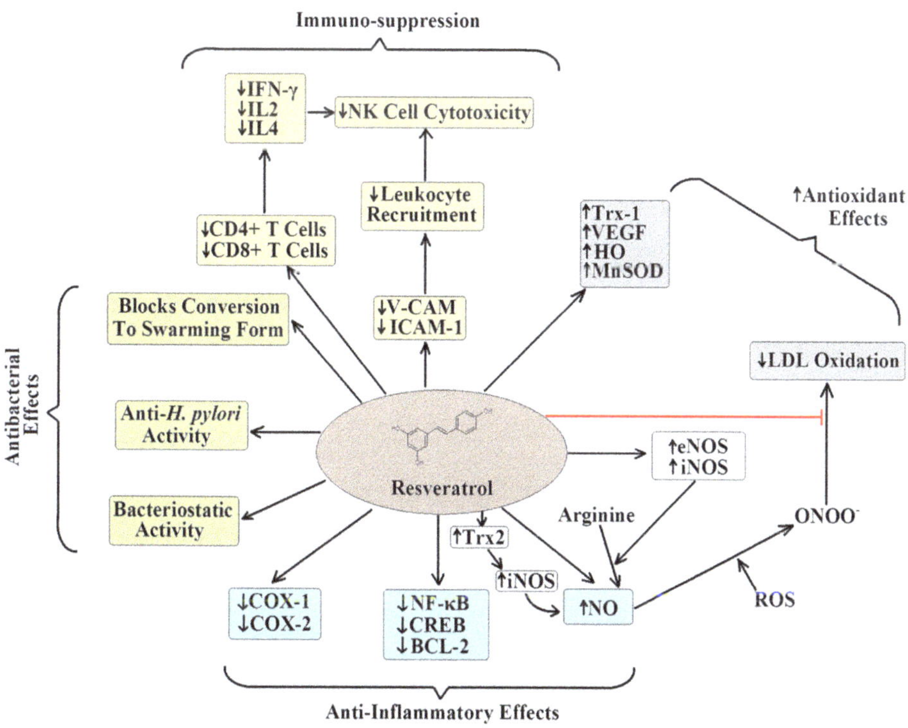

Figure 2.4. Known effects of resveratrol on the bacterial trigger(s) of MS (green), immune suppression (yellow) and direct anti-inflammatory affects (blue). Resveratrol also has antioxidant activity (grey) which may also affect MS progression.

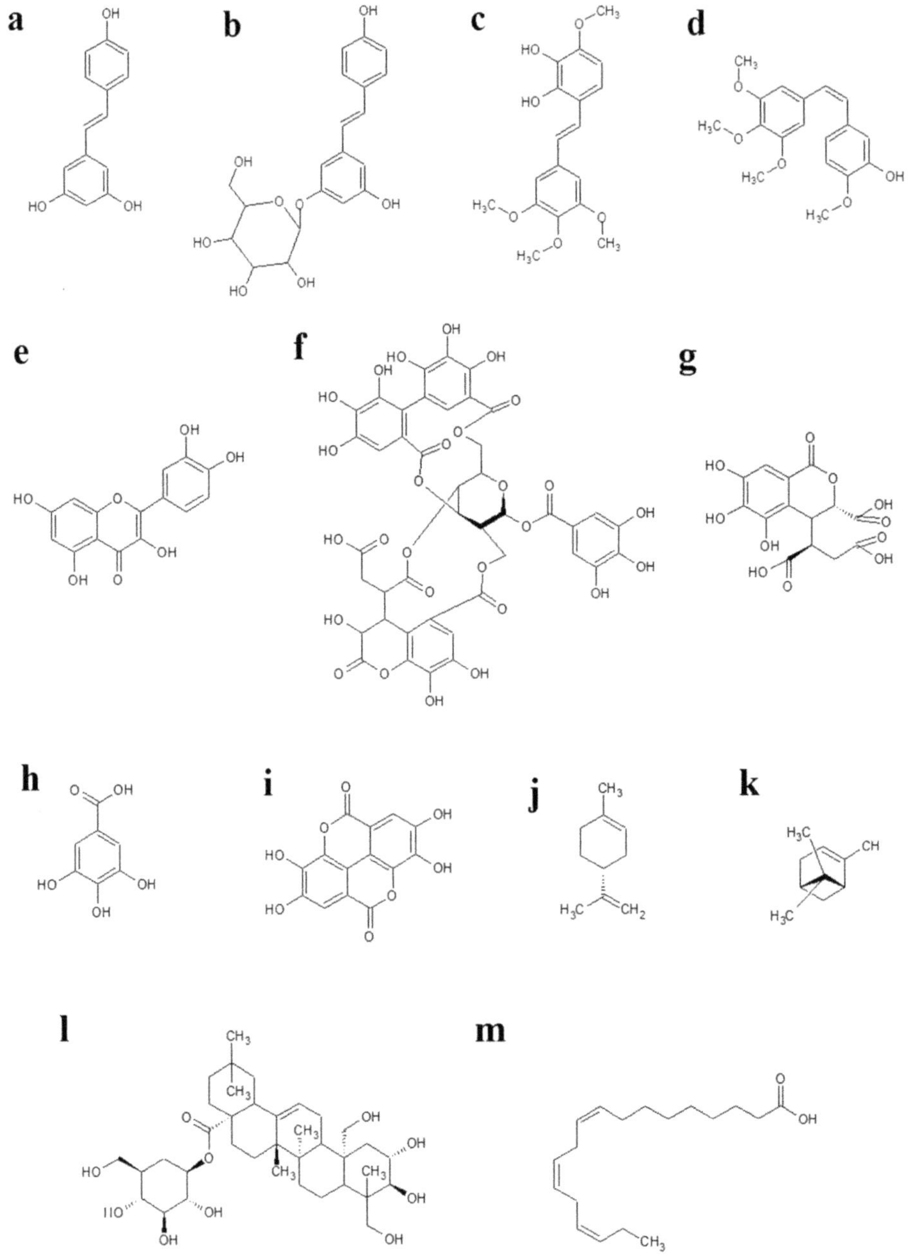

Figure 2.5. Chemical structures of (a) resveratrol; (b) piceid, (c) combretastatin A-1, (d) combretastatin A-4, (e) quercetin, (f) chebulagic acid, (g) chebulic acid, (h) gallic acid, (i) ellagic acid, (j) limonene, (k) α-pinene, (l) sericoside, (m) linolenic acid.

pro-inflammatory cytokines IFN-ϒ, IL2 and IL4 and therefore inhibits T cell maturation [75]. Additionally, resveratrol treatment down-regulates the inflammatory response by inhibiting cyclooxygenase enzymes [104, 105]. Furthermore, resveratrol decreases the transcription of pro-inflammatory mediators by decreasing the activity of NF-κβ and other cellular transcriptase enzymes [106, 107]. Any combinational therapy or extract containing resveratrol that is capable of inhibiting *Acinetobacter* spp. and/or *P. aeruginosa* growth would be likely to have anti-MS activity via several mechanisms (growth inhibition, colonisation blocking, cytokine production inhibition) and therefore would be particularly effective in treating MS.

Other stilbenes and stilbene glycosides also have bioactivities which would endow them with anti-MS properties. Piceid (2-[3-Hydroxy-5[(*E*)-2-(4-hydroxyphenyl) ethenyl] phenoxy]-6-(hydroxymethyl) oxane-3,4,5-triol) (figure 2.5(b)) is a resveratrol glycoside which may be hydrolysed *in vivo* to remove the glucose moiety, thereby releasing resveratrol. Piceid, and other glycosylated stilbenes can block inflammation by decreasing IL-17 production in stimulated human mononuclear cells [108]. Similarly, 2,3,4,5-tetrahydroxystilbene-2-O-β-D-glucoside (TSG) suppresses the induction of pro-inflammatory mediators by reducing the binding of NF-κB to DNA [109]. Interestingly, that study also detected TSG in numerous herbs used in traditional Chinese medicine (TCM) to treat inflammation. Combretastatins A-1 (figure 2.5(c)) and A-4 (figure 2.5(d)) are potent inhibitors of cancer cell progression. They induce apoptosis by binding intracellular tubulin and therefore disrupting microtubule formation [110]. Whilst there are a lack of studies examining the anti-inflammatory properties of the combretastatins, their mechanisms of inducing apoptosis in cancer cells indicates that they are also likely to have substantial anti-inflammatory activity. Combretastatins bind to the colchicine-binding site on the tubulin peptide, thereby inhibiting polymerisation via the same mechanism as colchicine [111]. It is thus likely that they may have similar anti-inflammatory activities and mechanisms to colchicine.

2.6.2 Polyphenolic compounds: flavonoids and tannins

Several other phytochemical classes also have significant anti-inflammatory properties. Many polyphenolic compounds modulate inflammatory pathways [112]. These compounds exert their anti-inflammatory effects by inhibiting cyclooxygenase and lipoxygenase enzymatic activity, thereby decreasing the synthesis of prostaglandins and leukotrienes and therefore the downstream release of cytokines [113, 114]. Quercetin (figure 2.5(e)) is a particularly potent inhibitor of both cyclooxygenase (COX) and lipoxygenase (LOX) enzymes, and substantially reduces eicosanoid biosynthesis [115]. It inhibits COX and LOX activities by down-regulating the expression of cyclooxygenase-2 (COX-2) and 5-lipoxygenase (5-LOX), tumor necrosis factor-alpha (TNF-α) and interleukin-6 (IL-6) [112]. This subsequently results in decreased production of the inflammatory mediators nitric oxide (NO) and prostaglandin E_2 (PGE_2). As mitogen-activated protein kinases (MAPKs) which regulate inflammatory and immune responses may be activated by the production of reactive oxygen species (ROS), the inhibition of ROS via quercetin may contribute to its anti-inflammatory activity. Furthermore, many flavonoids have antibacterial activity [112] and may therefore be useful in inhibiting the trigger mechanisms of MS.

Tannins also have potential in treating autoimmune inflammatory conditions including MS. Chebulagic acid functions via similar anti-inflammatory mechanisms as quercetin. It down-regulates COX-2 and LOX, and inhibits cytokine production and TNF-α and IL-6 expression in human lymphoblastic T lymphocytes, thereby decreasing chemotaxis [116–118]. Tannins are also potent inhibitors of bacterial growth and several tannins including chebulic acid (figure 2.5(g)), gallic acid (figure 2.5(h)) and ellagic acid (figure 2.5(i)) and their derivatives inhibit the growth of a broad range of bacterial pathogens [119, 120]. Therefore, tannins may also inhibit the trigger mechanisms of MS, although this has yet to be verified.

2.6.3 Terpenoids and non-polar anti-inflammatory plant compounds

Multiple terpenoids suppress NF-κB expression and therefore inhibit inflammation [121]. The monoterpenes limonene (figure 2.5(j)) and α-pinene (figure 2.5(k)) are particularly good inhibitors of NF-κB activity and function by binding directly to DNA and blocking transcription [122–125]. In addition, α-pinene also decreases inflammation by inhibiting p65 translocation into the nucleus in LPS-induced NF-κB signaling [124]. Many sesquiterpenes and sesquiterpene lactones also inhibit inflammation [121]. Although an extensive amount of study is still required in order to characterize the mechanisms of action of these compounds, it appears that inhibition of NF-κB activity is responsible. Some larger terpenoids also have good anti-inflammatory activity. The triterpenoidal saponin sericoside (figure 2.5(l)) decreases the extent and severity of colon inflammation colitis in an induced inflammatory bowel disease (IBD) experimental model by reducing neutrophil activation and infiltration into the colon mucosa [126]. Additionally, many terpenoids have potent antibacterial activity against a broad range of bacterial pathogens [112]. Whilst bacterial growth inhibitory activity has been reported for all classes of terpenoids, the monoterpenoids are generally the best bacterial growth inhibitors. Terpenoids may therefore also be useful in inhibiting the trigger mechanisms of MS, although further studies are required to confirm this. Unsaturated fatty acids hydrocarbons, including linolenic acid (figure 2.5(m)), also have substantial anti-inflammatory activity by blocking NF-κB activity [127].

2.7 Plant based approaches: Natural combination therapies

Plants have been used therapeutically by every civilisation, in some cases for thousands of years, and they continue to be the main therapeutic option for a large percentage of the world's population. Plants contain complex mixtures of secondary compounds and are essentially crude combinational therapies in their own right. They therefore have the potential to target several phases and processes of autoimmune diseases, including MS, concurrently. Plant chemotherapies are particularly useful against complex inflammatory diseases, which have many phases and therefore numerous therapeutic targets. Indeed, some plant medicines affect several phases of inflammatory disease progression concurrently. They may block the growth and infection of the antigenic bacterial triggers, modulate the immune response, or directly inhibit the inflammatory pathways. For example, extracts prepared from the bark of *Salix* spp., as well as salicylic acid (and acetosalicylic acid which may be derived from salicylic acid), have analgesic affects and alleviate the pain associated with inflammation [128, 129]. They also have effects on several inflammatory pathways, inhibiting cyclooxygenase activity, thereby decreasing prostaglandin levels. *Salix* spp. extracts, salicylic acid and acetosalicylic acid also inhibit several pro-inflammatory signalling pathways via inhibition of NF-κB, and therefore reduce polymorphonuclear leukocyte and macrophage migration [128]. Several other plant species are also well known for their uses to treat inflammatory disease (table 2.2). *Allium sativum* L. (garlic) and *Aloe vera* (L.) are naturalised globally, and are so widely used therapeutically, that it is no longer certain where their medicinal use originated.

2.7.1 The therapeutic effects of *Cannabis sativa* L.

Cannabis sativa is rich in bioactive secondary compounds including terpenoids, flavonoids and a diversity of cannabinoids (figure 2.6). Whilst *C. sativa* is best known for its psychotropic effects, it also has long been used in folk medicine for a variety of therapeutic purposes. Recent studies have reported that *C. sativa* is particularly useful as a symptomatic therapy for MS [166]. In particular, *C. sativa* and several of its chemical components (cannabinoids), are effective against several MS symptoms including spasticity, pain, ataxia, and frequent urination [166]. However, the use of medical marijuana is also associated with numerous side effects including dizziness and retarded memory. Given the severity of MS symptoms, it is likely that most sufferers would view these side effects as preferable to the symptoms of MS.

C. sativa and the several cannabinoids also directly affect inflammatory processes and may therefore function by pluripotent mechanisms. Interestingly, the anti-inflammatory compounds from *C. sativa* differ from the psychotropic components, negating concerns related to these aspects of MS therapy when using *C. sativa* compounds. Cannabidiol (the main non-psychoactive component of *C. sativa*) is particularly noteworthy. This compound has beneficial effects on at least two symptoms of inflammation (edema and hyperalgesia) and affects several inflammatory processes [137]. Oral administration in a murine model system induces substantial decreases in the levels of PGE2 and NO in the plasma, as well as decreasing cellular COX and NO synthase activities.

2.7.2 The anti-inflammatory effects of *Aloe vera* (L.) Burm.f.

A. vera leaf pulp, juice and extracts have several bioactivities that are beneficial in the treatment of MS (figure 2.7). *A. vera* leaves have immuno-regulatoratory activity and function as both immune-stimulants and immuno-suppressants [167]. The immunomodulatory properties of the polysaccharide acemannan have been particularly well studied. Acemannan treatment activates macrophages and induces antigen processing. Acemannan-activated macrophages secrete multiple cytokines

Table 2.2. Some notable plants used in traditional healing systems to treat and alleviate the symptoms of inflammation.

Plant species	Common name	Comments	Active compound(s) (if known)	Mechanism of action	References
Allium sativum L.	Garlic	*A. sativum* (and other related *Allium* spp.) are reputed to have anti-inflammatory, anticancer and antiviral activities.	High in sulfur containing compounds including alliin, ajoene, S-allyl cysteine etc. Also contains saponins and flavonoids in significant levels.	Suppresses inflammatory cytokine production	[130, 131]
Aloe vera (L.) Burm.f	Aloe vera, burns plant, Barbados aloe, common aloe	Multiple other Aloe species including *A. ferox, A. arborescens*, etc have similar therapetuic properties including anti-inflammatory, anticancer, antibacterial activities.	Anthraquinones, anthrones, flavonoids, phytosterols.	Acemannan activates macrophages and stimulates the secretion of IL-1, IL-6, inteferon, GM-CSF and TNF-α. The anthraquinones reduce TNF-α, IL-1, IL-2 and IL-2 receptor expression, whilst increasing IL-10 expression. B-sitosterol blocks prostacyclin and prostaglandin release. Aloesin inhibits COX-2	[132]
Boswellia spp.	Frankincense	Multiple species are known including *B. carterii, B, sacra, B. serratia.* All are known for a wide array of therapetuic properties including anti-inflammatory, anticancer and antibacterial activities.	Triterpenoids (including boswellic acids), flavonoids, monoterpenoids.	Inhibition of TNF-α, IL-1β, NO and MAP kinase	[63, 133–136]

Cannabis sativa L.	Cannabis, marijuana	The related species *C. indica* and *C. ruderalis* have similar phytochemistry and therapeutic properties.	Cannabinoids including tetrahydrocannabinol, cannabidiol, cannabinol.	Inhibits COX-2	[11, 137–139]
Capsicum spp.	Chilli pepper	There are multiple species and cultivars which vary widely in their intensity of taste and levels of active compounds.	Capsaicin, other capsaicinoids and carotenoids.	Inhibition of pro-inflammatory cytokines TNF-α and IL-1β. Also has analgesic effects	[140, 141]
Commiphora molmol (Nees) Engl.	Myrhh	Has a wide array of therapeutic properties including anti-inflammatory, anticancer and antibacterial activities.	m-Cresol, eugenol, sesquiteriterpenoids, lindestrene, furaneudesma-1,3-diene.	Has analgesic effects	[64, 142]
Curcuma longa L.	Turmeric	Used in Ayurveda to treat inflammation, cancer, cardiovascular and gastrointestinal disease. Also has antimicrobial properties.	Curcumin.	Inhibits COX, 5-lipoxygenase and glutathione-S-transferase. It also lowers histamine release.	[143, 144]
Gaultheria yunnanensis (Franch.)	Wintergreen	Used in TCM to treat rheumatoid arthritis.	Methyl salicylate glycosides.	Suppresses the pro-inflammatory cytokines TNF-α, IL-1β and IL-6.	[145, 146]
Glycyrrhiza glabra L.	Licorice, liquorice	Used in multiple Asian, northern African and European traditional healing systems to treat inflammation, chronic gastritis, jaundice, and rheumatism. Also has anti-infective properties.	Glycyrrhizin, glabbrene, glabridin, anthole and several phytoestrogens.	Suppresses pro-inflammatory cytokines.	[60, 147, 148]

(*Continued*)

Table 2.2. (*Continued*)

Plant species	Common name	Comments	Active compound(s) (if known)	Mechanism of action	References
Harpagophytum procumbens (Burch.) DC. ex Meisn.	Devil's claw	Used in multiple traditional African medicine systems to treat inflammation. Also has antimicrobial properties.	Verbascoside, leveosceptoside A, β-OH-verbascoside, martynoside.	Suppresses pro-inflammatory cytokines and inhibits cyclooxygenase expression.	[149–151]
Olea europaea L.	Olive	Has anti-inflammatory properties and lowers blood glucose and cholesterol. Also has antimicrobial activity.	Oleocanthal. Also contains flavonoids and terpenoids.	Inhibits the expression of pro-inflammatory enzymes	[152, 153]
Stephanotis mucronata Merr.	Shitaki-sou (Japanese)	Used in TCM for the treatment of rheumatoid arthritis.	Steroidal glycosides and saponins.	Immunomodulation	[154, 155]
Tabebuia impetiginosa (Mart. Ex DC.) Mattos	Pau d'arco (Portuguese), lapacho (Spanish), pink ipe, pink lapacho, pink trumpet tree	Used in Central and South American traditional medicine systems to treat inflammation, cancer, stomach disorders and microbial infections.	Lapachol and β-lapachone.	Suppresses the production of prostaglandin E2 and NO. It also blocks the expression of COX-2 and iNOS and activates Nrf2-dependent gene expression.	[156, 157]
Terminalia chebula Retz.	Black myrobalan, chebulic myroblan, inknut	Used to treat inflammation and tumours. Also used for the treatment of coughs and colds, digestive disorders, and as an antimicrobial treatment. Multiple other *Terminalia* spp. have similar therapeutic uses.	Rich in galloyl- and ellagi-tannins (including chebulis acid). Also contains substantial triterpenoid levels.	Inhibits iNOS and COX-2	[56, 158–160]

Vitis vinifera L.	Grape	Seed extracts and fruit skins have anti-inflammatory properties.	Resveratrol (and other stilbenoids), anthocyanins, hydroxycinnamic acids, tannins.	Suppresses the pro-inflammatory cytokines TNF-α and IL-6.	[161]
Withania somnifera (L.) Dunal	Ashwagandha (Indian), Indian ginseng, poison gooseberry, winter cherry.	Used in Ayurveda to treat inflammation and rheumatism, microbial diseases, gastrointestinal disease and a wide variety of other illness.	Alkaloids and steroidal lactones, including withaferin A.	Modulates COX-2 expression. Also inhibits the growth of the bacterial triggers of MS.	[162, 163]
Zingiber officinale Roscoe	Ginger	Has anti-inflammatory and antimicrobial properties.	Gingerol, flavonoids.	Immunomodulation. Inhibits PGE_2 production and decreases the levels of pro-inflammatory cytokines.	[143, 164, 165]

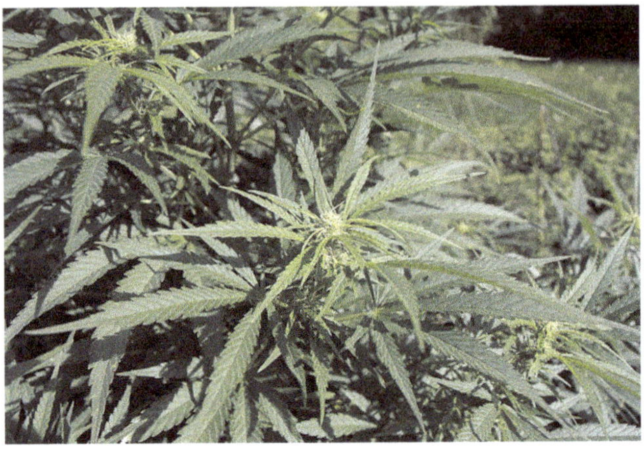

Figure 2.6. A photograph of a *Cannabis sativa* plant. This photograph is sourced from wiki commons (https://commons.wikimedia.org/wiki/File:Cannabis_sativa_plant_(4).JPG). It has been made freely available and is reproduced with here in accordance with all relevant permissions.

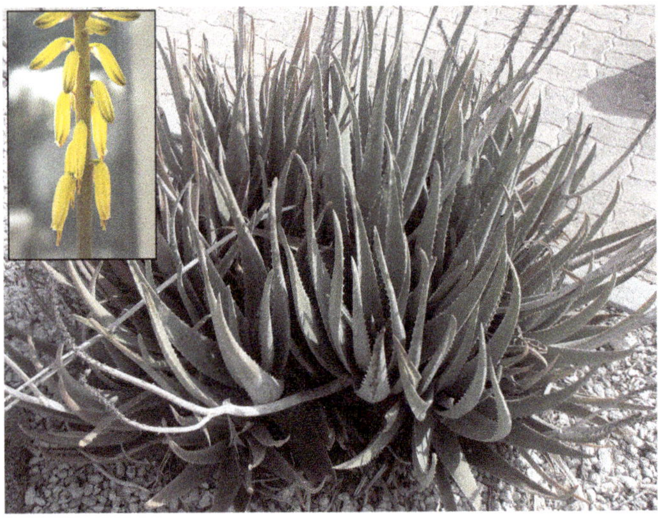

Figure 2.7. A photograph of *Aloe vera*. The photograph was taken by D J Midgley and is available from wiki commons for free use and distribution (https://en.wikipedia.org/wiki/Aloe_vera#/media/File:Aloe_vera_flower_inset.png). It has been made freely available by the photographer and is reproduced with here in accordance with all relevant permissions.

including IL-1, IL-6, interferon, GM-CSF and TNF-α, thereby inducing inflammation. Furthermore, acemannan also enhances the sensitivity of macrophages to IFN-γ and induces apoptosis by inhibiting the expression of Bcl-2 proteins. A number of smaller *A. vera* polyphenolic compounds also have immune-modulatory activity. Aloe emodin and other anthraquinone derivatives reduce the expression of receptors for the pro-inflammatory cytokines IL-1, IL-2 and IL-2 and therefore reduce inflammation.

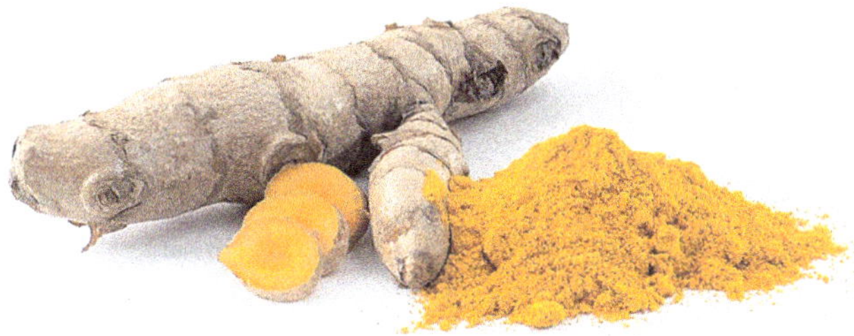

Figure 2.8. *Curcuma longa* L. roots and root powder. This photograph is available via wiki commons (https://en.wikipedia.org/wiki/Turmeric#/media/File:Curcuma_longa_roots.jpg). It has been made freely available by the photographer and is reproduced here in accordance with all relevant permissions.

A. vera leaves are rich in β-sitosterol which blocks the release of PGI2 and prostaglandin E2 (PGE2) from macrophages, thereby reducing vasodilation [167]. *A. vera* leaves also contain substantial levels of chromones which can inhibit COX-2 activity and the synthesis of thromboxane A2. These chromones inhibit inflammation and would therefore decrease neuronal myelin damage and the symptoms of MS. In contrast, *A. vera* anthraquinone components stimulate PGE2 release and therefore have pro-inflammatory effects. The release of chemotactic factors stimulate motality of leukocytes during inflammation. Thus, preventing the release of these factors or blocking their effects prevents inflammation and the associated tissue damage. Several *A. vera* anthraquinones decrease chemotaxis by inhibiting cytokine production and IL-2 mRNA expression in activated T lymphocytes. In particular, aloe emodin decreases plasma levels of IL-2 and TNF-α, whilst increasing IL-10 (which itself down-regulates IL-2 and TNF-α cytokine activity). Thus, *A. vera* contains compounds that target multiple aspects of inflammation. Furthermore, it is likely that the combined effects of these components provides greater efficacy than for the individual components alone, although studies are required to confirm this.

2.7.3 The anti-inflammatory activity of *Curcuma longa* L. (turmeric)

Turmeric is widely used in traditional Ayurvedic medicine to treat a wide variety of medical conditions including inflammation, gastrointestinal and cardiovascular disease, as well as cancer (figure 2.8). Curcumin is the main compound responsible for the anti-inflammatory activity of this plant [53, 168]. Curcumin has a wide range of effects that give it anti-inflammatory properties. Briefly, curcumin:

- Inhibits COX-2 [143], thereby decreasing the production of prostaglandins, prostacyclins and thromboxanes. Several prostaglandins have powerful pro-inflammatory properties. In particular, PGI2 and PGE2 are powerful vasodilators. Inhibiting their production inhibits the migration of T cells out of blood vessels into the surrounding tissue (including the CNS). Thus, inhibiting PGI2 and PGE2 production would directly inhibit neuronal myelin damage and the formation of CNS lesions.

- Inhibits the metabolism of arachidonic acid by lipoxygenase and the scavenging of free radicals [143]. It also inhibits the activity of glutathione-S-transferase. This would also inhibit neuronal myelin damage.
- Inhibits NF-κB (which controls cytokine transcription), profoundly affecting several inflammatory pathways, thereby decreasing the levels of pro-inflammatory cytokines. Furthermore, NF-κB also regulates several genes responsible for innate and adaptive immune responses, resulting in a down-regulation of the immune system.
- Decreases the expression of several pro-inflammatory cytokines including TNF-α, IL-1β, IL-6, which mediate the innate immune response. Decreasing the levels of these cytokines lessens the effects and severity of inflammation and would therefore decrease MS related myelin damage.
- Down-regulates protein kinase C, which mediates inflammation.

As curcumin targets multiple aspects of inflammation, it may be a particularly effective chemotherapy for the treatment of a variety of inflammatory diseases, including MS. However, curcumin has relatively low solubility, which impacts its bioavailability and clinical usefulness. There is substantial recent interest in the development of curcumin nano-formulations with improved bioavailability through combination with carriers [168]. If these formulations are ultimately successful in enhancing bioavailability, the use of curcumin may become far more common clinically. Interestingly, turmeric also substantially decreases histamine release [144], although this effect is less evident for pure curcumin.

2.7.4 The anti-inflammatory activity of Boswellia spp. (frankincense)

Multiple species of the genus *Boswellia* are used in traditional healing systems, for a wide array of therapeutic properties, including anti-inflammatory and antibacterial activities. Extracts from several species (including *B. carterii, B, sacra* (figure 2.9)*, B. serratia*) strongly inhibit the release of TNF-α, PGE2, IL-2, IL-1β, NO and MDA, as well as inhibiting MAP kinase [133–135]. Frankincense extracts and essential oils are also good inhibitors of COX-2 [136]. α-Pinene, linalool, and 1-octanol are major components of frankincense extracts and oils and each of these compounds inhibit

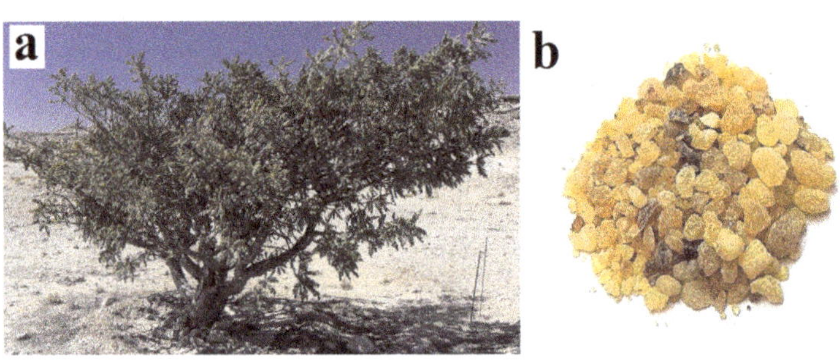

Figure 2.9. (a) *Boswellia sacra* Flueck. tree growing near Salalah, Oman, and (b) the oleoresin known as frankincense which is derived from the tree.

COX-2. Interestingly, a mixture of these three compounds is a substantially more potent inhibitor of COX-2 than the any of the compounds alone, highlighting the potential of developing a combinational therapy. Furthermore, *Boswellia* spp. extracts also have antibacterial activity against the bacterial triggers of several autoimmune inflammatory diseases, including the bacterial triggers of multiple sclerosis [63]. Therefore *Boswellia* spp. have multiple beneficial effects in the prevention and treatment of MS.

2.7.5 The anti-inflammatory effects of *Harpagophytum procumbens* Burch. (Devil's claw)

H. procumbens roots are effective in reducing the symptoms (pain, swelling, heat, redness) of inflammation and are recognised globally as an effective anti-inflammatory therapy [149]. The *H. procumbens* whole plant and fruiting body are shown in figure 2.10. Aqueous *H. procumbens* extracts suppress PGE2 and NO production by inhibiting the expression of COX-2 and nitric oxide synthase (iNOS) enzymes, without significantly affecting cellular viability [150]. Further studies have confirmed that *H. procumbens* root extracts significantly inhibit COX-2 and iNOS expression in murine macrophages by approximately 70% and 40%, respectively [151]. That study also reported substantial inhibition of NO, TNF-α and IL-6 (by approximately 20%, 45% and 32%, respectively, compared to the untreated control). Several *H. procumbens* extract components have been isolated and investigated for anti-inflammatory activities. Verbascoside and harpagoside were highlighted as the major anti-inflammatory constituents of *H. procumbens* roots. Interestingly, whilst pure verbascoside and harpagoside are potent anti-inflammatory mediators alone, the crude extract was substantially stronger than either pure component, indicating that the extracts may contain potentiating compounds that increase the efficacy of the anti-inflammatory compounds. Future studies to screen *H. procumbens* root extracts for potentiating compounds may identify combinations with greatly enhanced efficacy. If/when these potentiator compounds are identified, mixtures of verbascoside and/or harpagoside in combination with the potentiating compound(s)

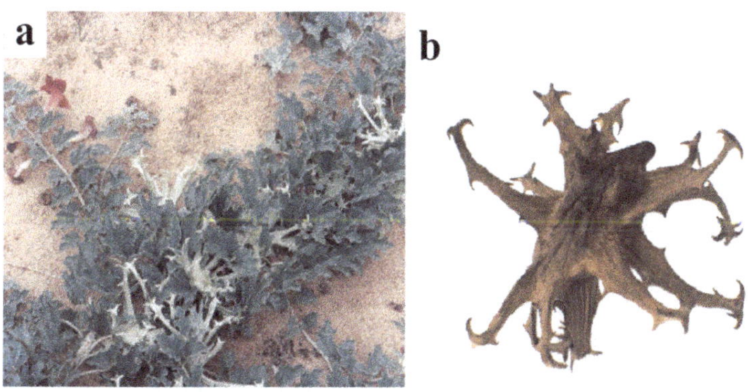

Figure 2.10. *Harpagophytum procumbens* (Burch.) DC. Ex Meisn. (a) Plant and (b) dried fruiting body, from which the plant takes its common name.

in defined ratios could be prepared and may be particularly effective as therapeutics against inflammatory diseases, including MS.

2.8 Conclusion

MS is a complex disease which may be triggered in genetically susceptible individuals who are exposed to *A. baylyi* and/or *P. aeruginosa*, inducing the synthesis of self-reactive antibodies. This manuscript reviews some of the early events in MS disease progression and highlights several targets for the development of drugs to prevent the onset and early stage progression of the disease. It is unlikely that any single drug will be completely effective at preventing the onset of MS due to the complexity of the triggering events and the later phase cascades. Instead, the use of combinational therapies may be a preferred treatment modality, especially combinations that inhibit the onset of the disease as well as treating the later symptoms. Bioactive plant extracts and pure compounds (including stilbenes) have pluripotent effects on inflammation and may therefore be particularly useful in targeting multiple phases of MS disease progression. Crude plant extracts (especially those containing stilbenes) have appeal in the treatment of chronic inflammatory diseases (including MS) for a number of reasons:

- There is less likelihood of developing resistant strains of bacteria as combinations contain multiple components that may inhibit bacterial growth by multiple mechanisms.
- Multiple phases of the disease etiology and progression may be targeted simultaneously with a single chemotherapeutic treatment.
- Plant based therapeutics are generally cost effective and easy to produce, thereby increasing their availability to a greater number of people afflicted with MS.

References

[1] Miller D H, Hammond S R, McLeod J G, Purdie G and Skegg D C 1990 Multiple sclerosis in Australia and New Zealand *J. Neurol. Neurosurg. Psychiatry* **53** 903–5

[2] Milo R and Kahana E 2010 Multiple sclerosis: Geoepidemiology, genetics and the environment *Autoimmun. Rev.* **9** A387–94

[3] Compston A, McDonald I, Noseworthy J, Lassmann H, Miller D, Smith K, Wekerle H and Confavreux C 2006 *McAlpine's Multiple Sclerosis* (Philadelphia, PA: Churchill Livingstone/Elsevier)

[4] World Health Organization and Multiple Sclerosis International Federation 2008 *Atlas: Multiple Sclerosis Resources in the World* (Geneva: World Health Organization) Available at: http://who.int/mental_health/neurology/en (Accessed August 2014)

[5] Compton A and Coles A 2008 Multiple sclerosis *Lancet* **372** 1502–17

[6] Lublin F D and Reingold S C 1996 Defining the clinical course of multiple sclerosis: results of an international survey. National Multiple Sclerosis Society (USA) Advisory Committee on Clinical Trials of New Agents in Multiple Sclerosis *Neurology* **46** 907–91

[7] Graham D J, Campen D, Hui R, Spence M, Cheetham C, Levy G, Shoor S and Ray W A 2005 Risk of acute myocardial infarction and sudden cardiac death in patients treated with

cyclo-oxygenase 2 selective and non-selective non-steriodal anti-inflammatory drugs: nested case-control study *Lancet* **365** 475–81

[8] Miller D H, Thompson A J, Morrissey S P, MacManus D G, Moore S G, Kendall B E, Moseley I F and McDonald W I 1992 High dose steroids in acute relapses of multiple sclerosis: MRI evidence for a possible mechanism of therapeutic effect *J. Neurol. Neurosurg. Psychiatry* **55** 450–3

[9] Saag K G, Koehnke R, Caldwell J R, Brasington R, Burmeister L F, Zimmerman B, Kohler J A and Furst D E 1994 Low dose long-term corticosteroid therapy in rheumatoid arthritis: an analysis of serious adverse events *Am. J. Med.* **96** 115–23

[10] Huntley A 2006 A review of the evidence for efficacy of complementary and alternative medicines in MS *Int. MS. J.* **13** 5–12

[11] Yadav V, Bever C, Bowen J, Bowling A, Weinstock-Guttman B, Cameron M, Bourdette D, Gronseth G S and Narayanaswami P 2014 Summary of evidence-based guideline: Complementary and alternative medicine in multiple sclerosis. Report of the Guideline Development Subcommittee of the American Academy of Neurology *Neurology* **82** 1083–92

[12] Compston A and Coles A 2008 Multiple sclerosis *Lancet* **372** 1502–17

[13] Bertolotto A and Gilli F 2008 Interferon-beta responders and non-responders. A biological approach *Neurol. Sci.* **29** S216–7

[14] Fox E J 2006 Management of worsening multiple sclerosis with mitoxantrone: A review *Clin. Ther.* **28** 461–74

[15] Balcer L J *et al* 2007 Natalizumab reduces visual loss in patients with relapsing multiple sclerosis *Neurology* **68** 1299–304

[16] Wiendl H and Kieseier B 2013 Multiple sclerosis: reprogramming the immune repertoire with alemtuzumab in MS *Nat. Rev. Neurol.* **9** 125

[17] McGinley M P, Moss B P and Cohen J A 2017 Safety of monoclonal antibodies for the treatment of multiple sclerosis *Expert Opin. Drug Saf.* **16** 89–100

[18] La Mantia L, Munari L M and Lovati R 2010 Glatiramer acetate for multiple sclerosis *The Cochrane Database Syst. Rev.* **5** CD004678

[19] Arnon R and Sela M 1999 The chemistry of the copaxone drug *Chem. Israel* **1** 12–7

[20] Sanford M 2014 Fingolimod: A review of its use in relapsing-remitting multiple sclerosis *Drugs* **74** 1411–33

[21] Vollmer T 2009 MS therapies in the pipeline: Teriflunomide *EMS News*

[22] Rashid T and Ebringer A 2012 Autoimmunity in rheumatic diseases is induced by microbial infections via crossreactivity or molecular mimicry *Autoimmune Dis.* **2012** 539282

[23] Ebringer A, Rashid T and Wilson C 2012 The role of Acinetobacter in the pathogenesis of multiple sclerosis examined by using Popper sequences *Med. Hypotheses* **78** 763–9

[24] Ebringer A, Hughes L, Rashid T and Wilson C 2005 Acinetobacter immune response in multiple sclerosis. Etiopathogenetic role and its possible use as a diagnostic marker *JAMA Neurol.* **62** 33–6

[25] Rashid T and Ebringer A 2011 Rheumatoid arthritis is caused by asymptomatic Proteus urinary tract infections *Clinical Management of Complicated Urinary Tract Infection* vol 11 ed A Nikibakhsh (London: In-Tech)

[26] Rashid T and Ebringer A 2007 Ankylosing spondylitis is linked to Klebsiella—the evidence *Clin. Rheumatol.* **26** 858–64

[27] Cock I E and Cheesman M J 2018 The potential of plants of the genus Syzygium (Myrtaceae) for the prevention and treatment of arthritic and autoimmune diseases

Bioactive Foods as Dietary Interventions for Arthritis and Related Inflammatory Diseases 2nd edn (Amsterdam: Elsevier) pp 401–24

[28] Ercolini A and Miller S 2009 The role of infections in autoimmune disease *Clin. Exp. Immunol.* **155** 1–15

[29] Kivity S, Agmon-Levin N, Blank M and Shoenfeld Y 2009 Infections and autoimmunity–friends or foes? *Trends Immunol.* **30** 409–14

[30] Zabriskie J B, Hsu K and Seegal B 1970 Heart-reactive antibody associated with rheumatic fever: characterization and diagnostic significance *Clin. Exp. Immunol.* **7** 147

[31] Courtney R, Sirdaarta J, Matthews B and Cock I 2015 Tannin components and inhibitory activity of Kakadu plum leaf extracts against microbial triggers of autoimmune inflammatory diseases *Pharmcogn. J.* **7** 18–31

[32] Ebringer A and Rashid T 2006 Rheumatoid arthritis is an autoimmune disease triggered by *Proteus* urinary tract infection *Clin. Dev. Immunol.* **13** 41–8

[33] Nepom G T, Byers P, Seyfried C, Healey L A, Wilske K R, Stage D and Nepom B S 1989 HLA genes associated with rheumatoid arthritis. Identification of susceptibility alleles using specific oligonucleotide probes *Arthritis Rheum.* **32** 15–21

[34] Rashid T and Ebringer A 2007 Ankylosing spondylitis is linked to *Klebsiella*—the evidence *Clin. Rheumatol.* **26** 858–64

[35] Ebringer A, Rashid T, Wilson C, Ptaszynska T and Fielder M 2006 Ankylosing Spondylitis, HLA-B27 and *Klebsiella*—an overview: proposal for early diagnosis and treatment *Curr. Rheumatol. Rev.* **2** 55–68

[36] Blankenberg-Sprenkels S, Fielder M, Feltkamp T, Tiwana H, Wilson C and Ebringer A 1998 Antibodies to *Klebsiella pneumoniae* in Dutch patients with ankylosing spondylitis and acute anterior uveitis and to *Proteus mirabilis* in rheumatoid arthritis *J. Rheumatol.* **25** 743–7

[37] Fielder M, Pirt S, Tarpey I, Wilson C, Cunningham P, Ettelaie C, Binder A, Bansal S and Ebringer A 1995 Molecular mimicry and ankylosing spondylitis: possible role of a novel sequence in pullulanase of *Klebsiella pneumoniae FEBS Lett.* **369** 243–8

[38] Schwimmbeck P L, Yu D T and Oldstone M B 1987 Autoantibodies to HLA B27 in the sera of HLA B27 patients with ankylosing spondylitis and Reiter's syndrome. Molecular mimicry with *Klebsiella pneumoniae* as potential mechanism of autoimmune disease *J. Exp. Med.* **166** 173–81

[39] Welsh J, Avakian H, Cowling P, Ebringer A, Wooley P, Panayi G and Ebringer R 1980 Ankylosing spondylitis, HLA-B27 and *Klebsiella*. I. Cross-reactivity studies with rabbit antisera *Br. J. Exp. Pathol.* **61** 85

[40] Lee C J, Wright M H, Arnold M S J, Greene A C and Cock I E 2016 Inhibition of *Streptococcus pyogenes* growth by native Australian plants: New approaches towards the management of impetigo, pharyngitis and rheumatic heart disease *Pharmacogn. Commun.* **6** 164

[41] Dinkla K, Rohde M, Jansen W T, Kaplan E L, Chhatwal G S and Talay S R 2003 Rheumatic fever–associated *Streptococcus pyogenes* isolates aggregate collagen *J. Clin. Invest.* **111** 1905

[42] Beermann C, Wunderli-Allenspach H, Groscurth P and Filgueira L 2000 Lipoproteins from *Borrelia burgdorferi* applied in liposomes and presented by dendritic cells induce CD8+ T-lymphocytes *in vitro Cell Immunol.* **201** 124–31

[43] Tellez M, Cooper J and Edmonds C 1992 Graves' ophthalmopathy in relation to cigarette smoking and ethnic origin *Clin. Endocrinol.* **36** 291–4

[44] Weetman A P 2000 Graves' disease *N. Engl. J. Med.* **343** 1236–48

[45] Kollef M H, West S, Davis D R and Winn R E 1991 Central and peripheral nervous system demyelination after infection with *Mycoplasma pneumoniae*: evidence of an autoimmune process *South Med. J.* **84** 1255–8

[46] Lee M N, Cha J H, Ahn H M, Yoo J H, Kim H S, Sohn S and Hong Y M 2011 *Mycoplasma pneumoniae* infection in patients with Kawasaki disease *Korean J. Pediatr.* **54** 123–7

[47] Wang J N, Wang S M, Liu C C and Wu J M 2001 *Mycoplasma pneumoniae* infection associated with Kawasaki disease *Acta Paediatr.* **90** 594–5

[48] Hughes L, Smith P, Bonell S, Natt R, Wilson C, Rashid T, Amor S, Thompson E, Croker J and Ebringer A 2003 Cross-reactivity between related sequences found in *Acinetobacter* sp., *Pseudomonas aeruginosa*, myelin basic protein and myelin oligodendrocyte glycoprotein in multiple sclerosis *J. Neuroimmunol.* **144** 105–15

[49] Hughes L E *et al* 2001 Antibody responses to *Acieitobacter* spp. and *Pseudomanas aeruginosa* in multiple sclerosis: Prospects for diagnosis using the myelin-*Acinetobacter*-neurofilament antibody index *Clin. Vaccine Immunol.* **8** 1181–8

[50] Gay D, Dick G and Upton G 1986 Multiple sclerosis associated with sinusitis: case-controlled study in general practice *Lancet* **1** 815–9

[51] Winstanley C, O'Brien S and Brockhurst M A 2016 *Pseudomonas aeruginosa* evolutionary adaption and diversification in cystic fibrosis chronic lung infections *Trends Microbiol.* **24** 32–337

[52] Weight S S, Purcell E M, Wilcox C, Brodericken M K and Finland M 1953 Antibiotic combinations and resistance to antibiotics. Development of resistance during repeated subcultures of *Staphylococci* and certain *Streptococci* on media containing penicillin, streptomycin, erythromycin, terramycin, and chloramphenicol used singly and in pairs *J. Lab. Clin. Med.* **42** 877–95

[53] Cock I E 2018 Is the pharmaceutical industry's preoccupation with the monotherapy drug model stifling the development of effective new drug therapies *Inflammopharmacology* **26** 861–79

[54] Cheesman M J, Ilanko A, Blonk B and Cock I E 2017 Developing new antimicrobial therapies: Are synergistic combinations of plant extracts/compounds with conventional antibiotics the solution? *Pharmacog. Rev.* **11** 57–72

[55] Sirdaarta J, Matthews B, White A and Cock I E 2015 GC-MS and LC-MS analysis of Kakadu plum fruit extracts displaying inhibitory activity against microbial triggers of multiple sclerosis *Pharmacog. Commun.* **5** 100–15

[56] Cock I E 2015 The medicinal properties and phytochemistry of plants of the genus *Terminalia* (Combretaceae) *Inflammopharmacology* **23** 203–29

[57] Winnett V, Boyer H, Sirdaarta J and Cock I E 2014 The potential of *Tasmannia lanceolata* as a natural preservative and medicinal agent: antimicrobial activity and toxicity *Pharmacog. Commun.* **4** 42–52

[58] Hart C, Ilanko P, Sirdaarta J, Rayan P, McDonnella P A and Cock I E 2014 *Tasmannia stipitata* as a functional food/natural preservative: Antimicrobial activity and toxicity *Pharmacog. Commun.* **4** 33–47

[59] Blonk B and Cock I E 2018 Interactive antimicrobial and toxicity profiles of *Scaevola spinescens* R. Br. extracts with conventional antibiotics *Pharmacog. J.* **10** 1024–35

[60] Maas H and Cock I E 2018 The interactive antimicrobial activity of *Glycyrrhiza glabra* L. root extracts and conventional antibiotics against some bacterial triggers of autoimmune inflammatory diseases *Pharmacog. Commun.* **8** 66–74

[61] Omer E, Elshamy A I, Nassar M, Shalom J, White A and Cock I E 2018 *Plantago squarrosa* Murray extracts inhibit the growth of some bacterial triggers of autoimmune diseases: GC–MS analysis of an inhibitory extract *Inflammopharmacology* **27** 373–85

[62] Hutchings A and Cock I E 2018 An interactive antimicrobial activity of Embelica officinalis Gaertn. fruit extracts and conventional antibiotics against some bacterial triggers of autoimmune inflammatory diseases *Pharmacog. J.* **10** 654–62

[63] Biggs I, Sirdaarta J, White A and Cock I E 2016 GC-MS analysis of frankincense extracts which inhibit the growth of bacterial triggers of selected autoimmune diseases *Pharmacog. Commun.* **6** 10–22

[64] Biggs I, Sirdaarta J, White A and Cock I E 2016 GC-MS analysis of *Commiphora molmol* oleo-resin extracts which inhibit the growth of bacterial triggers of selected autoimmune diseases *Pharmacog. J.* **8** 191–202

[65] Cock I E and Cheesman M J 2018 Plants of the genus *Syzygium* (Myrtaceae): A review on ethnobotany, medicinal properties, and phytochemistry *Bioactive Compounds of Medicinal Plants: Properties and Potential for Human Health* ed M R Goyal and A O Ayeleso (New York: Apple Academic)

[66] Logeswari P, Silambarasan S and Abraham J 2015 Synthesis of silver nanoparticles using plants extract and analysis of their antimicrobial property *J. Saudi Chem. Soc.* **19** 311–7

[67] Kazemian H, Ghafourian S, Heidari H, Amiri P, Yamchi J K, Shavalipour A, Houri H, Maleki A and Sadeghifard N 2015 Antibacterial, anti-swarming and anti-biofilm formation activities of *Chamaemelum nobile* against *Pseudomonas aeruginosa Rev. Soc. Bras. Med. Trop.* **48** 432–6

[68] Arokiyaraj S, Vincent S, Saravanan M, Lee Y, Oh Y K and Kim K H 2017 Green synthesis of silver nanoparticles using *Rheum palmatum* root extract and their antibacterial activity against *Staphylococcus aureus* and *Pseudomonas aeruginosa Artif. Cells Nanomed. Biotechnol.* **45** 372–9

[69] Mutembei J K, Kareru P G, Madivoli E S, Murigi M K, Karanja J, Cheruiyot K, Rechab S O and Maina E G 2018 Phytochemical and antimicrobial evaluation of selected medicinal plants in Meru community of Kenya *J. Med. Plant Econ. Dev.* **2** 1–4

[70] Kudumela R G and Masoko P 2018 *In vitro* assessment of selected medicinal plants used by the Bapedi community in South Africa for treatment of bacterial infections *J. Evid. Based Integrat. Med.* **23** 1–10

[71] Rashid T and Ebringer A 2011 Rheumatoid arthritis is caused by asymptomatic *Proteus* urinary tract infections *Clinical Management of Complicated Urinary Tract Infection* ed A Nikibakhsh (London: In-Tech)

[72] Manichanh C, Borruel N, Casellas F and Guarner F 2012 The gut microbiota in IBD *Nat. Rev. Gastroenterol. Hepatol.* **9** 599–608

[73] Sartor R B 2006 Mechanisms of disease: pathogenesis of Crohn's disease and ulcerative colitis *Nat. Clin. Pract. Gastroenterol. Hepatol.* **3** 390–407

[74] Stasi R, Sarpatwari A, Segal J B, Osborn J, Evangelista M L, Cooper N, Provan D, Newland A, Amadori S and Bussel J B 2009 Effects of eradication of *Helicobacter pylori* infection in patients with immune thrombocytopenic purpura: a systematic review *Blood* **113** 1231–40

[75] Cock I E 2014 The early stages of rheumatoid arthritis: New targets for the development of combinational drug therapies. *OA Arthritis* **2** 5
[76] Banin E, Hughes D and Kuipers O P 2017 Editorial: Bacterial pathogens, antibiotics and antibiotic resistance *FEMS Microbiol. Rev.* **41** 450–2
[77] Woessner D J and Dawson S 2012 The Giardia median body protein is a ventral disc protein that is critical for maintaining a domed disc conformation during attachment *Eukaryot. Cell* **11** 292–301
[78] Buret A G, Mitchell K, Muench D G and Scott K G E 2002 *Giardia lamblia* disrupts tight junctional ZO-1 and increases permeability in non-transformed human small intestinal epithelial monolayers: effects of epidermal growth factor *Parasitology* **125** 11–9
[79] Cain D W and Cidlowski J A 2017 Immune regulation by glucocorticoids *Nat. Rev. Immunol.* **17** 233
[80] Azzi J R, Sayegh M H and Mallat S G 2013 Calcineurin inhibitors: 40 years later, can't live without... *J. Immunol.* **191** 5785–91
[81] Focosi D, Maggi F, Pistello M, Boggi U and Scatena F 2011 Immunosuppressive monoclonal antibodies: current and next generation *Clin. Microbiol. Infect.* **17** 1759–68
[82] Zheng Y and Jiang Y 2015 mTOR inhibitors at a glance *Mol. Cell Pharmacol.* **7** 15
[83] Mimouni D and Nousari H C 2002 Inhibitors of purine and pyrimidine synthesis: mycophenolate, azathioprine, and leflunomide *Dermatol. Ther.* **15** 311–6
[84] Sultan B, Ramanathan M Jr, Lee J, May L and Lane A P 2013 Sinonasal epithelial cells synthesize active vitamin D, augmenting host innate immune function *Int. Forum Allergy Rhinol.* **3** 26–30
[85] Lin W C and Lin J Y 2011 Berberine down-regulates the Th1/Th2 cytokine gene expression ratio in mouse primary splenocytes in the absence or presence of lipopolysaccharide in a preventive manner *Int. Immunopharmacol.* **11** 1984–90
[86] Xu Y K, Liao S G, Na Z, Hu H B, Li Y and Luo H R 2012 Gelsemium alkaloids, immunosuppressive agents from *Gelsemium elegans Fitoterapia* **83** 1120–4
[87] Yum M K, Jung M Y, Cho D and Kim T S 2011 Suppression of dendritic cells' maturation and functions by daidzein, a phytoestrogen *Toxicol. Appl. Pharmacol.* **257** 174–81
[88] Lee J S *et al* 2007 Silibinin polarizes Th1/Th2 immune responses through the inhibition of immunostimulatory function of dendritic cells *J. Cell. Physiol.* **210** 385–97
[89] Liu S H, Lin C H, Hung S K, Chou J H, Chi C W and Fu S L 2010 Fisetin inhibits lipopolysaccharide-induced macrophage activation and dendritic cell maturation *J. Agric. Food Chem.* **58** 10831–9
[90] Yoshimura M, Akiyama H, Kondo K, Sakata K, Matsuoka H, Amakura Y, Teshima R and Yoshida T 2012 Immunological effects of oenothein B, an ellagitannin dimer, on dendritic cells *Int. J. Mol. Sci.* **14** 46–56
[91] Kim G Y, Kim K H, Lee S H, Yoon M S, Lee H J, Moon D O, Lee C M, Ahn S C, Park Y C and Park Y M 2005 Curcumin inhibits immunostimulatory function of dendritic cells: MAPKs and translocation of NF-κB as potential targets *J. Immunol.* **174** 8116–24
[92] Aherne S A and O'brien N M 2008 Modulation of cytokine production by plant sterols in stimulated human Jurkat T cells *Mol. Nutr. Food Res.* **52** 664–73
[93] Marotta F, Mao G S, Liu T, Chui D H, Lorenzetti A, Xiao Y and Marandola P 2006 Anti-inflammatory and neuroprotective effect of a phytoestrogen compound on rat microglia *Ann. N.Y. Acad. Sci.* **1089** 276–81

[94] Lau F C, Bielinski D F and Joseph J A 2007 Inhibitory effects of blueberry extract on the production of inflammatory mediators in lipopolysaccharide-activated BV2 microglia *J. Neurosci. Res.* **85** 1010–7

[95] Jin C Y, Lee J D, Park C, Choi Y H and Kim G Y 2007 Curcumin attenuates the release of pro-inflammatory cytokines in lipopolysaccharide-stimulated BV2 microglia 1 *Acta Pharmacol. Sin.* **28** 1645–51

[96] Kang G, Kong P J, Yuh Y J, Lim S Y, Yim S V, Chun W and Kim S S 2004 Curcumin suppresses lipopolysaccharide-induced cyclooxygenase-2 expression by inhibiting activator protein 1 and nuclear factor κB bindings in BV2 microglial cells *J. Pharmacol. Sci.* **94** 325–8

[97] Brück J *et al* 2017 Nutritional control of IL-23/Th17-mediated autoimmune disease through HO-1/STAT3 activation *Sci. Rep.* **7** 44482

[98] de Pascual-Teresa S 2014 Molecular mechanisms involved in the cardiovascular and neuroprotective effects of anthocyanins *Arch. Biochem. Biophys.* **559** 68–74

[99] Ahmed M E, Khan M M, Javed H, Vaibhav K, Khan A, Tabassum R, Ashafaq M, Islam F, Safhi M M and Islam F 2013 Amelioration of cognitive impairment and neurodegeneration by catechin hydrate in rat model of streptozotocin-induced experimental dementia of Alzheimer's type *Neurochem. Int.* **62** 492–501

[100] Lamy S, Saad A B, Zgheib A and Annabi B 2016 Olive oil compounds inhibit the paracrine regulation of TNF-α-induced endothelial cell migration through reduced glioblastoma cell cyclooxygenase-2 expression *J. Nutr. Biochem.* **27** 136–45

[101] Attiq A, Jalil J, Husain K B and Ahmad W 2018 Raging the war against inflammation with natural products *Front. Pharmacol.* **9** 976

[102] Maroon J C, Bost J W and Maroon A 2010 Natural anti-inflammatory agents for pain relief *Surg. Neurol. Int.* **1** 80

[103] Paulo L, Ferreira S, Gallardo E, Queiroz J A and Domingues F 2010 Antimicrobial activity and effects of resveratrol on human pathogenic bacteria *World J. Microbiol. Biotechnol.* **26** 1533–8

[104] Mukherjee D and Ahmad R 2018 Resveratrol attenuates nitrosodiethylamine-induced liver injury ain anti-inflammatory manner via regulating cyclooxygenase *J. Food Biochem.* **42** e12594

[105] Chen X, Lu J, An M, Ma Z, Zomg H and Yang J 2014 Anti-inflammatory effect of resveratrol on adjuvant arthritis rats with abnormal immunological function via the reduction of cyclooxygenase-2 and prostaglandin E_2 *Mol. Med. Rep.* **9** 2592–8

[106] Pan W, Yu H, Huang S and Zhu P 2016 Resveratrol protects against TNF-α-induced injury in human umbilical endothelial cells through promoting sirtuin-1-induced repression of NF-KB and p38 MAPK *PLoS One* **11** e0147034

[107] Bagul P K, Deepthi N, Sultana R and Banerjee S K 2015 Resveratrol ameliorates cardiac oxidative stress in diabetes through deacetylation of NFkB-p65 and histone 3 *J. Nutr. Biochem.* **26** 1298

[108] Lanzilli G and Cottarelli A *et al* 2012 Anti-inflammatory effect of resveratrol and polydatin by *in vitro* IL-17 modulation *Inflammation* **35** 240–8

[109] Huang C and Wang Y *et al* 2013 2-O-β-D-glucoside suppresses induction of pro-inflammatory factors by attenuating the binding activity of nuclear factor-κB in microglia *J. Neuroinflammation* **10** 129

[110] Dark G G, Hill S A, Prise V E, Tozer G M, Pettit G R and Chaplin D J 1997 Combretastatin A-4, an agent that displays potent and selective toxicity towards tumor vasculature *Cancer Res.* **57** 1829–34

[111] Bhardwaj S, Bakshi S, Chopra B, Dhingra A and Dhar K L 2010 Synthesis of combretastatin analogues with their potent anticancer activity *Int. J. Res. Pharm. Sci.* **1** 414–6

[112] Cock I E 2013 The phytochemistry and chemotherapeutic potential of *Tasmannia lanceolata* (Tasmanian pepper): A review *Pharmacog. Commun.* **3** 13–25

[113] Ferrandiz M L and Alcaraz M J 1991 Anti-inflammatory activity and inhibition of arachidonic acid metabolism by flavonoids *Agents Actions* **32** 283–8

[114] Laughton M J, Evans P J, Moroney M A, Hoult J R and Halliwell B 1991 Inhibition of mammalian 5 lipoxygenase and cyclo-oxygenase by flavonoids and phenolic dietary additives. Relationship to antioxidant activity and to iron ion-reducing ability *Biochem. Pharmacol.* **42** 1673–81

[115] Kim H P, Mani I, Iversen L and Ziboh V A 1998 Effects of naturally-occurring flavonoids and bioflavonoids on epidermal cyclooxygenase and lipoxygenase from guinea-pigs *Prostaglandins Leukot. Essent. Fatty Acids* **58** 17–24

[116] Das N D, Jung K H, Park J H, Choi M R, Lee H T, Kim M S, Lee S R and Chai Y G 2012 Proteomic analysis of *Terminalia chebula* extract-dependent changes in human lymphoblastic T cell protein expression *J. Med. Food* **15** 651–7

[117] Reddy D B and Reddanna P 2009 Chebulagic acid (CA) attenuates LPS-induced inflammation by suppressing NK-κB and MAPK avtivation in RAW 264.7 macrophages *Biochem. Biophys. Res. Commun.* **381** 112–7

[118] Reddy D B, Reddy T C, Jyotsna G, Sharan S, Priya N, Lakshmipathi V and Reddanna P 2009 Chebulagic acid, a COX-LOX dual inhibitor isolated from the fruits of *Terminalia chebula* Retz., induces apoptosis in COLO-205 cell line *J. Ethnopharmacol.* **124** 506–12

[119] McManus K, Wood A, Wright M H, Matthews B, Greene A C and Cock I E 2017 Terminalia ferdinandiana Excell. extracts inhibit the growth of body odour-forming bacteria *Int. J. Cosmet. Sci.* **39** 500–10

[120] Buzzini P, Arapitsas P, Goretti M, Branda E, Turchetti B, Pinelli P, Ieri F and Romani A 2008 Antimicrobial and antiviral activity of hydrolysable tannins *Mini Rev. Med. Chem.* **8** 1179–87

[121] Salminen A, Lehtonen M, Suuronen T, Kaarniranta K and Huuskonen J 2008 Terpenoids: Natural inhibitors of NF-κB signalling with anti-inflammatory and anticancer potential *Cell. Mol. Life Sci.* **65** 2979–99

[122] Berchtold C M, Chen K S, Miyamoto S and Gould M N 2005 Perillyl alcohol inhibits a calcium-dependent constitutive nuclear factor-kB pathway *Cancer Res.* **65** 8558–66

[123] Zhou J Y, Tang F D, Mao G G and Bian R L 2004 Effect of a-pinene on nuclear translocation of NF-kB in THP-1 cells *Acta Pharmacol. Sin.* **25** 480–4

[124] Lu X G, Zhan L B, Feng B A, Qu M Y, Yu L H and Xie J H 2004 Inhibition of growth and metastasis of human gastric cancer implanted in nude mice by d-limonene *World J. Gastroenterol.* **10** 2140–4

[125] Crowell P L 1999 Prevention and therapy of cancer by dietary monoterpenes *J. Nutr.* **129** 775S–8S

[126] Mochizuki M and Hasegawa N 2007 Anti-inflammatory effect of extract of *Terminalia sericea* roots in an experimental model of colitis *J. Health Sci.* **53** 329–31

[127] Ren J and Chung S H 2007 Anti-inflammatory effect of α-linolenic acid and its mode of action through the inhibition of nitric oxide production and inducible nitric oxide synthase gene expression via NF-κB and mitogen-activated protein kinase pathways *J. Agric. Food Chem.* **55** 5073–80

[128] Morris T, Stables M, Hobbs A, de Souza P, Colville-Nash P, Warner T, Newson J, Bellingan G and Gilroy D W 2009 Effects of low-dose aspirin on acute inflammatory responses in humans *J. Immunol.* **183** 2089–96

[129] Fiebich B L and Chrubasik S 2004 Effects of an ethanol *Salix* extract on the release of selected inflammatory mediators *in vitro Phytomed* **11** 135–8

[130] Capasso A 2013 Antioxidant action and therapeutic efficacy of *Allium sativum* L *Molecules* **18** 690–700

[131] Hodge G, Hodge S and Han P 2002 *Allium sativum* (garlic) suppresses leukocyte inflammatory cytokine production *in vitro*: Potential therapeutic use in the treatment of inflammatory bowel disease *Cytometry* **48** 209–15

[132] Cock I E 2016 The genus Aloe: Phytochemistry and therapeutic uses including treatments for gastrointestinal conditions and chronic inflammation *Novel Natural Products: Therapeutic Effects in Pain, Arthritis and Gastro-intestinal Diseases, Progress in Drug Research* vol 70 ed K D Rainsford *et al* (Basel: Springer) pp 179–235

[133] Su S *et al* 2015 Frankincense and myrrh suppress inflammation via regulation of the metabolic profiling and the MAPK signalling pathway *Sci. Rep.* **5** 13668

[134] Gayathri B, Manjula N, Vinaykumar K S, Lakshmi B S and Balakrishnan A 2007 Pure compound from *Boswellia serrata* extract exhibits anti-inflammatory property in human PBMCs and mouse macrophages through inhibition of TNFα, IL-1β, NO and MAP kinases *Int. Immunopharmacol.* **7** 473–82

[135] Banno N, Akihisa t, Yasukawa K, Tokuda H, Tabata K, Nakamura Y, Nishimura R, Kimura Y and Suzuki T 2006 Anti-inflammatory activities of the triterpene acids from the resin of *Boswellia carteri J. Ethnopharmacol.* **107** 249–53

[136] Li X J, Yang Y J, Li Y S, Zhang W K and Tang H B 2016 α-Pinene, linalool, and 1-octanol contribute to the topical anti-inflammatory and analgesic activities of frankincense by inhibiting COX-2 *J. Ethnopharmacol.* **179** 22–6

[137] Costa B, Colleoni M, Conti S, Parolaro D, Franke C, Trovato A E and Giagnoni G 2004 Oral anti-inflammatory activity of cannabidiol, a non-psychoactive constituent of cannabis, in acute carrageenan-induced inflammation in the rat paw *Naunyn Schmiedeberg's Arch. Pharmacol.* **369** 294–9

[138] Ruhaak L R, Felth J, Karlsson P C, Rafter J J, Verpoorte R and Bohlin L 2011 Evaluation of the cyclooxygenase inhibiting effects of six major cannabinoids isolated from *Cannabis sativa Biol. Pharm. Bull.* **34** 774–8

[139] Turner C E, Elshohly M A and Boeren E G 1980 Constituents of *Cannabis sativa* L. XVII. A review of the natural constituents *J. Nat. Prod.* **43** 169–234

[140] Hernández-Ortega M, Ortiz-Moreno A, Hernández-Navarro M D, Chamorro-Cevallos G, Dorantes-Alvarez L and Necoechea-Mondragón H 2012 Antioxidant, antinociceptive, and anti-inflammatory effects of carotenoids extracted from dried pepper (*Capsicum annuum* L.) *J. Biomed. Biotechnol.* **2012** 524019

[141] Spiller F, Alves M K, Vieira S M, Carvalho T A, Leite C E, Lunardelli A, Poloni J A, Cunha F Q and de Oliveira J R 2008 Anti-inflammatory effects of red pepper (*Capsicum*

baccatum) on carrageenan- and antigen-induced inflammation *J. Pharm. Pharmacol.* **60** 473–8
[142] Mohamed A A, Ali S I, El-Baz F K, Hegazy A K and Kord M A 2014 Chemical composition of essential oil and antimicrobial activities of crude extracts of *Commiphora myrrha* resin *Ind. Crops Prod.* **57** 10–6
[143] Ramadan G, Al-Kahtani M A and El-Sayed W M 2014 Anti-inflammatory and antioxidant properties of *Curcuma longa* (Tumeric) versus *Zingiber officinale* (Ginger) rhizomes in rat adjuvant-induced arthritis *Inflammation* **34** 291–301
[144] Akram M, Shahab-Uddin A A, Usmanghani K, Hannan A, Mohiuddin E and Asif M 2010 *Curcuma longa* and curcumin: a review article *Rom. J. Biol. Plant Biol.* **55** 65–70
[145] Zhang D, Liu R, Sun L, Huang C, Wang C, Zhang D M, Zhang T T and Du G H 2011 Anti-inflammatory activity of methyl salicylate glycosides isolated from *Gaultheria yunnanensis* (Franch.) Rehder *Molecules* **16** 3875–84
[146] Xiong Y, Xiao B, Ma X, Li C, Zheng J and Ye J 2009 Effects of *Gaultheria yunnanensis* on adjuvant arthritis in rats *Chin. J. Chin. Mater. Med.* **34** 2516–9
[147] Liu Z, Zhong J Y, Gao E N and Yang H 2014 Effects of glycyrrhizin and licorice flavonoids on LPS-induced cytokines expression in macrophages *Chin. J. Chin. Mater. Med.* **39** 3841–5
[148] Xie Y C, Dong X W, Wu X M, Yan X F and Xie Q M 2009 Inhibitory effect of flavonoids extracted from licorice on lipopolysaccharide-induced acute pulmonary inflammation in mice *Int. Immunopharmacol.* **9** 194–200
[149] Van Wyk B E, van Oudtshoorn B and Gericke N 2009 *Medicinal Plants of South Africa* 2nd edn (Pretoria: Briza Publications) pp 162–3
[150] Jang M H, Lim S, Han S M, Park H J, Shin I, Kim J W, Kim N J, Lee J S, Kim K A and Kim C J 2003 *Harpagophytum procumbens* suppresses lipopolysaccharide-stimulated expressions of cyclooxygenase-2 and inducible nitric oxide synthase in fibroblast cell line L929 *J. Pharmacol. Sci.* **93** 367–71
[151] Gyurkovska V, Alipieva K, Maciul A, Dimitrova P, Ivanovska N, Haas C, Bley T and Georgiev M 2011 Anti-inflammatory activity of Devil's claw *in vitro* systems and their active constituents *Food Chem.* **125** 171–8
[152] Süntar I, Akkol E K and Baykal T 2010 Assessment of anti-inflammatory and antiociceptive activities of *Olea europaea* L *J. Med. Food* **13** 352–6
[153] El S N and Karakaya S 2009 Olive tree (*Olea europaea*) leaves: potential beneficial effects on human health *Nutr. Rev.* **11** 632–8
[154] Li X Y, Zong S L, Chen F Y, Xu S F and Ye Y P 2012 Three novel immunosuppressive steroidal glycosides from the stems of *Stephanotis mucronata Nat. Prod. Commun.* **7** 1269–70
[155] Ye Y, Chen F, Sun H, Li X and Xu S 2008 Stemucronatoside K, a novel C21 steroidal glycoside from *Stephanotis mucronata*, inhibited the cellular and humoral immune response in mice *Int. Immunopharmacol.* **8** 1231–8
[156] Richter M, Winkel A F, Schummer D, Gerlitz M, de Hoop M, Brunner B, Glien M and Schmoll D 2014 Pau d-arco activates Nrf2-dependent gene expression via the MEK/ERK-pathway *J. Toxicol. Sci.* **2** 353–61
[157] Byeon S E, Chung J Y, Lee Y G, Kim B H, Kim K H and Cho J Y 2008 *In vitro* and *in vivo* anti-inflammatory effects of taheebo, a water extract from the inner bark of *Tabebuia avellanedae J. Ethnopharmacol.* **119** 145–52

[158] Mandeville A and Cock I E 2018 Terminalia chebula Retz. fruit extracts inhibit bacterial triggers of some autoimmune diseases and potentiate the activity of tetracycline *Indian J. Microbiol.* **58** 496–506

[159] Kim S J, Sancheti S A, Sancheti S S, Um B H, Yu S M and Seo S Y 2010 Effect of 1,2,3,4,6-penta-O-galloyl-beta-D-glucose on elastase and hyaluronidase activities and its type II collagen expression *Acta Pol. Pharm.* **67** 145–50

[160] Yang M H, Ali Z, Khan I A and Khan S I 2014 Anti-inflammatory activity of constituents isolated from *Terminalia chebula Nat. Prod. Commun.* **9** 965–8

[161] Terra X *et al* 2009 Grape-seed procyanidins prevent low-grade inflammation by modulating cytokine expression in rats fed a high-fat diet *J. Nutr. Biochem.* **20** 210–8

[162] Lai W, Chen J, Cock I E and Cheesman M J 2018 The interactive antimicrobial activity of Withania somnifera (L.) Dunal root extracts and conventional antibiotics against some bacterial triggers of autoimmune inflammatory diseases *Pharmacog. Commun.* **8** 86–92

[163] Kim J H and Kim S J 2014 Overexpression of microRNA-25 by withaferin A induces cyclooxygenase-2 expression in rabbit articular chondrocytes *J. Pharmacol. Sci.* **125** 83–90

[164] Adel S P R and Prakash J 2010 Chemical composition and antioxidant properties of ginger root (*Zingiber officinale*) *J. Med. Plant Res.* **4** 2674–9

[165] Grzanna R, Lindmark L and Frondoza C G 2005 Ginger—An herbal medicinal product with broad anti-inflammatory actions *J. Med. Food* **8** 125–32

[166] Yadav V, Bever C, Bowen J, Bolwing A, Weinstock-Guttman B, Cameron M, Bourdette D, Gronseth G S and Narayanaswami P 2014 Summary of evidence-based guideline: Complementary and alternative medicine in multiple sclerosis. Report of the Guideline Development Subcommittee of the American Academy of Neurology *Neurology.* **82** 1083–92

[167] Cock I E 2015 The genus Aloe: Phytochemistry and therapeutic uses including treatments for gastrointestinal conditions and chronic inflammation *Novel Natural Products: Therapeutic Effects in Pain, Arthritis and Gastro-intestinal Diseases, Progress in Drug Research* vol 70 ed K D Rainsford *et al* (Basel: Springer) pp 179–235

[168] Jurenka J S 2009 Anti-inflammatory properties of curcumin, a major constituent of *Curcuma longa*: A review of preclinical and clinical research *Altern. Med. Rev.* **14** 141–53

IOP Publishing

Neurological Disorders and Imaging Physics, Volume 2
Engineering and clinical perspectives of multiple sclerosis
Ayman El-Baz and Jasjit S Suri

Chapter 3

Advanced technique for characterization of balance disorders in multiple sclerosis: posturography

Hua Cao, Laurent Peyrodie and Olivier Agnani

Balance impairment is one of the most common symptoms in people with multiple sclerosis (MS), even found in the early stages. In this chapter, we present an advanced technique to characterize balance disorders in MS using a static force platform, called static posturography. Many linear (temporal and spectral) parameters and nonlinear indicators can be extracted from the stabilometric signals and are able to provide new diagnostic elements for the management, in particular with the possibility of predicting disability progression, and to improve the understanding of the mechanisms involved in the system for balance regulation in MS.

3.1 Introduction

3.1.1 Generalities on MS

3.1.1.1 Definition

Multiple sclerosis (MS) is a common chronic inflammatory disease of the central nervous system (CNS) that usually develops by relapses [1]. It is characterized by myelin and axon involvement (figure 3.1). This axonal damage can be primitive or secondary. The demyelination lesions are disseminated in the white matter of the CNS. The set of clinical symptoms is related to the localization of lesions, which explains their diversity. Remyelination made possible by oligodendrocytes, explains the possibility of recovery after a relapse. MS is the most common multifocal, diffuse and disability-causing neurological disorder of young people between the ages of 20 and 40 [2]. It mainly affects female subjects (sex ratio = 3 to 1). The prevalence is estimated at 95 per 100 000 and the incidence varies between 4 and 8 per 100 000 [3].

doi:10.1088/978-0-7503-1762-7ch3

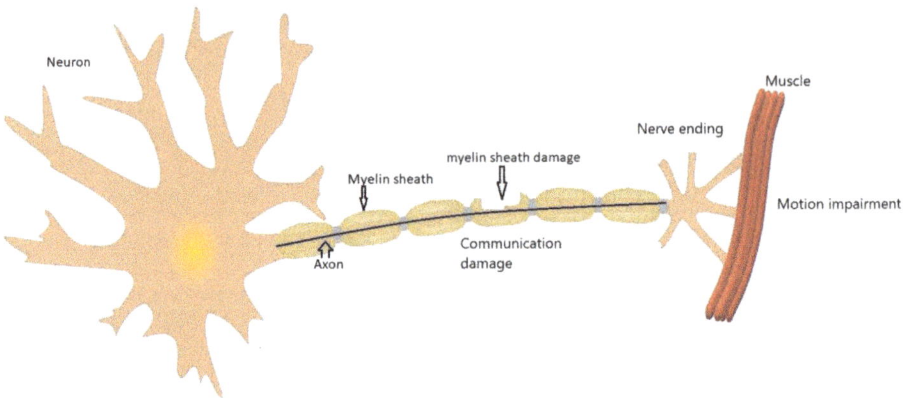

Figure 3.1. Demyelination related to MS.

3.1.1.2 Clinical forms

The disease has different clinical forms and their terminology has changed recently. Two forms of MS are currently defined in which the notion of clinical relapse or MRI activity are integrated. The concept of aggravation of disability is also taken into consideration over a given period of time (6 months, one year …) [4]. The relapsing-remitting form starts with a clinically isolated active or inactive syndrome depending on the MRI activity at the time of the clinical event, it is characterized exclusively by inflammatory events and can leave sequelae (potentially stable between two episodes) and starts usually around 30 years old. It represents 85% of the initial forms of the disease. The progressive form also includes subtypes: active with or without progression, inactive with or without progression. The secondarily progressive form is the late natural evolution of the previous form, it can affect all subjects initially remittent in a mean time of 15–20 years. The primary progressive form is characterized by an evolution present from the beginning of the disease, without relapses and affects 15% of the subjects. It starts on average around 40 years old [5].

3.1.1.3 Etiology

The etiology of MS is currently unknown but is nevertheless considered multifactorial. Genetic factors are present: Caucasian population, concordance of 30% in monozygotic twins against 2%–3% in heterozygotic twins, susceptibility genes (linked to the HLA group). Environmental factors are also advanced as well as a viral infection with EBV, smoking, vitamin D deficiency and low sunlight, obesity. Some authors argue that excessive hygiene during childhood increases the risk and that some infantile parasitic infections have a protective effect [6]. The median age in all forms is 32 for a sex ratio of 0.75 for female subjects. There is a North–South gradient and MS is more common when one moves away from the Equator (MS is twice as prevalent in the Scandinavian countries as in the Mediterranean countries).

3.1.1.4 Diagnosis

Diagnosis is based on modified McDonald's criteria [5, 7] that associate clinical and neuroradiological criteria. It is thus demonstrated as spatial (location of lesions and

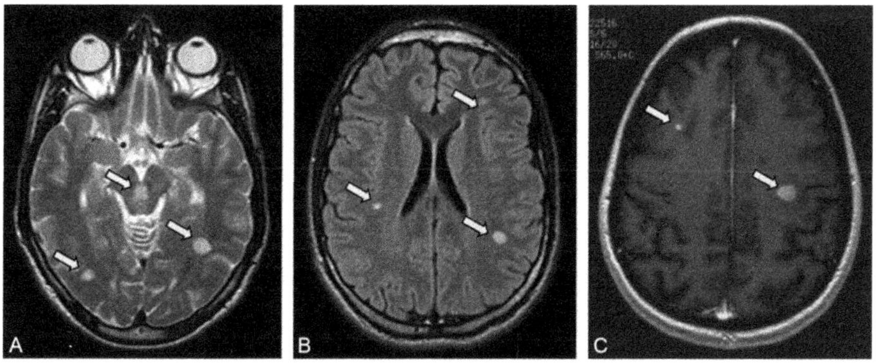

Figure 3.2. Brain Imaging and CNS Inflammation.

multiple clinical symptoms) and temporal (time-onset of new symptoms or changes in lesion MRI activity) [8]. Encephalic or medullary MRI reveals the location and activity of the various lesions (figure 3.2). These lesions generally have an ovoid aspect, they sit within the white matter in different places: near the ventricles, in the cerebellum or the brainstem, in the spinal cord. These multiple localizations and their modification of appearance over time explain the variety of clinical signs observed in patients and the chronological sequence of impairments. The analysis of the cerebrospinal fluid (CSF) is not systematic but confirms the presence of inflammatory phenomena in the CNS, it is based on the abnormal presence of immunoglobulin G (IgG).

The evolution of MS is unpredictable and varies greatly from one subject to another [9]. There is a multiplicity and a polymorphism of clinical signs: patients present or associate motor, sensory, visual, cognitive, bladder and urinary disorders.

3.1.1.5 Assessment of disability in MS

The disability assessment scale that is predominantly used and specifically adapted to MS is the Expanded Disability Status Scale (EDSS) (figure 3.3). This scale is composed of two parts: A first, rated from 0 to 4, takes into account the functional parameters specified by the neurological examination, a second part rated from 4 to 10 takes into account the ambulatory capacities of the patient (perimeter of walking with or without technical assistance) [10, 11].

3.1.2 Clinical signs

3.1.2.1 Motor impairments

They are characterized by muscular deficits and gait disturbances (limitation of walking perimeter, mowing, stepping), disorders of balance, mono or paraparesis and more rarely hemiparesis. All of these signs are related to the degradation of the pyramidal pathways.

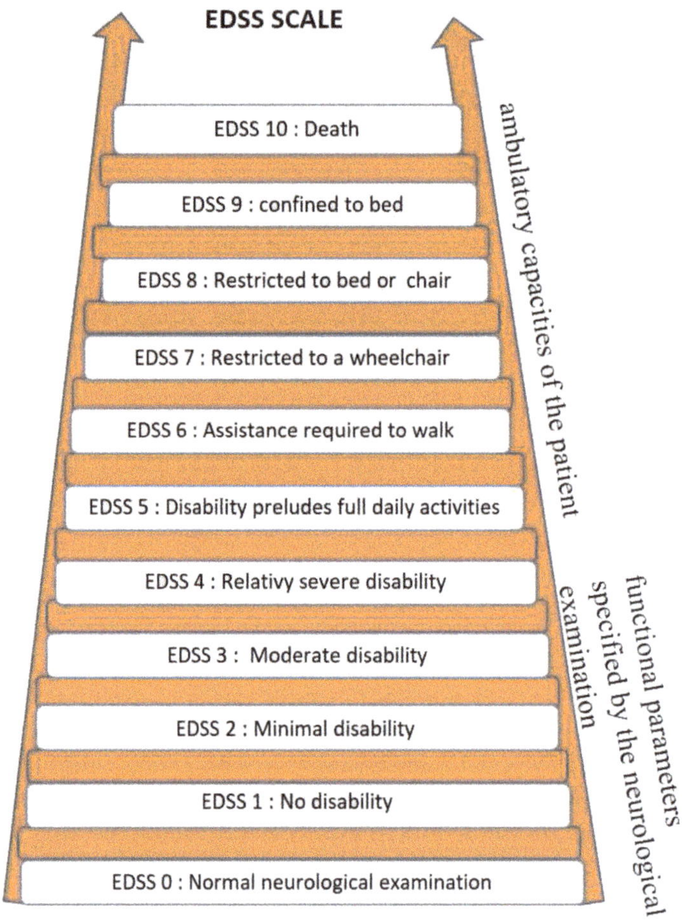

Figure 3.3. Expanded Disability Status Scale.

3.1.2.2 Optic neuritis

These signs reveal the disease in a quarter of the cases, especially in young adults. It leads to a decrease in visual acuity that sets in a few hours to a few days and is associated in 80% of cases to periorbital pain increased by the mobilization of eyeballs. The recovery of the visual function is complete in 80% of the cases in 6 months, nevertheless after recovery and during an effort or during the increase of body temperature, there can occur a transient decrease of the visual acuity of a few minutes (Uhthoff phenomenon).

3.1.2.3 Orthopedic disorders

The presence of orthopedic disorders is often described in MS as a compensation mechanism for balance disorders. They originate from excessive stressing of predominantly proximal tendino-muscular structures in response to distal deficits and will also lead to increased anticipatory postural adjustments [12].

3.1.2.4 Balance disorders

Balance disorders are common in MS with a prevalence of between 18% and 63% according to the authors [13–16]. These disorders are related to lesions of the central nervous system that affect the sensorimotor functions responsible for postural control [17, 18].

3.1.2.5 Fatigue and cognitive impairment

The frequency of cognitive impairment in MS ranges from 40% to 60% [19]. These disorders are found in undeveloped forms of the disease, with low levels of neurological functional impairment (EDSS < 3.5) [20], very recent evolution times [21], 'benign' forms [22] and in clinically isolated syndromes [23]. Fatigue and cognitive impairment (deficits in attention and concentration) affect postural balance [24, 25]. These postural disorders are reported by patients even before being detected by clinical examination [25–27].

3.1.3 Central regulation of balance in MS

3.1.3.1 General

Balance is a set of complex, referenced activities whose quality depends directly on neurophysiological and biomechanical mechanisms. Postural control regulates the position and orientation of the body in space and results from the central integration of visual, somesthetic and vestibular information [28]. The equilibration quality of a subject is related to the correlation of these three types of signals and leads to the construction of a unified reference [29]. This unification contributes to the development of internal models of spatial representation that are continuously updated according to environmental constraints [30]. These models respond to a complex, plastic stochastic neuronal process that can simulate sensorimotor behaviors through the knowledge of the physical characteristics of the body, the outside world and their interactions [31]. They make it possible to anticipate the consequences of a motor act and to determine the orders necessary to achieve performance [32]. Whatever its origin, any difficulty of central multi-sensory integration impacts the construction of these models [33]. As a motor task, posture is automatically regulated at the subcortical level by groups of spinal motoneurons and also requires the cognitive abilities of the subject [34, 35]. The level of cognitive solicitation is proportional to the complexity of the motor task performed, it involves the cortical structures involved in the motor attention within the pre-motor cortex [35] and in the 3D spatial representation of the body located in the parietal lobe [36, 37].

3.1.3.2 Neurophysiological point of view [38, 39]

Visual affiliation and ocular motricity

Gaze stabilization is ensured by reflexes of vestibular origin (vestibulo-ocular reflex and optokinetic reflex) and part of the vestibular messages reach via the posterior longitudinal strip and the thalamus to the vestibular cortex corresponding to the areas 5 and 7 located in the parietal posterior cortex. This zone ensures the conscious perception of the movements of the head in space. Movement vision involves the detection of moving forms and objects, the perception of eye tracking, and the perception of the movement itself. The detection of moving objects is ensured by the main optical channel and is transmitted to the neurons of the V5 which encode the displacement. At the next cortical level, the upper medio-temporal area (MTS) has plurimodal neurons: visual, proprioceptive, and vestibular. They project on the posterior parietal cortex (areas 5 and 7).

The ocular pursuit of an object in motion involves the participation of the fovea and takes the main optical pathway to the parietal cortex (areas 7a and 7b), this system can detect slow movements (ranging from 0.1 to 1 Hz). The perception of one's own movement makes use of the accessory optical system and allows the detection of a modification of the environment with respect to a stable subject, or of the subject with respect to a stable environment. This type of message merges into the cerebellum with vestibular messages, and produces the appropriate postural corrections. A copy of this 'fusion' is sent to the parietal cortex via the thalamus.

Proprioceptive afferents

These rely on the participation of proprioceptive receptors and more specifically the Muscle spindles (Ms) and the Golgi organs. Ms are placed in parallel with muscle fibers, code for stretching, and contribute to the conscious perception of movement. Their stimulation via the lemniscal pathway activates neurons of the area 3a by a double component (change of position of the limb and speed of displacement). The Golgi receptors are placed in the tendons, in series with the muscle fibers. They measure the force or its abrupt increase. The messages are then conveyed by the type 1b fibers and exert, via an inter neuron, an inhibition of α motoneurons. Joint receptors also intervene by informing the nerve centers on the static or dynamic spatial position of the segment (stereognosis).

Vestibular afferents

The vestibular receptors work as accelerometers and encode the second derivative of the displacements. The semi-circular channels detect the angular accelerations in the three planes of space: the horizontal (or lateral) channel is sensitive to accelerations detected in the horizontal plane, the posterior channel codes accelerations in the frontal (or transverse) plane and the upper (or anterior) channel of the sagittal plane. Otolithic organs (utricle and saccule) measure linear accelerations: the utricle detects the horizontal accelerations while the saccule detects the vertical accelerations. They constitute (especially with regard to the saccule) a gravity sensor and detect the static inclination of the head. Information from the vestibular system is transmitted via the vestibular nerve (VIII) to the vestibular nuclei of the brainstem.

Stabilization of the cervico-cephalic segment takes place via the vestibulo-spinal pathway (and its interactions with the α and γ motor neurons), to which are added information from the proprioceptive receptors of the neck muscles intended for the vestibular nuclei, the nucleus red and some reticular nuclei.

3.1.3.3 Biomechanical point of view

Mechanical model and postural strategy:

The human bipodal task has long been modeled as an inverted pendulum oscillating around its base of support [40–42]. Currently, this notion is moving towards another model: the double inverted pendulum to explain the compensatory role of the lumbo-pelvic region [43]. Various strategies are developed and controlled by the central nervous system (CNS) to stabilize the body position in orthostatic condition. The ankle strategy is the most commonly used: it is the most economical and effective solution because of the high concentration of mechanical sensors sitting in the distal muscles. The hip strategy is more expensive in terms of energy because it is less 'reactive'. Finally, the lowering of the center of mass allows a relative stabilization when the two previous strategies prove to be ineffective [44].

Distal control, center of mass (COM) and center of pressure (COP):

Many papers emphasize the importance of distal control when the equilibrium conditions of a subject are disturbed, as such, a fundamental role played by the muscular couples: anterior tibial and soleus (which ensure stability on the axis anteroposterior) on the one hand, posterior tibial and fibular (which control the medio-lateral axis) on the other hand [43, 45]. From a biomechanical point of view, the main challenge is to ensure the concordance between the respective positions of the center of mass (COM) and the center of pressure (COP), the shift of the COM with respect to the COP generates the implementation of permanent muscular tension which leads to an increase in joint constraints. The perpetuation of these constraints leads to painful conflicts and early degenerative phenomena [42, 44].

Muscular viscoelasticity and MS:

In MS the modification of viscoelastic properties and disturbances of sensorimotor control does not allow optimal stabilization of the body in space [46]. The muscular energy demand is markedly increased, especially on pelvic stabilizing muscles, quadriceps and the tibialis anterior/soleus pair [47].

3.1.3.4 Assessment of balance disorders

Assessments of balance disorders is usually based on validated clinical tests and the most widely used in the literature are the Berg balance test (BBS), the Dynamic Gait Index (DGI), the Dizziness Handicap Inventory (DHI) and the Activities-specific balance confidence (ABC) [27]. Nevertheless, these evaluations remain subjective with inter and intra-examiner variability [24]. For a decade, instrumental analyzes have been developed that allow the oscillations of a standing subject to be accurately analyzed by recording the displacement of the Center of Pressure on a force platform [48].

3.1.4 Instrumental analysis

In recent years, posturography has attracted a great deal of interest among re-educators and neurologists, but in early-stage multiple sclerosis the literature remains poor with regard to the instrumental study of somesthetic disorders. Two authors, Jackson [49] (concerning changes in perception of vertical and subjective horizontal in MS patients versus a control population) and Nelson [14] (about vestibular deficits and their sensory compensations highlighted on a dynamic platform) in 1995, studied the MS population on the strength platform. Some studies have analyzed postural regulation in multiple sclerosis, including Soyuer [50] in 2006. But little work has been done on proprioceptive disorders in MS, Frzosic *et al* [51] in 2000, Wildener *et al* [52, 53], more recently (2009), examined a study of this type. The existence of correlations between the posturometric signal (nonlinear analysis) and the EDSS score has been demonstrated [54]. It is clear from the literature that MS subjects experience a decrease in walking speed, step length, and increased double support time. Decrease in walking speed is very often associated with decreased hip and knee extension, plantar flexion, and propulsive force. This association evolves proportionally with the level of disability [55]. There is also an alteration of anticipated postural adjustments [56] and a significant increase in the risk of falling [57]. All of these phenomena increase fatigue in proportion to the disturbances related to insufficient motor control [58, 59]. In MS, proprioceptive disorders of the lower limbs associated with the presence of spasticity require the intervention of the paraplegral muscles to maintain the erect posture. This mode of compensation ensured by the spine results in an increase of the oscillations of the trunk along the medio-lateral axis [60]. More generally, studies carried out on subjects with low back pain, have shown a relation between lumbar pain and the increase of the amplitude of the oscillations recorded in orthostatic condition: the pain is generating postural disturbances and the converse is also true [59]. Experimentally, the pain caused by the triceps suraux influences the postural regulation and especially, the anticipated postural adjustments [61]. More generally, the compensations put in place by the CNS to maintain a stable erected posture are not limited to the pelvis and the lumbar region, in fact the intermediate joints and especially the knee will also experience a modification of the constraints. Biomechanical adaptations of the lower limb have been known for more than half a century but are still relevant [62].

3.2 Technical materials in posturography

3.2.1 Center of pressure versus center of gravity

The gravity line of the body corresponds to the vertical line going through the center of gravity (COG) of the human body or barycenter of the masses of all the segments that constitute the body. The center of mass (COM) is generally considered to be coincident with the (COG) of the human body [63]. In a standing posture, COG is located within the human body about 3 cm below the 3rd lumbar vertebrae. In static balance, the body, could be considered as a rigid solid that oscillates around the ankle joint. In this case, the body is only exposed to the actions of the gravitational force, applied at COG, and the ground reaction of the support, applied at center of pressure (COP); COP is the barycentre of the vertical forces applied to the ground (figure 3.4). Thus, the projection of the COG on the ground represents a

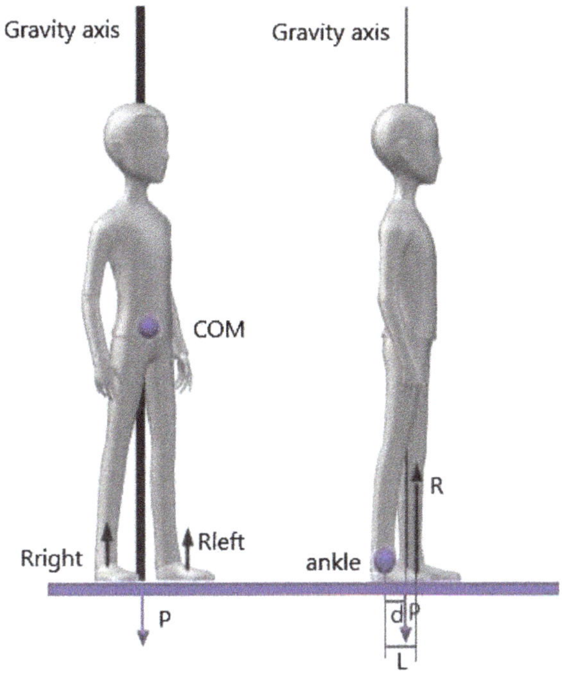

Figure 3.4. Estimation of static balance forces, (a) assuming the points of application of ground reaction forces distributed over both feet (R_{right}, R_{left}) and gravity P, (b) with a single point of application of the total ground reaction force which is the COP, the body is considered as a rigid stem whose point of support on the ground is the anchor, D distance between the COP and ankle and d distance between the COG and ankle.

downwardly directed vertical force whose amplitude reflects the weight of the body. This force is opposed to an equivalent vertical upwardly directed reaction force component whose point of application to the ground is called the center of pressure (COP) [64]. Balance is achieved when the gravitational and reaction forces of the ground as well as the moments around the ankle axis are balanced. The body's center of gravity is then projected into its sustaining polygon, which is the figure obtained by joining the most distant points of support as illustrated in figure 3.4. For a man, its surface is the area including area of each foot completed with the area between the two feet. The COP is considered as a variable controlled by the neurological system. Indeed, the COP is proportional to the moment of force applied to the ankles and therefore to the muscular forces required to stabilize the vertical stance [65, 66]. The COM is considered by several authors as the variable controlled by the COP [67]. Thus, analysis of the temporal structure of the COP and/or the COM could give some information on the control mechanisms of the postural system and on the nature of postural oscillations. Studies, carried out on the two components COM and COP, have shown that the oscillations of the two signals of the COM and COP are in constant phase shift once the postural system is stabilized [68, 69]. But as long as the system is unstable, the COP moves faster and further to the right, left, forward and backward as if it tries to bring the COM back and keep it near its average position. In fact, the COP's movements stabilize the COM. Some authors studied the difference between COM and COP signals and asserted that this difference could be associated with joint stiffness of the ankles. Force platforms measure COP variation during time.

3.2.2 Force platforms

Static posturography is performed using a force platform (figure 3.5), consisting of a non-deformable plate on which the subject must remain as static as possible. The force sensors are transmitting to a computer in real time, the evolution of the position of the COP is displayed as summarized in figure 3.6. This plot, the statokinesigram, allows an automated determination of the orthostatic balance parameters.

In contrast, dynamic posturography is performed using a mobile toggle platform (platform resting on a cylinder portion) equipped with an inclination sensor that analyzes the subject's ability to maintain balance on a spontaneously unstable basis. As the platform has only one degree of freedom of movement, the antero-posterior balance (AP) and the lateral balance (ML) are analyzed successively according to the orientation of the subject in relation to the axis of rotation of the cylinder. The length of the path of the platform pivot over a given time period characterizes the dynamic balancing performance. The frequency analysis of the platform oscillations makes it possible to consider the balancing strategies used by the patient.

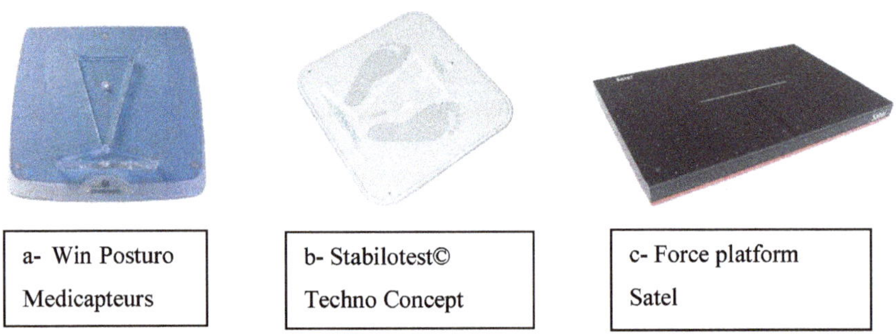

Figure 3.5. Example of static force platforms: (a) [https://www.medicapteurs.com/produits/winposturo] © Medicapteurs; (b) [http://www.technoconcept.fr] © TECHNO CONCEPT; (c) [http://www.satel-posture.com] © SATEL.

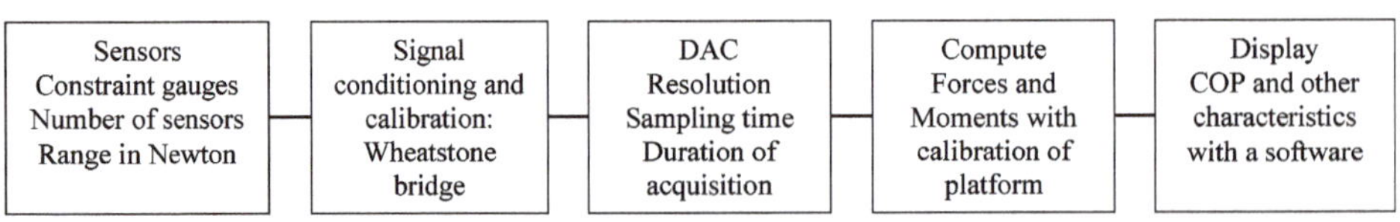

Figure 3.6. Acquisition and display of balance with a force platform.

3.2.2.1 Principle

A dynamometric force platform provides six components: three for the forces (F_X, F_Y, F_Z) and three for the moments of force (M_X, M_Y and M_Z) resulting from the forces and moments applied to its upper plate. A force platform generally consists of two rigid, non-deformable structures connected by force sensors. The lower recessed structure serves as a rigid frame. The upper surface is a tray that supports the supports. It returns forces fully and without delay to the sensors, which are the essential elements of force platforms. They can be classified according to the sensors used to measure forces.

3.2.2.2 Types of force platforms

Strain gauge: strain gauges are sensing devices that change resistance at their output terminals when stretched or compressed. They are constituted by a length of conductor arranged in a zigzag pattern on a membrane. They offer good accuracy for a reasonable cost, but range is limited. They are therefore the most widespread:

Principal manufacturers: AMTI [https://www.amti.biz/fps-guide_fr.aspx], Bertec [https://www.bertec.com/], Kyowa-Dengyo [http://www.kyowa-ei.com/].

Piezo-electric: piezo-electric are sensing devices that generate a voltage at their output terminals when stretched or compressed. Frequency and amplitude of voltage will characterize the answer of the sensor. They offer good accuracy and an important range of measure but the cost still high.

Principal manufacturer: Kistler [https://www.kistler.com/].

Figure 3.6 summarizes the different components and their characteristics to estimate the COP.

For example, Satel platform has four constraint gauges and a 16 bit DAC with a sampling frequency of 40Hz; Stabilotest© has three constraint gauges and a 16 bit CAN with a sampling frequency in the range 5–40 Hz.

3.2.2.3 Remarks on acquisition data parameters

The choice of a 16 bit (2 bytes) resolution seems to have become the standard. The sampling frequency and acquisition duration time are the subject of a significant amount of discussion in the literature. For example, the choice of a duration of 51.4 s, with a sampling frequency of 40 Hz, parameters that are recommended in France, consists in obtaining a file of 2048 points equivalent to 2^{11}. This choice is guided to facilitate the processing of the DAC and the acceleration of post processing too. However, one may wonder about the duration of registration and sampling frequency, which seem to be more imposed here by technical consideration than by clinical practice. The future representations of the signals, the computations performed on the basis of these measurements, and therefore the diagnostic considerations will follow from the duration time and especially the sampling frequency at which the COP is acquired. Thus, many authors have studied the breadth of information contained in the acquired data set and have discussed the influence of the number of points required to visualize and have a significant calculation [70], Satel platform, 40 Hz, 51.2 s. We can also find with the same acquisition parameters a study dealing with the Sample Entropy, but the influence of the number of points on the results is not discussed, this study is done on a Medicapteurs platform [71].

Some authors use a frequency data acquisition of 30 Hz to calculate the frequency parameters with a duration of 60 s of record [72], others use a duration of 30 s with a sampling of 100 Hz [73], Zebris platform, for the same parameters computed. For non-linear parameters like entropy, some authors used 1 KHz frequency [74], AMTI platform, or 100 Hz over a duration of 20 s for a dynamic task [75] on SwayStar TM platform.

Finally, a publication mentions a comparative study of estimating non-linear parameters such as Sample entropy and RQA variable with various sampling frequencies results [76], Bertec platform, acquisition frequency 100 Hz. The authors show that the sampling frequency chosen for the computations, under the experimental conditions of their study, seem to have a limited influence. However, it is practically impossible to compared objectively all these studies, because they were carried out on various machines, with various experimental conditions depending on the disease.

In fact, the problem can be summarized as follows: if we simply want to read the stabilogram or make simple calculations called linear here, the frequency does not need to be very high compared to the underlying slow dynamics of COP. In France, in addition to 40 Hz, the 100 Hz frequency is also becoming a standard sampling frequency. Several statements on the still debated issue of stabilometry standardization were agreed upon by the International Society of Posture & Gait Research Standardization Committee [73]. A set of metrological characteristics for stabilometric platforms was defined, relying both on practice and experimental verification. It was agreed that, to obtain appropriate accuracy and sensitivity, for example in the Romberg Test, the acquisition interval should not be less than 25 s, the sampling frequency should be at least 50 Hz. After careful consideration it was decided that the recommendations made in the previous Standardization proposal in 1983 regarding environmental conditions should be maintained.

The upgrade to 100 Hz allows a more accurate spectral analysis and increases the possible range of spectrum studies. The idea, that seems to be the more interesting, is based on the statement that 1 kHz sampling has become a standard for DACs, and that the explosion of memory capacities of electronic systems allows more important information to be stored. In this context, a 16 bit DAC, with fe = 1 kHz and then under-sampling the signal to recover all the possibilities between 40 Hz and 500 Hz on the post-processing seems to be the more adapted. Thus the acquired data will allow one to validate the theoretical assumptions coming from new non-linear type analysis methods that require a lot of points and could be adapted to future other data-based investigations.

In summary, the minimum of the published standards must be respected when choosing the sampling frequency. A minimum of 100 Hz for data acquisition in the clinical setting should allow mathematically correct analyses with more advanced algorithms, especially if you want to explore frequencies above 20 Hz or use more complex filtering methods.

For research activities, the choice of manufacturers who offer custom assembly at the level of sensor types, DAC and a sampling frequency of 1 kHz should give a finer tune in the indicators definition.

One of the most important points that emerged from this brief study is that a multi-machine clinical study should be carried out with a shared protocol to propose international standards in the interpretation of posturometric measurements.

3.2.2.4 Estimated measures with platform force

Statokinesigram: this displays the sampled location of the COP in relation to a reference frame with its origin located in the center of the platform. In figure 3.7, the representation of the subject's feet is on the scale of his shoe size.

Standardized representations are obtained from the statokinesigram:

- Normalized ellipse, it represents the area in which 95% of the most centered points of the sampling are located.
- Normalized circle, it represents the position statistically determined from the 20% of the most frequently encountered patients (core of the Standards).
- Force histogram.

From these standardized representations, a set of measures can be deduced that are used to establish the care. To facilitate this diagnosis, the manufacturers, in France, propose to compare the patient's values with the normalized values [77] defined by the association Posture and Balance [78].

Surface

From 95% of the successive positions of the COP recorded during the whole time of acquisition, a statistical measurement of the surface, expressed in mm^2, of the confidence ellipse is performed (table 3.1). 5% of the most extreme points, resulting from poorly controlled swings, are eliminated. Most posturologists agree that this parameter is one of the most relevant to quantify an individual's ability to balance under static conditions.

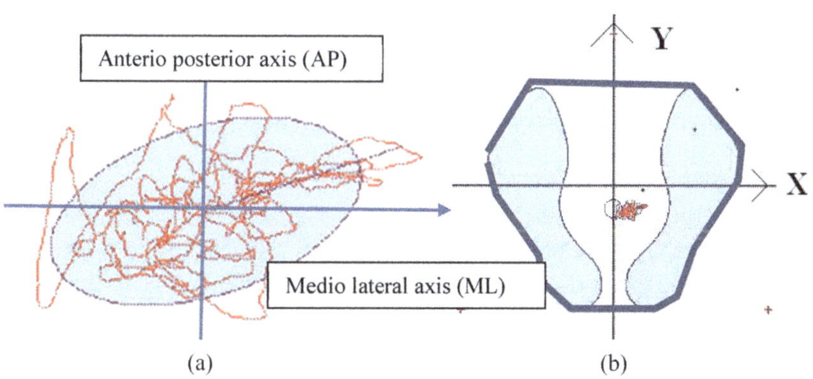

Figure 3.7. (a) Statokinesigram with normalized ellipse, (b) sustentation polygon with so-called statokinesigram.

Table 3.1. Normalized parameter (Norm 85) for surface of the ellipse.

Surface (mm^2)	Open eyes	Closed eyes
Average	91	225
Limite inf.	39	79
Limite sup.	210	638

Table 3.2. Normalized parameter (Norm 85) for Length of statokinesigram.

Length (mm)	Open yes	closed eyes
Average	429	613
Limit inf.	307	346
Limit sup.	599	880

Table 3.3. Normalized parameter (Norm 85) for LFS.

LFS	Open eyes	Closed eyes
Average	1	1
Limit inf.	0.72	0.7
Limit sup.	1.39	1.44

Length
The total length of the statokinesigram represents the distance travelled by the pressure centre throughout the examination (table 3.2).

LFS
The parameter LFS (Length according to Surface), reflects the amount of energy spent by a person controlling his orthostatic balance. The value of the LFS increases when the difficulty of standing upright is modifying by changing one of the inputs of the postural system (eyes closed for example) (table 3.3).

VFY:
Standard deviation of the velocity of the COP displacement as a function of the mean *Y*-position reflects the postural tone of certain muscles in the posterior cavity and their viscoelastic properties. In the elderly, a significant change in the VFY often indicates a change in the equilibration strategy, such as a shift from ankle to hip strategy (table 3.4).

Table 3.4. Normalized parameter (Norm 85) for VFY.

VFY	Open eyes	Closed eyes
Average	0	0
Limit inf.	−2.61	−4.73
Limit sup.	3.59	4.86

Table 3.5. Normalized parameter (Norm 85) for Romberg ratio.

Romberg ratio	Open eyes	Closed eyes
Average	0.862	2.88
Limit inf.	0.33	1.12
Limit sup.	2.37	6.77

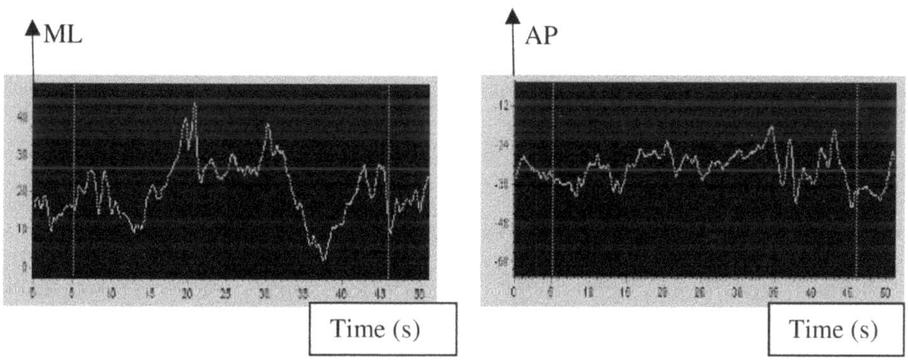

Figure 3.8. *X*-direction (ML) and *Y*-direction (AP) stabilograms from SATEL.

Romberg ratio

It is the ratio, expressed as a percentage, of the surface with eyes closed, to the surface with eyes open. This quotient is used to assess the quality of the visual input and its relative importance compared to other inputs in the system (table 3.5).

The stabilogram: the right–left and front–back stabilograms represent the vector components of the patient's oscillations throughout the examination. On the stabilogram there are cursors indicating the synchronisation with programmed stimulation (figure 3.8).

X_{mean}: projection on the *X*-axis (left and right subject axis) of the average position of the pressure centre expressed in mm. It indicates the average value of the patient's right/left balance movements.

Y_{mean}: projection on the Y-axis (antero-posterior axis of the subject) of the mean position of the pressure centre expressed in mm. It indicates the average value of the forward/backward balancing movements

When these values exceed certain standard values, there is an asymmetry in postural tonicity that can lead to a postural deficiency syndrome. When these values exceed certain standard values, there is an asymmetry in postural tonicity that can lead to a postural deficiency syndrome. In particular, it is known that tonicity changes with age. For example, a young adult would normally stand in forward positions, while at about 60, the average Y would first move back, then move forward depending on the degree of inclination of the trunk.

FFT (fast Fourier transform): to assess the proportion of the different frequency bands of postural oscillations in the statokinesigram, a frequency analysis can be performed. Each of these bands involves the use of a specific postural control loop. The slow frequencies correspond to control loops with a visual or vestibular starting point. The higher frequencies correspond to regulation loops with a plantar or proprioceptive muscle skin starting point.

In figure 3.9, three frequency bands are delimited by the two vertical lines. Those cursors could be moved manually with the mouse. Spectral energies in each band could be estimated in percentages too.

Correlations

The inter-correlation function compares the antero-posterior oscillations with the right–left oscillations. If the shape of the curve representing this function is clearly sinusoidal, the right–left and forward–back oscillations are no longer independent since they share a common periodicity.

3.3 Analysis methods in posturography

As explained in section 3.1, MS patients experience balance deficits in the ML and/or AP direction(s) in quiet standing [17, 46, 73]. The directional control impairment has been further observed in the right side and backward diagonal (backward-right and backward-left) directions in individuals with MS [79]. In recent years,

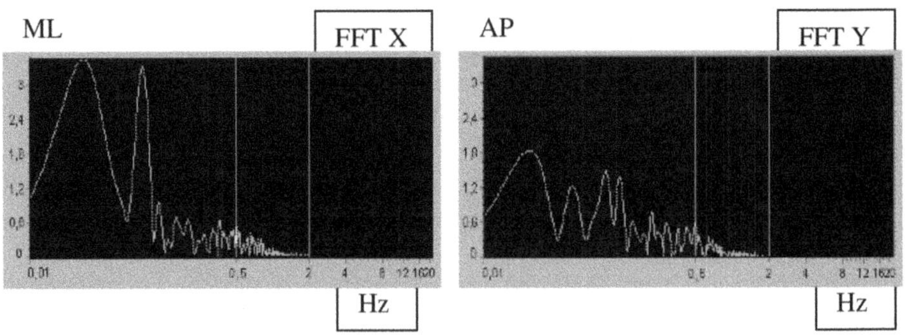

Figure 3.9. FFT X and FFT Y from SATEL.

posturography has become a popular and advanced technique to evaluated balance impairment in people with MS. Moreover, numerous linear and non-linear analysis methods have been proposed to explore in depth characteristics of the stabilograms of MS patients.

3.3.1 Linear analysis

3.3.1.1 Time domain

Time-domain measures extracted from the stabilograms are associated with the displacement of the COP in the ML and AP directions. In addition to the surface of the confidence ellipse (or the sway area) and the total length of the COP path (or the total excursion) indicated previously in the section 3.2, several other parameters can be found in the literature [80–82], such as:

- the mean velocity (or the sway rate): defined as the total length of the COP path divided by the total testing time;
- the ML and AP ranges: defined as the differences between the maximum and the minimum COP values along the ML and AP axes, respectively;
- the root-mean-square (RMS) distances from the mean COP in the ML and AP directions: defined as the statistical standard deviations of all COP values along the ML and AP axes, respectively;
- the total excursions in the ML and AP directions: defined as the total distances that the COP traveled along the AP and ML axes, respectively;
- the mean velocities in the ML and AP directions: defined as the total excursions in the ML and AP directions, respectively, divided by the total testing time.

Numerous studies have shown that the amplitude and the velocity of postural sway were significantly greater in MS patients compared to healthy subjects under the condition of EO or EC [26, 46, 73]. In addition, some studies have found greater postural sway in patients with a greater EDSS score compared to those with a smaller EDSS score [83, 84], although differences in some temporal measures were not significant.

3.3.1.2 Frequency domain

In addition to analysis of the ML and AP sway in time domain, several studies have focused on their frequency content and spectral characteristics [85, 86]. For this, the power spectrum, describing the distribution of power into the signal's frequency components, needs to be calculated for the COP signal in the ML or AP direction by FFT. As a few investigations of the body sway using frequency analysis approach have reported that different frequencies are associated with different regulations in MS [87], the COP power spectrum could be divided into several frequency bands in order to be further explored [88]. Kanekar *et al* have reported [89] that the MS group showed a significant decrease in the magnitude of COP power spectrum in the low frequency band and a pattern of increase in the medium and high frequency bands in the ML direction.

Furthermore, many spectral parameters are used to characterize the postural stability for the ML and AP directions [82, 90], such as:

- the total power: defined as the integrated area of the power spectrum;
- the median power frequency: defined as the frequency at which the power spectrum is divided into two equal energy regions;
- the 95% power frequency: defined as the frequency below which 95% of the total power is present;
- the centroidal frequency (or the zero crossing frequency): defined as the square root of the ratio of the second to the zeroth spectral moments.

3.3.2 Nonlinear analysis

In addition to the classical parameters indicated previously, many nonlinear methods have been applied to the postural signals in order to better analyze human static stability.

3.3.2.1 Methods used to analyze postural stability in MS

Entropy analysis

Approximate entropy (ApEn) is a nonlinear dynamic parameter used to quantify the amount of regularity and the unpredictability of fluctuations in a time series [74]. As a non-negative number, ApEn reflects the occurrence of new information in the time series. Since the presence of repetitive fluctuation patterns renders a time series more predictable than the one in which such patterns are absent, a time series containing many repetitive patterns has a relatively smaller ApEn and a more complex (i.e. less predictable) process has a higher ApEn.

The algorithm for computing ApEn has been published [91, 92]. Given a sequence S_N, consisting of N measurements equally spaced in time, its ApEn is defined as follows:

$$ApEn(S_N, m, r) = ln\left[\frac{C_m(r)}{C_{m+1}(r)}\right], \tag{3.1}$$

where m specifies the pattern length and r defines the similarity criterion. Two subsequences (or patterns) of m measurements, beginning at different intervals within S_N, are considered similar if the difference between any pair of corresponding measurements in the patterns is less than the tolerance r. The quantities $C_m(r)$ and $C_{m+1}(r)$ indicate the prevalence of repetitive patterns of length m and that of length $m + 1$, respectively.

Therefore, smaller values of ApEn reflect a greater likelihood that similar patterns of measurements will be followed by additional similar measurements. On the other hand, if the time series is highly irregular, the occurrence of similar patterns will not be predictive for the following measurements, and ApEn will be relatively large. It should be noted that ApEn is not well suited for analysis of the short and noisy datasets and may lead to inconsistent results. For this reason, the sample entropy (SampEn) has been introduced to avoid bias due to the shortening of the data.

SampEn is a measure basically quantifying the irregularity of a time series. For a given embedding dimension (m), tolerance (r) and number of data points (N), we take the negative logarithm of the probability that if the distance between two template vectors of length m is less than r then the distance between two template vectors of length $m + 1$ is also less than r.

$$\text{SampEn}(m, r, N) = -\log(A(r)/B(r)) \tag{3.2}$$

where $A(r)$ is the total number of template matches in a $(m + 1)$-dimensional phase space within a distance tolerance r, and $B(r)$ is the one in a m-dimensional phase space [71]. An increase in SampEn implies a higher level of disorder and unpredictability in a time series.

Manor *et al* studied the SampEn associated with the COP displacements in older adults during quiet standing [93]. They related the parameter SampEn to the complexity of postural sway, and consequently to the adaptive capacity of the postural control system to cognitive and other stressors.

Huisinga *et al* found that patients with MS exhibit increased regularity (decreased ApEn) during standing compared to healthy controls [94], while we observed a significant increase in SampEn between the healthy subjects and the MS patients in EO and EC [95]. Christopher *et al* reported that the ApEn and the SampEn (algorithms typically used to quantify the entropy of COP) might yield very different results, particularly when sampling frequency and noise are different [74].

Recurrence quantification analysis

Recurrence quantification analysis (RQA), developed by Zbilut and Webber [96, 97], is a method of nonlinear analysis to investigate and characterize the recurrence behavior (e.g. the number and duration of recurrences) of the phase space trajectory of dynamical systems, based on the recurrence plot (RP).

The RP is a black and white plot showing the times when a phase space trajectory of the system visits roughly the same region in the phase space [98]. As shown in figure 3.10, an RP revealing a behavior of the phase space trajectory is composed of single dots and lines which can be horizontal, vertical, or parallel to the mean diagonal (also known as line of identity, LOI) [99]. Generally, each black dot in such a plot represents a recurrent point. Among the lines in the RP, the diagonal lines (lines parallel to the LOI) represent periodic recurrent structures of the dynamical system, whereas the horizontal and vertical lines represent the segments of the phase space trajectory which remain in the same phase space area for a while. Since the RP is usually symmetric with respect to the LOI, each horizontal line corresponds to a certain vertical line. For this reason, the horizontal lines are often ignored and only the vertical lines are considered in the RQA.

The RQA quantifies the small-scale structures in RPs of dynamical systems, and can provide useful information even for short non-stationary data. To analyze a dynamical system, represented by a time series, using the RQA, a reconstructed phase space is first required and usually established by means of a time delay

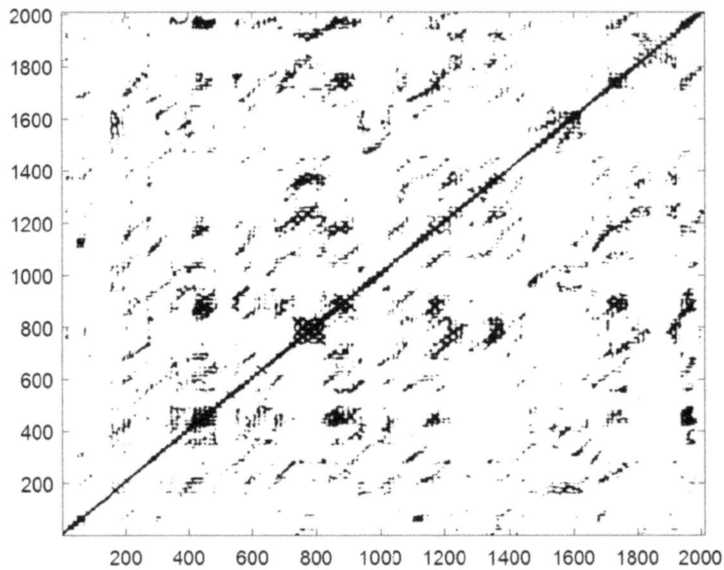

Figure 3.10. Recurrence plot of the COP signal of a MS participant with EDSS = 2.0 (black dot: recurrent point).

embedding where two embedding parameters (the embedding dimension and the time delay) have to be chosen appropriately [96, 97, 98]. Because the information about the original data series is transmitted to the vectors in the reconstructed phase space, the recurrence of states of the dynamical system can be identified by comparing the states at any two different times so that an RP can be constructed for the system. With the help of the RP, several measures of complexity can be estimated as follows [98].

The recurrence rate (RR) or the percentage of recurrence (%Rec), is the simplest RQA measure, which is the density of recurrence points in an RP:

$$RR = \frac{1}{N^2} \sum_{i,j=1}^{N} R(i, j), \tag{3.3}$$

where N represents the number of considered states and $R(i, j)$ is equal to 0 or 1. If the states of a system at two different times i and j are similar, $R(i, j) = 1$. Otherwise, $R(i, j) = 0$. This measure reflects the probability that a specific state recurs in the phase space, and corresponds to the correlation sum, where the LOI is excluded during the computation.

In order to explore the distribution of recurrence points in the RP, two RQA measures called determinism (DET) and laminarity (LAM) have been further proposed to reflect the numbers of recurrence points which form diagonal lines and vertical lines, respectively.

$$\mathrm{DET} = \frac{\sum_{l=l_{\min}}^{N} l \bullet P(l)}{\sum_{l=1}^{N} l \bullet P(l)}, \tag{3.4}$$

$$\mathrm{LAM} = \frac{\sum_{v=v_{\min}}^{N} v \bullet P(v)}{\sum_{v=1}^{N} v \bullet P(v)}, \tag{3.5}$$

where $P(l)$ represents the frequency distribution of the lengths l of the diagonal lines (with the minimal length l_{min}) and $P(v)$ represents the frequency distribution of the lengths v of the vertical lines (with the minimal length v_{min}). The determinism is related to the predictability of the dynamical system, whereas the laminarity is related to the number of laminar phases in the system.

In addition, the averaged diagonal line length (L) and the average length of the vertical lines (known as the trapping time, TT) in the RP can be also determined from the RP.

$$L = \frac{\sum_{l=l_{\min}}^{N} l \bullet P(l)}{\sum_{l=l_{\min}}^{N} P(l)} \tag{3.6}$$

$$TT = \frac{\sum_{v=v_{\min}}^{N} v \bullet P(v)}{\sum_{v=v_{\min}}^{N} P(v)} \tag{3.7}$$

The averaged diagonal line length reflects the predictability time of the dynamical system, while the trapping time reflects the laminarity time of the system.

The maximal diagonal line length (L_{max}) and its inverse, called divergence (DIV)

$$\mathrm{DIV} = \frac{1}{L_{\max}} \tag{3.8}$$

are two RQA measures as well. L_{max} is the length of the longest diagonal in the RP. The smaller L_{max} the more divergent the trajectories. Although there is a relationship between the largest positive Lyapunov exponent and L_{max}, [99] this relationship is not as simple as stated in the literature, but even more complex.

The Shannon entropy (ShanEn) represents the probability of finding a diagonal of a given length

$$\mathrm{ShanEn} = -\sum_{l=l_{\min}}^{N} p(l) \bullet \ln(p(l)), \tag{3.9}$$

where l_{min} represents the minimal diagonal length, and $p(l)$ represents the probability of a diagonal line of length l in the RP. This entropy can be estimated from the frequency distribution $P(l)$ with

$$p(l) = \frac{P(l)}{\sum_{l=l_{\min}}^{N} P(l)}, \tag{3.10}$$

and reflects the complexity of deterministic structures in the system. However, this parameter is sensitive to the bin number of the processor and may differ for different data preparations or different realizations of a process.

The trend is another RQA measure, which is a linear regression coefficient of the relationship between the recurrence point density in a line parallel to the LOI and its distance to the LOI. Considering the recurrence rate in a diagonal line parallel to LOI of distance k (RR_k):

$$\mathrm{RR}_k = \frac{1}{N-k} \sum_{j-i=k}^{N-k} R(i, j), \tag{3.11}$$

the trend (TND) is defined by

$$\mathrm{TND} = \frac{\sum_{i=1}^{\tilde{N}} (i - \tilde{N}/2)(RR_i - \langle RR_i \rangle)}{\sum_{i=1}^{\tilde{N}} (i - \tilde{N}/2)^2}, \tag{3.12}$$

where <·> gives the average value and Ñ <N. The edges of the RP should be excluded during the TND computation because recurrence point densities are too low in the edges. This measure provides information about the stationarity of the dynamical system.

RQA has been widely used in biomedical research and applied to different kinds of clinical data, including the posturographic signal. Negahban *et al* have observed [76] that as the postural conditions became more difficult, COP time series of both MS and control groups became less regular (lower recurrence rate), less complex (lower RQA entropy), and less nonstationary (lower trend). In addition, when cognitive conditions became more difficult (from a single postural task to a dual postural-cognitive task), COP time series became less regular (lower recurrence rate in the AP direction and lower determinism in both directions), less complex (lower RQA entropy in the AP direction), and less nonstationary (lower trend in the AP direction). Their results have shown that, although the MS patients and the control group had a similar dynamical structure, their nonlinear behavior was different under some experimental conditions.

In our previous study [100], the EDSS score was estimated from two linear parameters, the length and the surface, and four RQA parameters: percentage of recurrence, Shannon entropy, mean diagonal line length and trapping time. Moreover, all four RQA parameters were calculated for position, instantaneous velocity and acceleration of the COP in order to select the most accurate method for estimating the EDSS. The results demonstrated that estimations of EDSS from the surface, the percentage of recurrence and the mean diagonal line length of the position, best agreed with clinical scores. Then, this EDSS modeling strategy was evaluated using both mono- and multi-dimensional RQAs [101]. These studies have emphasized the possibility of distinguishing EDSS scores using postural sway and RQA parameters, and suggested that the posturographic signal's mono-dimensional RQA is a more pertinent method to quantify disability in MS than the multi-dimensional RQA.

3.3.2.2 Other methods in the literature

Some other non-linear analysis methods can be also found in the literature to analyze the COP signal. Although they have not yet been used to analyze postural stability in MS, they could be able to provide some other useful information linked to MS in the future.

Fractal dimension approach

Fractal dimension analysis (FDA) is used to quantify the complexity of a system. When the COP trajectory is analyzed during a quiet stance, a change in fractal dimension (FD) may reflect a change in postural control strategies for maintaining body balance. Previous studies [102, 103] reported that FDA is a reliable method to provide us with specific characteristics of human postural control.

FD of COP signal can be computed using the box-counting algorithm [104]. To calculate the FD for a given set, we first cover the set with a grid and count how many boxes of the grid are covering part of the set. Then we do the same thing but using a finer grid with smaller boxes. By shrinking the size of the grid repeatedly, we end up more accurately capturing the structure of the pattern.

If $N(\varepsilon)$ represents the number of boxes (of grid size ε) needed to fully cover the set, then the box-counting dimension is defined as follows:

$$FD = \lim_{\varepsilon \to 0} \frac{\log(N(\varepsilon))}{\log(1/\varepsilon)}. \tag{3.13}$$

Thus, FD is the slope of the plot $\log(N(\varepsilon))$ versus $\log(1/\varepsilon)$. In a two-dimensional picture, the FD value ranges from 0 to 2 and is higher when the set (or picture) is more complex [105].

Empirical mode decomposition processing method

Empirical mode decomposition (EMD) is an adaptive time–frequency analysis method. The principle of this method is to decompose a signal into a set of band-limited elementary signals, called intrinsic mode functions (IMFs), which represent the oscillatory modes embedded in the signal [106]. This technique allows extracting from the signal all IMFs with different frequencies. Breaking down biomedical signals into various components, EMD can be compared with other analysis methods such as Fourier transform and wavelet transform. However, these two methods need some predefined basis functions to decompose a signal, while the EMD method does not require a prior known basis. Since the decomposition is based on the local characteristic time scale of the data, it can be applied to nonlinear and nonstationary processes. EMD obtains much better temporal and frequency resolutions compared to Fourier and wavelet analyses [107, 108].

Detrended fluctuation analysis

Detrended fluctuation analysis (DFA) is a method to determine the statistical self-affinity of a signal. It is useful to analyze time series that appear to be long-memory processes or $1/f$ noise [109]. Briefly, the integrated time series of length N is divided into intervals of equal length n without overlapping. In each interval of length n, a least squares line fitted to the data is subtracted. Next, the root-mean-square fluctuation of this integrated and detrended time series is calculated by

$$F(n) = \sqrt{\frac{1}{N} \sum_{k=1}^{N} [y(k) - y_n(k)]^2}. \tag{3.14}$$

A linear relationship on a log–log plot indicates the presence of power law (fractal) scaling. Under such conditions, the fluctuations can be characterized by a scaling exponent α, the slope of the line relating log ($F(n)$) to log(n) [110]. When the DFA coefficients α are > 0.5, they indicate a more structured signal with long-term correlations, and thus low variability. When $\alpha < 0.5$, the signal has negative correlations, and $\alpha = 0.5$ indicates a non-correlated random series.

3.4 Conclusion

In this chapter, we presented an advanced technique to characterize balance disorders in MS using a static force platform, called static posturography, including the introduction to this technique, the machines used in the clinic, the linear (temporal and spectral) parameters and the new nonlinear indicators extracted from the stabilometric signals, as well as the links with the clinic in the context of MS. The data from the posturographic analysis inform clinicians about the postural control strategies developed by MS patients.

The advantage of posturography lies in its simplicity of implementation for clinicians and its character with very little restriction for MS patients (short duration, non-invasive, …) regarding its clinically proven performance. The use of new indicators opens up new perspectives for posturography in MS. It would be able to provide new diagnostic elements for the management, in particular with the possibility of predicting the evolution of the EDSS score, and thus improve the understanding of the mechanisms involved in the system for balance regulation in MS.

References

[1] Compston A and Coles A 2008 Multiple sclerosis *Lancet* **372** 1502–17

[2] Confavreux C and Vukusic S 2006 Natural history of multiple sclerosis: a unifying concept *Brain J. Neurol.* **129** 606–16

[3] Fromont A, Binquet C, Clerc L and Moreau T 2009 Epidemiology of multiple sclerosis: the special situation in France *Rev. Neurol.* **165** 671–5

[4] Barkhof F, Filipi M, Miller D H, Scheltens P, Campi A and Polman C H *et al* 1997 Comparison of MRI criteria at first presentation to predict conversion to clinically definite multiple sclerosis *Brain* **120** 2059–69

[5] Polman C H, Reingold S C, Banwell B, Clanet M, Cohen J A and Filipi M *et al* 2011 Diagnostic criteria for multiple sclerosis: 2010 revisions to the McDonald criteria *Ann. Neurol.* **69** 292–302

[6] Lucchinetti C F, Popescu B F G, Bunyan R F, Moll N M, Roemer S F and Lassman H *et al* 2011 Inflammatory cortical demyelinisation in early multiple sclerosis *N. Engl. J. Med.* **365** 2188–97

[7] Polman C H *et al* 2005 Diagnostic criteria for multiple sclerosis: 2005 revisions to the MacDonald *Ann. Neurol.* **58** 840–6

[8] Nylander A and Hafler D A 2012 Multiple sclerosis *J. Clin. Invest.* **122** 1180–8

[9] De Seze J, Mackowiak A, Stojkovic T, Ferriby D, Hautecoeur P and Vermersch P 2002 Primary progressive forms of multiple sclerosis: application of the new diagnostic criteria *Rev. Neurol.* **158** 341–5

[10] Kurtzke J F 1983 Rating neurologic impairment in multiple sclerosis: an expanded disability status scale (EDSS) *Neurology* **33** 1444–52

[11] Brochet B 2009 Place de l'EDSS dans l'évaluation précoce du handicap (Assessing incapacity at early stages of multiple sclerosis using the EDSS) *Rev. Neurol.* **165** S173–9

[12] Rougier P, Thoumie P, Cantalloube S and Lamotte D 2007 Quelles stratégies motrices de compensation les patients souffrant de sclérose en plaques sont-ils capables de développer pour contrôler leur équilibre? *Rev. Neurol.* **63** 1054–64

[13] Grenman R 1985 Involvement of the audiovestibular system in multiple sclerosis. An otoneurologic and audiologic study *Acta Otolaryngol. Suppl.* **420** 1–95

[14] Nelson S R, Di Fabio R P and Anderson J H 1995 Vestibular and sensory interaction deficits assessed by dynamic platform posturography in patients with multiple sclerosis *Ann. Otol. Rhinol. Laryngol.* **104** 62–8

[15] Williams N P, Roland P S and Yellin W 1997 Vestibular evaluation in patients with early multiple sclerosis *Am. J. Otol.* **18** 93–100

[16] Finlayson M, Guglielmello L and Liefer K 2001 Describing and predicting the possession of assistive devices among persons with multiple sclerosis *Am. J. Occup. Ther.* **55** 545–51

[17] Chung L H, Remelius J G, Van Emmerik R E and Kent-Braun J A 2008 Leg power asymmetry and postural control in women with multiple sclerosis *Med. Sci. Sports Exerc.* **40** 1717–24

[18] Cameron Michelle H and Lord S 2010 Postural control in multiple sclerosis: implications for fall prevention *Curr. Neurol. Neurosci. Rep.* **10** 407–12

[19] Chiaravalloti N D and DeLuca J 2008 Cognitive impairment in multiple sclerosis *Lancet Neurol.* **7** 1139–51

[20] Ruggieri R M, Palermo R, Vitello G, Gennuso M, Settipani N and Piccoli F 2003 Cognitive impairment in patients suffering from relapsing-remitting multiple sclerosis with EDSS < or = 3.5 *Acta Neurol. Scand.* **108** 323–6

[21] Olivares T, Nieto A, Sanchez M P, Wollmann T, Hernandez M A and Barroso J 2005 Pattern of neuropsychological impairment in the early phase of relapsing-remitting multiple sclerosis *Mult. Scler.* **11** 191–7

[22] Amato M P, Zipoli V and Portaccio E 2006 Multiple sclerosis-related cognitive changes: a review of cross-sectional and longitudinal studies *J. Neurol. Sci.* **245** 41–6

[23] Glanz B I, Holland C M, Gauthier S A, Amunwa E L, Liptak Z, Houtchens M K, Sperling R A, Khoury S J, Guttmann C R and Weiner H L 2007 Cognitive dysfunction in patients

with clinically isolated syndromes or newly diagnosed multiple sclerosis *Mult. Scler.* **13** 1004–10
[24] Fjeldstad C, Pardo G, Frederiksen C, Bemben D and Bemben M 2009 Assessment of postural balance in multiple sclerosis *Int. J. MS Care* **11** 1–5
[25] Karst G M, Venema D M, Roehrs T G and Tyler A E 2005 Center of pressure measures during standing tasks in minimally impaired persons with multiple sclerosis *J. Neurol. Phys. Ther.* **29** 170–80
[26] Martin C L, Phillips B A and Kilpatrick T J *et al* 2006 Gait and balance impairment in early multiple sclerosis in the absence of clinical disability *Mult. Scler.* **12** 620–8
[27] Cattaneo D, Jonsdottir J, Zocchi M and Regola A 2007 Effects of balance exercises on people with multiple sclerosis: a pilot study *Clin. Rehabil.* **21** 771–81
[28] Lacour M, Bernard-Demanze L and Dumitrescu M 2009 Postural control, aging, and attention resources: models and posture-analysis methods *Neurophysiol. Clin.* **160** 411–21
[29] Lacour M, Barthelemy J, Borel L, Magnan J, Xerri C, Chays A and Ouaknine M 1997 Sensory strategies in human postural control before and after unilateral vestibular neurotomy *Exp. Brain Res.* **115** 300–10
[30] Wolpert D M, Ghahramani Z and Jordan M I 1995 An internal model for sensorimotor integration *Science* **269** 1880–2
[31] Gómez-Pinilla F, Ying Z, Roy R R, Molteni R and Edgerton V R 2002 Voluntary exercise induces a BDNF-mediated mechanism that promotes neuroplasticity *J. Neurophysiol.* **88** 2187–95
[32] Chabeauti P Y, Assaïante C and Vaugoyeau M 2012 Extreme short-term environmental constraints do not update internal models of action as assessed from motor imagery in adults *Neuroscience* **222** 69–74
[33] Lacour M and Borel L 1993 Vestibular control of posture and gait *Arch. Ital. Biol.* **131** 81–104
[34] Lajoie Y, Teasdale N, Bard C and Fleury M 1993 Attentional demands for static and dynamic equilibrium *Exp. Brain Res.* **97** 139–44
[35] Rushworth M F S, Johansen-Berg H, Göbel S M and Devlin J T 2003 The left parietal and premotor cortices: motor attention and selection *NeuroImage.* **20** S89–100
[36] Their P and Karnath P O 1997 *Parietal Lobe Contribution to Orientation in 3D Space* (Heidelberg: Springer)
[37] Michel C, Rosseti Y, Rode G and Tlikete C 2003 After-effects of visuo-manual adaptation to prisms on body posture in normal subjects *Exp. Brain Res.* **148** 219–26
[38] Berthoz A 1997 *Le sens du movement* (Paris: Odile Jacob)
[39] Bioulac B, Burbaud P, Cazalets J-R and Gross C 2005 Fonctions motrices *EMC-Kinésithérapie* **4** 183–233
[40] Gagey P M, Baron J B and Ushio N 1980 Introduction to clinical posturology *Agressologie* **21** 119–23
[41] Collins J J and De Luca C J 1993 Open-loop and Closed-loop control of posture: a random-walk analysis of center of pressure trajectory *Exp. Brain Res.* **95** 308–18
[42] Rougier P 2005 Compatibility of postural behavior induced by two aspects of visual feedback: time delay and scale display *Exp. Brain Res.* **165** 193–202
[43] Suzuki Y, Nomura T, Casadio M and Morasso P 2012 Intermittent control with ankle, hip and mixed strategies Turing quiet standing: a theoretical proposal based on a double inverted pendulum model *J. Theor. Biol.* **310** 55–79

[44] Berger L, Chuzel M, Buisson G and Rougier P 2005 Undisturbed upright stance control in the elderly: Part 1. age-related changes in undisturbed upright stance control *J. Mot. Behav.* **37** 348–58
[45] Van Der Kooij H and De Vlugt E 2007 Postural responses evoked by platform perturbations are dominated by continuous feedback *J. Neurophysiol.* **98** 730–43
[46] Sosnoff J J, Shin S and Motl R W 2010 Multiple sclerosis and postural control: the role of spasticity *Arch. Phys. Med. Rehabil.* **91** 93–9
[47] Wurdeman S R, Huisinga J M, Filipi M and Stergiou N 2013 Multiple sclerosis alters the mechanical work performed on the body's center of mass during gait *J. Appl. Biomech.* **29** 435–42
[48] Broglio S P, Sosnoff J J, Rosengren K S and McShane K 2009 A comparison of balance performance: computerized dynamic posturography and a random motion platform *Arch. Phys. Med. Rehabil.* **90** 145–50
[49] Jackson R T, Epstein C M and De l'Aune W R 1995 Abnormalities in posturography and estimations of visual vertical and horizontal in multiple sclerosis *Am. J. Otol.* **16** 88–93
[50] Soyuer F, Mirza M and Erkorkmaz U 2006 Balance performance in three form of multiple sclerosis *Neurol. Res.* **28** 555–62
[51] Frzovic D, Morris M E and Vowels L 2000 Clinical tests of standing balance: performance of persons with multiple sclerosis *Arch. Phys. Med. Rehabil.* **81** 215–21
[52] Widener G L, Allen D O and Gibson-Horn C 2009 Balance-based torso-weighting in a patient with ataxia and multiple sclerosis: a case report *J. Neurol. Phys. Ther.* **32** 139–46
[53] Widener G L, Allen D O and Gibson-Horn C 2009 Balance-based torso-weighting may enhance balance in persons with multiple sclerosis: preliminary evidence *Arch. Phys. Med. Rehabil.* **90** 602–9
[54] Peyrodie L, Boudet S, Pinti A, Cavillon F, Agnani O and Gallois. P 2010 Corrélation entre l'analyse de données posturologiques et le score EDSS dans la sclérose en plaques *Sci. Technol. Handicap* **4** 55–72
[55] Kelleher K J, Spence W, Solomodis S and Apatsidis D 2010 The characterisation of gait pattern of people with multiple sclerosis *Disabil. Rehabil.* **32** 1242–50
[56] Krishnan V, Kanekar N and Aruin A S 2012 Anticipatory postural adjustments in individuals with multiple sclerosis *Neurosci. Lett.* **506** 256–60
[57] Martin C L, Phillips B A, Kilpatrick T J, Butzkueven H, Tubridy N, Mac Donald E and Galea M P 2006 Gait and balance impairment in early multiple sclerosis in the absence of clinical disability *Mult. Scler.* **12** 620–8
[58] Andreasen A K, Jakobsen J, Petersen T and Andersen H 2009 Fatigued patients with multiple sclerosis have impaired central muscle activation *Mult. Scler.* **15** 818–27
[59] Findling O, Seliner J, Meïer N, Allum J H, Vibert D, Lienert C and Mattle H P 2011 Trunk sway in middly disabled multiple sclerosis patients with and without impairment *Exp. Brain Res.* **213** 363–70
[60] Della Volpe R, Popa T, Ginanneschi F, Spidalieri R, Mazzochio R and Rossi A 2006 Changes in coordination of postural control during dynamic stance in chronic low back pain patients *Gait Posture* **24** 349–55
[61] Hirata R P, Arendt-Nielsen L and Graven-Nielsen T 2010 Experimental calf muscle pain attenuates the postural stability during quiet stance and perturbation *Clin. Biomech.* **25** 931–7

[62] Inman V 1969 The influence of the foot and ankle complex on the proximal skeletal structures *Artif. Limbs* **13** 59–65

[63] Gagey P M and Weber B 1999 Stabilométrie *Posturologie: régulation et dérèglements de la station debout* (Paris: Masson) pp 45–59

[64] Massion J 1992 Movement, posture and equilibrium: interaction and coordination *Prog. Neurobiol.* **38** 35–56

[65] Pai Y C and Patton J 1997 Center of mass velocity-position predictions for balance control *J. Biomech.* **30** 347–54

[66] Sinha T and Maki B E 1996 Effect of forward lean on postural ankle dynamics *IEEE Trans. Rehabil. Eng.* **4** 348–59

[67] Dietz V 1992 Human neuronal control of automatic functional movements: Interaction between central programs and afferent input *Physiol. Rev.* **72** 33–69

[68] Winter D A, Patla A E, Prince F, Ishac M and Gielo-Perczak K 1998 Stiffness control of balance in quiet standing *J. Neurophysiol.* **80** 1211–21

[69] Gagey P M, Bizzo G, Debruille O and Lacroix D 1985 *The one Hertz phenomenon Vestibular and Visual Control on Posture and Locomotor Equilibrium* ed M Igarashi and F O Black (Basel: Karger) pp 89–92

[70] Cao H, Agnani O, Peyrodie L, Boudet S and Donzé C 2013 Automatic assessment of expanded disability status scale (EDSS) in multiple sclerosis using a decision tree *Engineering* **5** 566–9

[71] Ramdani S, Seigle B, Lagarde J, Bouchara F and Bernard P L 2009 On the use of sample entropy to analyze human postural sway data *Med. Eng. Phys.* **31** 1023–31

[72] Nagymáté G and Kiss R M 2016 Parameter reduction in the frequency analysis of center of pressure in stabilometry *Period. Polytech. Mech. Eng.* **60** 238–46

[73] Morrison S, Ryndersb C A and Sosnoff J J 2016 Deficits in medio-lateral balance control and the implications for falls in individuals with multiple sclerosis *Gait Posture* **49** 148–54

[74] Rhea C K, Silver T A, Hong S L, Ryu J H and Studenka B E *et al* 2011 Noise and complexity in human postural control: interpreting the different estimations of entropy *PLoS One* **6** e17696

[75] Corporaal S H, Gensicke H, Kuhle J, Kappos L, Allum J H and Yaldizli Ö 2013 Balance control in multiple sclerosis: Correlations of trunk sway during stance and gait tests with disease severity *Gait Posture* **37** 55–60

[76] Negahban H, Sanjari M A, Mofateh R and Parnianpour M 2013 Nonlinear dynamical structure of sway path during standing in patients with multiple sclerosis and in healthy controls is affected by changes in sensory input and cognitive load *Neurosci. Lett.* **553** 126–31

[77] Bizzo G, Guillet N, Patat A and Gagey P M 1985 Specifications for building a vertical force platform designed for clinical stabilometry *Med. Biol. Eng. Comput.* **23** 474–6

[78] AFP 1985 *Normes* 85 Editées par l'Association Posture et Équilibre, 66, rue de Lisbonne 75008 Paris

[79] Ganesan M, Kanekar N and Aruin A S 2015 Direction-specific impairments of limits of stability in individuals with multiple sclerosis *Ann. Phys. Rehabil. Med.* **58** 145–50

[80] Lawson T, Morrison A, Blaxland S, Wenman M, Schmidt C G and Hunt M A 2015 Laboratory-based measurement of standing balance in individuals with knee osteoarthritis: A systematic review *Clin. Biomech.* **30** 330–42

[81] Maki B E, Holliday P J and Fernie G R 1990 Aging and postural control: A comparison of spontaneous- and induced-sway balance tests *J. Am. Geriatr. Soc.* **38** 1–9

[82] Prieto T E, Myklebust J B, Hoffmann R G, Lovett E G and Myklebust B M 1996 Measures of postural steadiness: differences between healthy young and elderly adults *IEEE Trans. Biomed. Eng.* **43** 956–66

[83] Boes M K, Sosnoff J J, Socie M J, Sandroff B M, Pula J H and Motl R W 2012 Postural control in multiple sclerosis: effects of disability status and dual task *J. Neurol. Sci.* **315** 44–8

[84] Kalron A, Givon U, Frid L, Dolev M and Achiron A 2016 Static posturography and falls according to pyramidal, sensory and cerebellar functional systems in people with multiple sclerosis *PLoS One* **11** e0164467

[85] Laboissière R, Letievant J C, Ionescu E, Barraud P A, Mazzuca M and Cian C 2015 Relationship between spectral characteristics of spontaneous postural sway and motion sickness susceptibility *PLoS One* **10** e0144466

[86] Salsabili H, Bahrpeyma F, Esteki A, Karimzadeh M and Ghomashchi H 2013 Spectral characteristics of postural sway in diabetic neuropathy patients participating in balance training *J. Diabetes Metab. Disord.* **12** 29

[87] Nagy E, Toth K, Janositz G, Kovacs G, Feher-Kiss A, Angyan L and Horvath G 2004 Postural control in athletes participating in an ironman triathlon *Eur. J. Appl. Physiol.* **92** 407–13

[88] Alpini D, Berardino F D, Mattei V, Caputo D, Schalek P and Cesarani A 2012 Characteristics of multiple sclerosis patient stance control disorders, measured by means of posturography and related to brainstem lesions *Audiol. Res.* **2** e9

[89] Kanekar N, Lee Y J and Aruin A S 2014 Frequency analysis approach to study balance control in individuals with multiple sclerosis *J. Neurosci. Methods* **222** 91–6

[90] Pan Y T, Yoon H U and Hur P 2017 A portable sensory augmentation device for balance rehabilitation using fingertip skin stretch feedback *IEEE Trans. Neural Syst. Rehabil. Eng.* **25** 28–36

[91] Pincus S M 1991 Approximate entropy as a measure of system complexity *Proc. Natl Acad. Sci. USA* **88** 2297–301

[92] Ho K K L, Moody G B, Peng C K, Mietus J E, Larson M G, Levy D and Goldberger A L 1997 Predicting survival in heart failure case and control subjects by use of fully automated methods for deriving nonlinear and conventional indices of heart rate dynamics *Circulation* **96** 842–8

[93] Manor B, Costa M D, Hu K, Newton E, Starobinets O, Kang H G, Peng C K, Novak V and Lipsitz L A 2010 Physiological complexity and system adaptability: evidence from postural control dynamics of older adults *J. Appl. Physiol.* **109** 1786–91

[94] Huisinga J M, Yentes J M, Filipi M L and Stergiou N 2012 Postural control strategy during standing is altered in patients with multiple sclerosis *Neurosci. Lett.* **524** 124–8

[95] Cao H, Peyrodie L, Agnani O and Donzé C 2016 Nonlinear analysis of postural sway in multiple sclerosis *Int. J. Biomed Biol. Eng.* **10**

[96] Zbilut J P and Webber C L 1992 Embedding and delays as derived from quantification of recurrence plot *Phys. Lett.* A **171** 199–203

[97] Webber C L and Zbilut J P 1994 Dynamical assessment of physiological systems and states using recurrence plot strategies *J. Appl. Physiol.* **76** 965–73

[98] Marwan N, Carmenromano M, Thiel M and Kurths J 2007 Recurrence plots for the analysis of complex systems *Phys. Rep.* **438** 237–329

[99] Eckmann J P, Kamphorst S O and Ruelle D 1987 Recurrence plots of dynamical systems *Europhys. Lett.* **5** 973–7

[100] Cao H, Peyrodie L, Boudet S, Cavillon F, Agnani O, Hautecoeur P and Donzé C 2013 Expanded Disability Status Scale (EDSS) estimation in multiple sclerosis from posturographic data *Gait Posture* **37** 242–5

[101] Cao H, Peyrodie L, Agnani O, Cavillon F, Hautecoeur P and Donzé C 2015 Evaluation of an Expanded Disability Status Scale (EDSS) modeling strategy in multiple sclerosis *Med. Biol. Eng. Comput.* **53** 1141–51

[102] Doyle T L, Newton R U and Burnett A F 2005 Reliability of traditional and fractal dimension measures of quiet stance center of pressure in young, healthy people *Arch. Phys. Med. Rehabil.* **86** 2034–40

[103] Myklebust J B, Prieto T and Myklebust B 1995 Evaluation of nonlinear dynamics in postural steadiness time series *Ann. Biomed. Eng.* **23** 711–9

[104] Feder J 1988 *Fractals* (New York: Plenum)

[105] Cimolin V, Galli M, Rigoldi C, Grugni G, Vismara L, Mainardi L and Capodaglio P 2011 Fractal dimension approach in postural control of subjects with Prader-Willi Syndrome *J. Neuroeng. Rehabil.* **8** 45

[106] Huang N E, Shen Z, Long S R, Wu M C, Shih H H and Zheng Q *et al* 1998 The empirical mode decomposition and the Hilbert spectrum for nonlinear and non-stationary time series analysis *Proc. R. Soc. A Math. Phys. Eng. Sci.* **454** 903–95

[107] Labate D, Foresta F L, Occhiuto G, Morabito F C, Lay-Ekuakille A and Vergallo P 2013 Empirical mode decomposition vs. wavelet decomposition for the extraction of respiratory signal from single-channel ECG: A comparison *IEEE Sens. J.* **13** 2666–74

[108] Liang H, Bressler S L, Desimone R and Fries P 2005 Empirical mode decomposition: a method for analyzing neural data *Neurocomputing* **65–66** 801–7

[109] Peng C K, Havlin S, Stanley H E and Goldberger A L 1995 Quantification of scaling exponents and crossover phenomena in nonstationary heartbeat time series *Chaos* **5** 82–7

[110] Zhou J, Manor B, Liu D, Hu K, Zhang J and Fang J 2013 The complexity of standing postural control in older adults: a modified detrended fluctuation analysis based upon the empirical mode decomposition algorithm *PLoS One* **8** e62585

IOP Publishing

Neurological Disorders and Imaging Physics, Volume 2
Engineering and clinical perspectives of multiple sclerosis
Ayman El-Baz and Jasjit S Suri

Chapter 4

Recent developments in the understanding and assessment of hope and psycho-emotional expressions of illness for people with Multiple Sclerosis

Andy Soundy

There is a need to consolidate recent developments in the area of hope, psychological adaptation and emotions as factors which are central to understanding the experience of illness. One-way research has achieved this through a deeper understanding of illness narrative master plots (common stories of illness). This chapter provides an overview of the most recent developments in the concept of hope, psychological adaptation and illness narratives master plots for people who have a clinical diagnosis of multiple sclerosis (MS). The chapter introduces; (1) understanding generalised hope for chronic illness, (2) the factors that influence hope, (3) the model of emotional adjustment and hope (MEAH) and (4) illness narrative master plots and how they are mapped on to the MEAH.

4.1 Introduction

This chapter considers several different aspects relating to hope. These different aspects include:

(a) understanding generalised hope for individuals with chronic illness;
(b) the factors that influence hope;
(c) the model of emotional adjustment and hope (MEAH);
(d) illness narrative master plots and how they are mapped on to the MEAH.

4.1.1 Understanding generalised hope for individuals with chronic illness

Hope is generated in suffering. Marcel [1] uses the idea of captivity to define hope stating '*the truth is that there can be strictly speaking no hope except when the temptation to despair exits. Hope is the act by which this temptation is actively or*

doi:10.1088/978-0-7503-1762-7ch4

victoriously overcome.' (p 36). Viewing hope in this way can illustrate hope as a posture and mode of experiencing oneself in relationship to time, events and one's experience of reality [2]. It also illustrates the emotional dimension of hope [3] and the nature of hope being expressed within a spectrum [4]. This is opposed to considering hope as a motive for the attainment of a particular goal, which Synder and colleagues [5] identify as particularised hopes. Particularised hopes are specific hopes that relate to goals and include agency (energy or motivation to undertake a task, activity or goal) and pathway (routes for how the hope will be achieved) as enabling factors. Generalised hopes, in contrast, reflect hope as a posture and illustrate the experience of one's life within levels that distinguishes the value of meaning for the individual. Both types of hope include: (a) the focus towards the future and the belief that changes in the future are possible and can add value to life, and (b) that hope includes both cognitive and affective components [6]. Generalised hopes refer to a positive orientation towards life, but should not be confused with optimism. The optimist believes good rather than bad things will occur in one's life, whereas the hopeful person has an understanding and recognition that life may not work out as planned [7]. Acceptance of risk that there may be disappointment despite one's effort is likely central to the application of both types of hope [8, 9]. Further to this, acceptance that what is hoped for may not occur is central to the ability to adjust and reconsider one's generalised hopes [9].

The meaning and purpose of life is often challenged following the onset of a chronic illness. Marcel [1] identifies different levels of hope within the idea of generalised hope. The levels of hope describe the different ways meaning is found by people in living. The levels of hope enable a clear way to understand what aspects of living are hoped for and are distinguished according to the importance or necessity an individual places on achieving the hope. The levels of generalised hopes exist from superficial hopes to deeper integral hopes that include the individual's social identities, relationships, careers, security and a need to relieve suffering. The importance and need to achieve what is hoped for can be extremely intense. For instance, the need to reduce the pain levels experienced from an illness may be so great that it dominates an individual's decision making, actions and interactions. This could be true for other symptoms of the illness that have the greatest impact on an individual's bio-psychosocial well-being. If and when suffering becomes manageable, the individual may be affected by considering the perceived loss created by illness from their present situation to their past situation. The loss can mean that specific social identities are ended, such as being a father or mother, a provider (gained through meaningful employment) like an accountant or football player. The impact of this is often described as relative and unique, for instance, one individual may perceive and experience a great need to return to work the way it used to be. This need and hope could be so important that steps are taken regardless of health or ability to achieve it. For example, it would be unacceptable for an individual to seek an alternative hope or even modify what is hoped for because the loss is very personal and significant.

The ability to adapt hope also may be too difficult within the present situation. However, another individual may be able to embrace the change and consider the perceived loss as an opportunity. As hopes that result from loss are relative, the significance an individual places towards any particular level of hope can be unique. Thus, what is perceived as incredibly important for one patient may not be so important to another patient. A motivating factor that may drive this is located in an individual's need to restore purpose and meaning in their life, which is relative to how they derive it within their unique situation.

What is clear from chronic illness literature is that the impact of an illness may prevent hope and create an inability to (re)establish hope across all the different levels of hope. Thus, when hope is compromised the meaning and value in living can be questioned and hopes are often directed at ways the individual can re-establish those aspects of living which enable a sense of purpose, meaning and value. It is clear that when hope is challenged psychological and emotional adaptation is required, but there are factors which exist to interrupt this process. See figure 4.1 for a framework which enables hope.

4.1.2 The factors that influence hope

Factors which generate and challenge hope in patients with chronic neurological disease have been identified by previous research [10]. This section uses these established factors as a guide to identify the main and most significant variables which can impact on a patient's hope, both in terms of enabling and disabling hope.

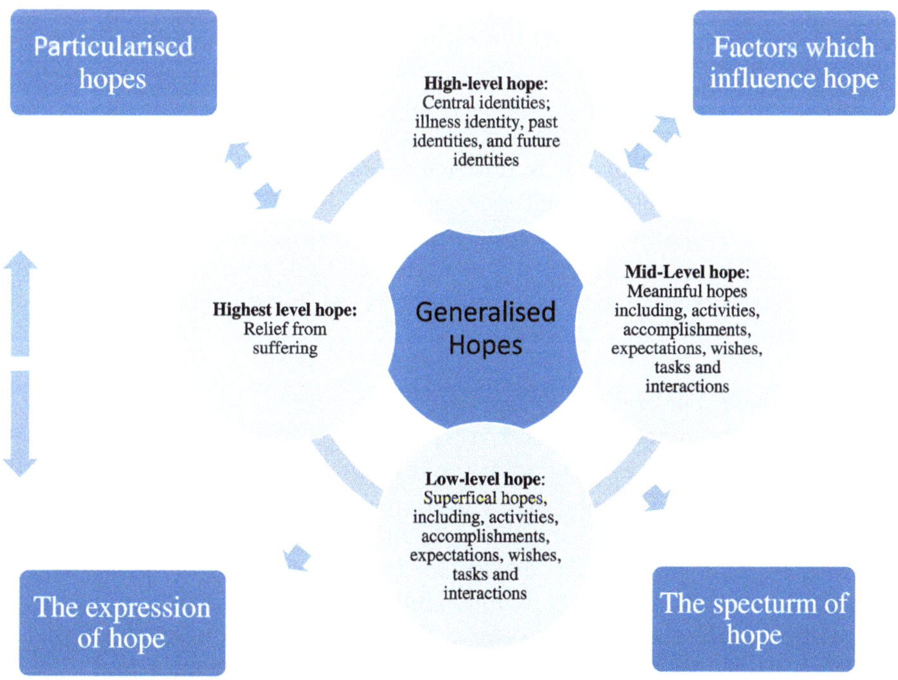

Figure 4.1. A framework for understanding hope in chronic illness.

4.1.2.1 Factors which enable hope

4.1.2.1.1 Goals used within rehabilitation

For goal setting to enable hope goals must be attainable, tailored, negotiated and meaningful [10]. Recent research has highlighted the importance of personally meaningful goals for individuals with MS. Meaning can be derived from the different levels of hope and these levels need to be understood for each patient, for instance, if relief from suffering is present there may be little or no opportunity to consider lower levels of hope. Thus, understanding the patient and what they are hoping for in terms of the levels of hope is important to establishing what is meaningful as a goal for them. This may have an implication for what assessment tool is used to identify change. Often well-known or used scales may not be capturing the change occurring during a rehabilitation intervention for people with MS [11]. For example, the Bathel Index has been reported as falling short of capturing meaningful change during rehabilitation [12]. It may be that a tool is used to understand the levels of hope that is important for the patient before setting goals. The process of enabling hope may be supported by shared decision making. Review evidence [13] has highlighted that whilst staff often see the benefit of shared decision making, the time required for such an approach often acted as a barrier to using it. However, patients frequently perceived a greater sense of control of their treatment and ownership over their goals if shared decision making was employed.

4.1.2.1.2 Mastery experiences within rehabilitation setting

The rehabilitation process provides access to a rich learning environment and enables a process of achieving and mastering tasks and meaningful activities [10]. These aspects are critical for establishing a patient's self-efficacy or their ability to be confident about tasks attempted during rehabilitation. By increasing a patient's self-efficacy, improvements across physical, cognitive and social functioning have been observed [14]. Personal competence is essential to the resilience of individuals with MS [15] and to building self-efficacy [16]. This is likely achieved through group encouragement and social comparison. Importantly, self-efficacy appraisals, self-esteem and perceived control [17] are often identified mechanisms of positive change for mental well-being and such concepts are significantly associated with hope [18].

4.1.2.1.3 Psychological needs of adaptation

The following psychological needs of adaptation have been identified in patients [19]: (a) the cognitive needs for adaptation; this requires an ability to recognise the change and losses that are occurring. The ability to recognise change is related to the ability an individual has of acknowledging change or loss in their present circumstances. This requires an ability to adapt and come to terms with the change. (b) The psychological need of having hope in the possibility of a variety of outcomes that could occur in the future. There is a need to understand that the future has become to some extent uncontrollable, unknown or uncertain. The idea of possibility is in contrast to future hopes being certain or finalised. The need for hope in possibility is contrasted to 'unrealistic hopes' identified about a patient by a healthcare professional (HCP) [9]. A critical difference for the HCP is the importance of seeing a patient's perspective, listening to their expressions of hope and allowing hopes to remain in place. This is important because a direct challenge to the hopes a patient has is unlikely to result in change. (c) The internal need for action. Dufault and Martocchio [3] identify the concept of psychological action, which is a process that involves coping strategies, reality testing and physical or social action which involves the practical steps that allow the hope to be realised. Individuals are required to consider how they take ownership of the need for taking action which is combined with understanding that they have the internal resources needed to do this. A further understanding of this need can be, according to Dufault and Martocchio [3], identified as spiritual action and focus and awareness of God using prayer or participating in spiritual and religious activities and practices. The internal need for action enables independence, autonomy and purpose whilst preserving a patient's integrity and dignity. (d) An ability to take action which enables and preserves independence and allows continuation of living. When a patient's desired independence is not possible, it may defer to the preservation of dignity.

4.1.2.1.4 Healthcare professional's attitude and advice

Review evidence [20] has identified the variation of interactional experiences between HCPs and patients. Positive experiences are reported most often when HCPs can see patients quickly or efficiently and identify problems whilst acknowledging the limitations of science. Negative experiences reported frequently included not receiving information about what is happening from the doctor or being left with unanswered questions following an encounter with a HCP. In some examples, no diagnosis could be given or the wrong diagnosis was identified. The most influential factors which impacted on the patient–clinician relationship (and most likely impacted on hope) included the inability to provide choice when considering procedures and rehabilitation and identify the aspects which matter to them. Further, individuals identified difficulties including; (a) the continuity of care, (b) the need for support from family members, (c) insensitive delivery of information (casual delivery of information, patronising or dismissive comments, judgemental or flippant remarks) and (d) a paternalistic approach to care. Patients highlighted the importance of comfort and emotional support, often highly valuing clinicians who would just listen. Words of encouragement used by HCPs influence the individual's ability to cope [20].

4.1.2.1.5 Patient support network

Review [21] evidence has identified that the provision of support is a key factor that moderates negative psychological well-being following the impact of MS. A consistent relationship was found from this review across 12 studies (12/14 within the review). This identified a significant positive association between perceived support and positive psychological adaption. Changes in the relationships with others often occur and are important, as relationships are considered as a high or critical level of hope [10] and this is particularly important for preventing depression and anxiety in people with MS [22]. The most prominent changes in relationships include losing friends, family death or children growing older [23]. Changes in relationships can aid hope when individuals create and strengthen social ties with existing individuals or when new friendships are formed. However, the relationships may have a negative impact on hope when reduced relatedness occurs between the patients and their friends. It is important to consider the relative importance of who is supporting the patient. The extent to which MS groups provide emotional support has been questioned [23]. However, positive evidence is available for the benefits of groups on hope and other psychological constructs like isolation and a sense of belonging [24, 25].

4.1.2.2 Factors which challenge hope

4.1.2.2.1 Physical factors

The greater the duration of the illness and the more severe or progressive the MS is for a patient, the lower the health-related quality of life that is reported [26]. Further, individuals with MS who have a greater perceived disability are likely to experience greater depression and deterioration in mental well-being [22]. Thus, hope is clearly impacted by the types and/or symptoms of MS on an individual. Specific time points during MS have been identified as central to challenging an individual's hope. These include: at disease onset, during exacerbations, whilst waiting for change to occur, where there is a failure to achieve a goal, during experiences of slowing improvement, and at discharge with the withdrawal of support [10].

4.1.2.2.2 Psychosocial and emotional factors

Hope is impacted by psychological, emotional and social well-being. It is also impacted by experiences of isolation [10]. Negative emotions may prevent any psychological distance from an MS related event [4] and create an inability to cope and be hopeful. It is important to understand that negative emotions have been negatively associated with resilient behaviours and an individual's ability to cope [16]. In addition, emotional suppression [27] could impact an individual's ability to be hopeful. For instance, to express despair can be frowned upon or be perceived as socially unacceptable [28]. Positive emotions are likely generated from being in a meaningful and purposeful environment and being able to access higher levels of hope. The reason for this is due to the reciprocal relationship between positive emotions and meaningful activities being undertaken [29].

4.1.3 The model of emotional adjustment and hope (MEAH)

The MEAH was identified as a way to capture the expressions and experiences of loss or change that are a direct result of MS [20]. The model is represented by combining the hope and adaptation scale with the circumplex model of affect [20]. This combination resulted in a graphical representation of the experience or story being shared by a patient [30].

4.1.3.1 The hope and adaptation scale

The hope and adaptation scale provides an assessment of a loss that a patient is finding difficult to adapt to. The named loss or change is then assessed across two dimensions: (a) the dichotomy of hope and adaptation, and (b) the circumplex model of affect.

4.1.3.1.1 The dichotomy of hope

Hope has previously been considered as a dichotomy [4] and represented as a concept that exists externally to the person. Thus, if it is currently absent in someone it should be able to be obtained [7]. The dichotomy of hope can be illustrated by the certainty by which hope is expected, from complete certainty, through possibility towards complete hopelessness. These distinct points have been identified as critical within hope literature for individuals with chronic illness [4]. The dichotomy of hope provides an illustration of the range and limits of hope. The uppermost limit of hope identified on a continuum is concrete hope. This type of hope is considered as a solid and definite wish or expectation. Within chronic neurological illnesses concrete hope is often combined with an idea of restoration of one's former self [4]. The danger with this form of hope is that it can be expressed as an uncompressing position which can be regarded by HCPs as problematic. At the midpoint of the dichotomy of hope is hope in possibility [4]. Hope in possibility represents a patient who has been able to reconcile their present circumstances to what their future may have been. It is a form of hope that enables personal integrity to be maintained. The idea of possibility simultaneously incorporates an acknowledgement that what is hoped for is not possible, allowing the patient a defiant attitude. Thus, the emotion associated with the idea of hope in possibility is generally more pleasant or positive. This contrasts to the idea of uncertainty about a particular outcome which is generally considered or associated with more unpleasant or negative emotional states. This difference can be illustrated by identifying that in one way people can be confident in what they hope for, however, on the other hand, people can lack certainty about what is hoped for [7]. Hope in possibility may allow a patient to retain their sense of social identity. This may be important for allowing hope in the future and bringing less suffering now [31]. Hope in possibility could be considered as a mode of thinking that enables a continuation of agency for living. The final point on the dichotomy of hope is the experience of no hope. The experience of no hope may be considered as hopelessness and represents the lowest point on the continuum of hope. Lynch [31] states that there are three powerful feelings associated with hopelessness. These feelings include a sense of the impossible, a sense of what they face is too much or too great to be handled by themselves and, finally, a sense that trying is futile.

4.1.3.1.2 Adaptation

The adaptation scale in the hope and adaptation scale (based on the MEAH) [20] provides an illustration of how an individual expresses their response to a difficulty. This response is illustrated by contrasts which can be seen as extremes. At one end of the response individuals may completely embrace the difficulty but, at the other end, individuals may reject or deny the difficulty.

The complete embracement of the difficulty can be found in expressions of an individual that life could not be better. In fact, the individual may express that they would not want to change the difficulty or experience. An underlying aspect of this reaction is represented by a very positive acceptance of the difficulty. Acceptance is a multidimensional concept and the ability to accept prognosis doesn't mean a patient will accept a loss of their social identity. Acceptance has been associated with a decrease in negative emotions [32]. As such, this will likely lead an individual to recognise a need to take action and begin a search–learning process. This is considered essential for psychological adaptation in people with MS [19]. One value of acceptance has been identified as the reduction in need or the wish to defy or resist the experience of change generated by MS [20]. Thus, as there is movement away from the positive embracement, the idea of acceptance becomes more prominent. A mid-point on the spectrum of the adaptation scale is acknowledgement. This is a simple recognition of what has happened and illustrates that individuals have identified what has happened on some level. Finally, at the other end of the scale, is rejection or denial. This represents an inability to accept what has happened or reject the difficulty experienced.

4.1.3.1.3 The circumplex model of affect

A broad range of feelings and emotions accompany the hoping process. This is referred to as the affective dimension of hope [3]. Emotional responses often are reactions to the sense of personal significance related to hope for a particular outcome and feelings related to the confidence and or uncertainty regarding attaining that outcome. It has been identified that hope can be difficult to control. Hope can be more like a passion and can appear irrational if strong feelings are associated with it [7]. The losses which are a direct result of MS are often associated with specific and often strong emotions. Specific emotions felt by a patient following chronic or palliative illness or symptoms change will clearly influence their subsequent decision making and responses to illness [33] and their agency and ability to defy the constantly changing illness. Review [20] evidence has identified grouped emotional expressions as part of the experience of living with MS. This evidence identified one consistently pleasant emotion; relief (identified in 16/47 studies). Relief was most often related to the difficulty experienced not being worse. However, far more apparent, were unpleasant activated emotions such as panic, fear or being scared (19/47), anger (15/47) or frustration (18/47) and deactivated unpleasant emotions such as sadness (12/47), depression (12/47), pessimism (7/47), or feeling upset (14/47). It is important to note that hope is particularly affected by experiences of anxiety, fear, grief and loneliness [10, 34]. If patients feel overwhelmed with fear or worry and powerless within the experience of illness, the cognitions expressed by them may be more likely to lead to a succumbing illness response, dominated by an inability to access coping resources [35]. The way the HAS is able to capture these emotions is through the circumplex model of affect [36]. This model provides a spectrum of emotions and maps the experiences of difficulties

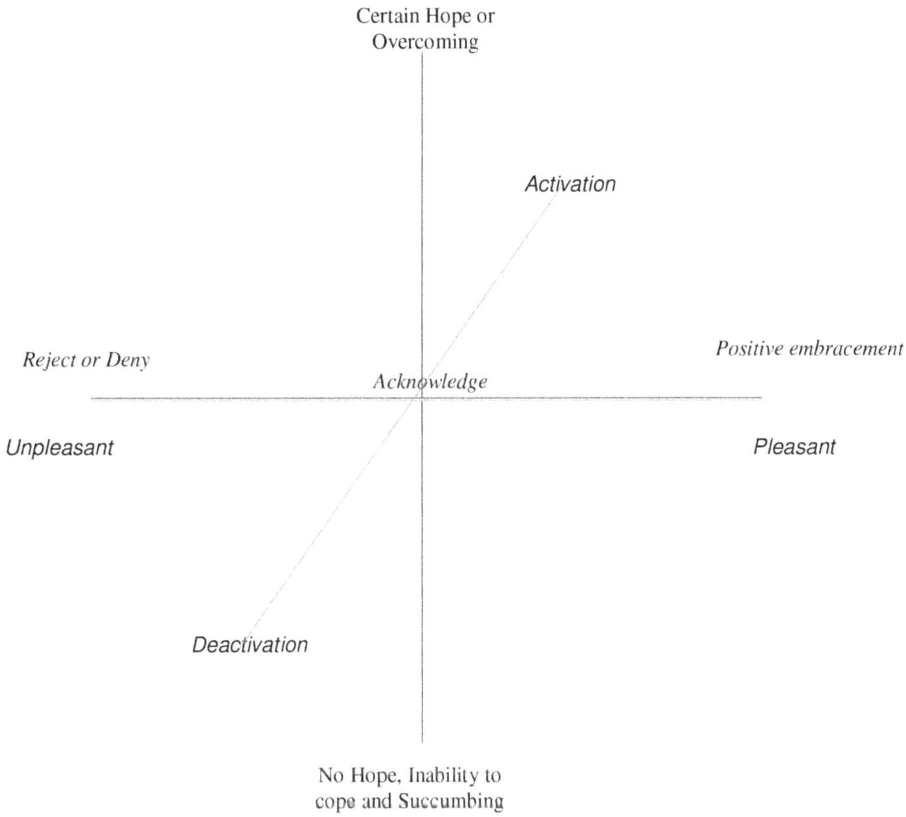

Figure 4.2. The model of emotional adjustment and hope (MEAH; adapted from [20]).

like injuries, illness and change on to a spectrum. Figure 4.2 illustrates how the hope and adaptation scale and the circumplex model of affect are combined to illustrate the MEAH.

4.1.4 Illness narratives and how they are mapped onto the MEAH

In order to understand the MEAH in the context of the expression of illness, an understanding of illness narratives is required. Illness narratives reflect stories told by patients about their experience of illness, they contain a plot that reveals a beginning, middle and end. The term narrative most often is a reference to at least one character who experiences at least one event. However, many narratives will bring together multiple events which are identified around a sequence of events. HCPs can use illness narratives as a way to help patients manage their illness. Illness narratives have been associated with a greater level of emotional support and can aid behaviour change [37]. This is important as emotional support is consistently associated with more positive psychological adaptation and hope in individuals with chronic illness [38].

Table 4.1. Illustrating 13 common illness narrative master plots.

Master plot or type	Definition and use in illness
Restitution	The restitution narrative is told by a patient who identifies the hope of being restored to his or her previous state of health and identity.
Heroic	The heroic or epic narratives are associated with maintaining or defending existing social values. It can be considered as a challenge that has been taken on and met. It may be regarded as implicit through actions that are described or explicitly identified through a fight or battle against what is happening, and the difficulty experienced.
Detective	The detective narrative revolves around a search for answers that explore the mystery of the illness. This can involve a search for a cure or treatments which can help maintain the life of the individual.
Comedy	A comedy provides the patient with an opportunity to observe illness in a different light.
Ironic or Satirical	An ironic or satirical narrative provides the patient with an opportunity to present other outcomes that are apparent.
Detached	The Disembodied or detached narratives document the events of life in a third party, with an emotionally flat dialogue. These narratives can lack any attempt to evaluate the meaning of illness to the patient.
Romantic	The romantic narrative is associated with a struggle for personal meaning, it details a contrast that was involved, it highlights a struggle and what has been overcome.
Quest	The quest narrative suggests that patients accept their illness and seek to use it.
Supernatural	The supernatural intervention identifies God as an ally in the experience of illness, where salvation is offered. It illustrates an ability to view the experience differently and can identify gains.
Didactic	The didactic narrative is illustrated by a patient who identifies the lessons that have been learnt following the experience of illness.
Sad or Tragic narrative	A sad narrative represents the idea of loss and a disease that is out of the patient's control, as more distance is put between the narrator and their desired goal. A tragic narrative is more severe and regressive and illustrates an inevitable outcome.
Chaos	This narrative is an expression of loss, leaving no distance from the experience, where the future is empty.

Illness narrative master plots are common stories of illness which are meaningful to the patient. The narratives have a recognisable structure and have a common or identifiable plot. An overview of 13 common illness narrative master plots has been developed by Soundy *et al* [4]. Table 4.1 provides a definition of each of these 13 master plots. However, this should not be considered an exhaustive list. Rather those identified should be considered as an example.

The different master plots illustrate the varied impact of an illness on a patient. Such plots focus on key psychological attributes including psycho-emotional adaptation to illness, the patient's expression of hope related to their situation and a focus of events in relationship to time. The reference to time indicates psychological adaptation to what life was like in the past, what it is currently like, and can reflect hope regarding what the future will be like and whether that is acceptable or not [4]. Some illness narrative master plots have a very distinct representation of this. For instance, the chaos illness narrative master plot is located in the past, it illustrates hopelessness and an inability to adapt to the change as a result of the illness and symptoms. The narrative is illustrative of great loss and emotional turmoil. In contrast, the restitution illness narrative master plot is firmly focused on future and often a concrete hope of restoration to a former self is identified. There appears to be an inability to accept an alternative version of the future. Thus, illness narrative master plots provide an idea of how an individual may consider time within their story. Time has been identified as an important dimension of hope [3]. The two narratives identified above provide an example of the expression of illness as a representation of impact of change following the illness. Whilst narratives can be distinctly different, they can be specific and relate to specific levels of hope. Thus, individuals may tell different narrative master plots in relationship to different difficulties or challenges experienced. Different and seemingly contrasting illness narrative master plots can be told simultaneously by a patient and are an important process as they reflect key stages in illness adaptation, expressions of hope and illustrations of coping processes [10]. It is important to note that access to different and altering stories can provide patients with an opportunity to evolve their story and adapt by listening to peers' stories [25].

Certain illness narrative master plots can be difficult to hear or can be denied by others [39]. Patients and HCPs need to have an awareness of the psychological meaning behind a patient's narrative master plots. The MEAH provides a way to understand this and uses this meaning as an intervention for patients. For instance, each of the scales of the MEAH can be used to ask questions about a patient's story. Alternatively, it can be seen through the MEAH that by offering, hearing or learning about different stories of illness a patient can adapt in their well-being by redefining their own story of illness.

Recent research [30] has identified that narratives master plots can be mapped onto the MEAH (see figure 4.3). By mapping narrative master plots patients, HCPs and researchers may be able to capture underlying psychological and emotional responses to illness. This enables a consideration of how plots vary across time, what plots may be dominant for particular conditions or time following illness symptom change and how, and if, particular master plots are associated with one another. There is also a need to use the understanding of emotive and cognitive components of different master plots to target psychological interventions e.g., the emotional reaction expressed by a patient may be that of fear of what is happening which may cause them to want to escape or deny their circumstances [29]. In addition, understanding the cognitive processes of adaptation and hope may provide a point of discussion from where psychological intervention can begin. HCPs should be able to map the patient's response on a session-by-session basis e.g. HCPs by their responses have an opportunity to aid a patient's mood. For instance, a poor choice

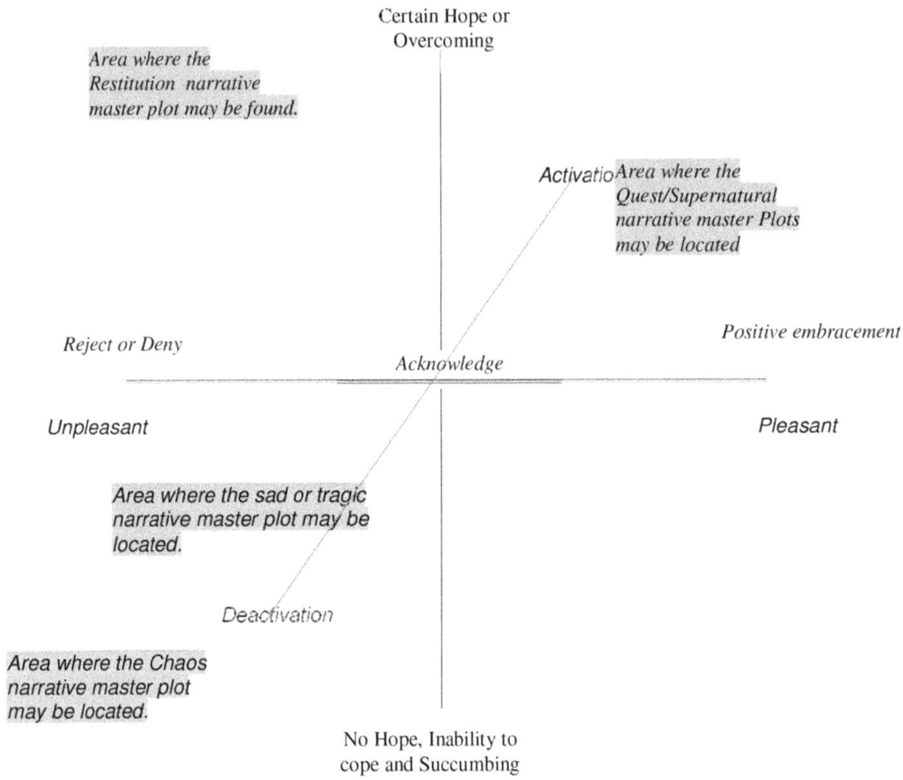

Figure 4.3. Examples of specific illness narrative master plots mapped on to the MEAH.

of words and an inability to listen may generate negative moods from interactions and be regarded as a perceived threat by an HCP. The mapping of illness narratives may provide greater clues to how particular narratives are dominant or become dominant in a patient. It will likely provide an insight into how changeable certain master plots of individuals with MS are.

4.1.4.1 The need to understand how narrative master plots illustrate psycho-emotional adaptation.

Illness narrative master plots are recognisable stories that people, tell, hear and want to listen to. The MEAH provides evidence that listening to a patient's story, encouraging a patient to share their story and actively seeking other stories will often have a positive psychological benefit. The HCP can seek to further understand the psychological well-being of a patient with MS by using the MEAH as a psychological assessment tool. The assessment undertaken using the MEAH can determine a course of action to be taken.

4.1.5 limitations

This work is currently limited by its focus on the development and analysis of the constructs defined by the MEAH. Alternative insights and understandings of these constructs are possible. Caution is required when considering the applicability of these results into all settings and areas of MS. Further research is needed to understand a deeper application of the MEAH as an assessment outcome and as a basis for providing an intervention.

4.1.6 Conclusion

HCPs should consider the importance of hope and the factors which influence hope within their practice. Illness narrative master plots provide one way to achieve this. The MEAH provides a psychological assessment tool and can also be used for a psychological intervention. Further research is warranted to establish the parameters for this.

References

[1] Marcel G 1951 *Homo Viator: Introduction to a Metaphysics of Hope* ed E Crawford Trans. (Chicago, IL: Henry Regnery) pp 29–31

[2] Barnard D 1995 Chronic illness and the dynamics of hoping *Chronic Illness from Experience to Policy* ed S K Toombs, D Barnard and R A Carson (Bloomington, IN: Indiana University Press) pp 38–57

[3] Dufault K J and Martocchio B C 1985 Hope: Its spheres and dimensions *Nurs. Clin. North Am.* **20** 379–91

[4] Soundy A, Smith B, Dawes H, Pall H, Gimbrere K and Ramsay J 2013 Patient's expression of hope and illness narratives in three neurological conditions: a meta-ethnography *Health Psychol. Rev.* **7** 177–201

[5] Synder C R, Lopez S J, Shorey H S, Rand K L and Feldman D B 2003 Hope theory, measrements, and application to school psychology *Sch. Psychol. Q.* **18** 122–39

[6] Dorsett P 2010 The importance of hope in coping with severe acquired disability *Aust. Soc. Work* **63** 83–102

[7] O'Hara D 2013 *Hope in Counselling and Psychotherapy* (London: Sage)

[8] Van Hooft S 2011 *Hope* (Durham: Acumen)

[9] Soundy A, Smith B, Butler M, Minns Lowe C, Dawes H and Winward C H 2010 A qualitative study in neurological physiotherapy and hope: Beyond physical improvement *Physiother. Theory Pract.* **26** 79–88

[10] Soundy A, Stubbs B, Freeman P, Coffee P and Roskell C 2014 Factors influencing patients' hope in stroke and spinal cord injury: A narrative review *Int. J. Ther. Rehabil.* **21** 210–8

[11] Rannisto M, Rosti-Otajarvi E, Mantynen A, Koivisto K, Huhtala H and Hamalainen P 2015 The use of goal attainment scales in neuropsychological rehabilitation in multiple sclerosis *Disabil. Rehabil.* **37** 1984–91

[12] Khan F, Pallant J F and Turner-Stokes L 2008 Use of goal attainment scaling in inpatient rehabilitation for persons with multiple sclerosis *Arch. Phys. Med. Rehabil.* **89** 652–9

[13] Rose A, Rosewilliam S and Soundy A 2017 Shared decision making within goal setting in rehabilitation settings: A systematic review *Patient Educ. Couns.* **100** 65–75

[14] Schmitt M M, Goverover Y, DeLuca J and Chiaravalloti N 2014 Self-efficacy as a predictor of self-reported physical, cognitive, and social functioning in multiple sclerosis *Rehabil. Psychol.* **59** 27–34

[15] Tan-Kristanto S and Kiropoulos L A 2015 Resilience, self-efficacy, coping styles and depressive and anxiety symptoms in those newly diagnosed with multiple sclerosis *Psychol. Health Med.* **20** 635–45
[16] Black R and Dorstyn D 2015 A biopsychosocial model of resilience for multiple sclerosis *J. Health Psychol.* **20** 1434–44
[17] Thoits P A 2011 Mechanisms linking social ties and support to physical and mental health *J. Health Soc. Behav.* **52** 145–61
[18] Foote A W, Piazza D, Holcombe J, Paul P and Daffin P 1990 Hope, self-esteem and social support in persons with multiple sclerosis *J. Neurosci. Nurs.* **22** 155–9
[19] Soundy A and Elder T 2017 Developing and applying the theory of psychological adjustments needs in patients with multiple sclerosis *Multiple Sclerosis: Food and Lifestyle in Neurological Autoimmune* ed R Watson (New York: Elsevier)
[20] Soundy A, Roskell C, Adams R, Elder T and Dawes H 2016 Understanding health care professional-patient interactions in Multiple Sclerosis: A systematic review and thematic synthesis *Open J. Ther. Rehabil.* **4** 187–217
[21] Dennison L, Moss-Morris R and Chalder T 2009 A review of psychological correlates of adjustment in patients with multiple sclerosis *Clin. Psychol. Rev.* **29** 141–53
[22] Lewis V M, Williams K, KoKo C, Woolmore J, Jones C and Powell T 2017 Disability, depression and suicide ideation in people with multiple sclerosis *J. Affect. Disord.* **208** 662–9
[23] Fong T, Finlayson M and Peacock N 2006 The social experience of aging with a chronic illness: Perspectives of older adults with multiple sclerosis *Disabil. Rehabil.* **28** 695–705
[24] Horton S, MacDonald D J and Erickson K *et al* 2015 A qualitative investigation of exercising with MS and the impact on the spousal relationship *Eur. Rev. Aging Phys. Act.* **12** 3
[25] Soundy A, Dawes H, Collett J, Coe S and Rosewilliam S 2018 Understanding the importance of illness narratives in people with multiple sclerosis who participated in an exercise rehabilitation trial; a qualitative study *Arch. Physiother. Rehabil.* **1** 1–20
[26] Benito-León J, Morales J M and Rivera-Navarro J 2002 Health-related quality of life and its relationship to cognitive emotional functioning in multiple sclerosis patients *Eur. J. Neurol.* **9** 497–502
[27] Peña-Sarrionandia A, Mikolajczak M and Gross J J 2015 Integrating emotion regulation and emotional intelligence traditions: a meta-analysis *Front. Psychol.* **6** 160
[28] Little M and Sayers E-J 2004 While there's life…: hope and the experience of cancer *Soc. Sci. Med.* **59** 1329–37
[29] Fredrickson B L 2004 The broaden-and-build theory of positive emotions *Philos. Trans. R. Soc. B: Biol. Sci.* **359** 1367–78
[30] Soundy A 2018 Psycho-emotional content of illness narrative master plots for people with chronic illness: Implications for assessment *World J. Psychiatry* **8** 79–82
[31] Lynch S J 1974 *Images of Hope. Imagination as a Healer for the Hopeless* (Notre Dame, IN: Notre Dame Press)
[32] Sin N L and Lyubomirsky S 2009 Enhancing well being and alleviating depressive symptoms with positive psychology interventions: A practice friendly meta analysis *J. Clin. Psychol.* **65** 467–87
[33] Lerner J S, Li Y, Valdesolo P and Kassam K S 2015 Emotion and decision making *Annu. Rev. Psychol.* **66** 799–823
[34] Duggleby W, Holtslander L, Kylma J, Duncan V, Hammond C and Williams A 2010 Metasynthesis of hope experience of family caregivers of persons with chronic illness *Qual. Health Res.* **20** 148–58

[35] Soundy A and Condon N 2015 Patients experiences of maintaining mental well-being and hope within motor neuron disease: a thematic synthesis *Front. Psychol.* **6** 606
[36] Russell J A 1980 A circumplex model of affect *J. Pers. Soc. Psychol.* **39** 1161–78
[37] Lucius-Hoene G, Thiele U, Breuning M and Haug S 2011 Doctors' voices in patients' narratives: coping with emotions in storytelling *Chronic Illn.* **8** 163–75
[38] Boinon D, Sultan S, Charles C, Stulz A, Guillemeau C, Delaloge S and Dauchy S 2014 Changes in psychological adjustment over the course of treatment for breast cancer: The predictive role of social sharing and social support *Psycho-Oncology* **23** 291–8
[39] Norrick N R 2015 The dark side of tellability *Narrative Inquiry* **15** 323–43

IOP Publishing

Neurological Disorders and Imaging Physics, Volume 2
Engineering and clinical perspectives of multiple sclerosis
Ayman El-Baz and Jasjit S Suri

Chapter 5

Multiple sclerosis symptoms

Khadije Janalipour

Multiple sclerosis (MS) is a progressive chronic neurologic disorder which topically causes the destruction and inflammation of the myelin sheath in the brain and the spinal cord. MS is a chronic, immune-mediated disease that affects the central nervous system (CNS) which includes the brain, spinal cord, and optic nerves is diagnosed most commonly in young adults.

5.1 Introduction

Multiple sclerosis (MS) is one of the most common diseases of the central nervous system. MS is not considered a genetic disease in the classic sense because it usually occurs sporadically. However, population and family studies are consistent with a principal pathogenic role for genetic risk factors in MS etiology. This genetic component is indicated primarily by the increased relative risk to siblings of affected individuals compared with the general population [1]. It is characterized by a huge interindividual variability of clinical symptoms and an unpredictable course ranging from asymptomatic sequelae to severe disability. Early initiation of treatment has proved effective in delaying the second neurological episode and reducing long-term disability [2]. It is therefore mandatory to identify as early as possible patients who may develop the disease. Prevalence varies (<1 to 193 per 100 000) depending on ethnic and geographical variables [3]. There are no reasons for MS incidence, however, there is a combination of environmental and hereditary factors including pollution, viral and bacterial infections, and stress may be included. There are many factors that may be responsible for MS and these factors can be summarized into: microbial, viral and other infections. MS is not a genetic disease although there a lot of genetic changes that are responsible for MS symptoms. MS increases among the family of an MS patient, however, MS rate increases to 30% in identical twins with a rate of 5% in nonidentical twins. Therefore, the biomarkers of the damage to the central nervous system are being extensively sought, to allow prediction and follow-up of the disease course. The body's actions and reactions to outside stimuli involve

doi:10.1088/978-0-7503-1762-7ch5

a lightning-quick and complicated process in which the body receives those stimuli through the various senses. This ongoing process depends on the coordinated transmission of nerve impulses from one nerve cell to the next. Nerve impulses pass along nerve fibers that connect at the synapse [4].

Multiple sclerosis (MS) is a chronic, immune-mediated disease that affects the central nervous system (CNS)—which includes the brain, spinal cord, and optic nerves—and is diagnosed most commonly in young adults. Although a specific cause of MS has not yet been determined, several theories are plausible. MS generally is considered to be an autoimmune disease in which—for unknown reasons—the body's own immune system begins to attack normal body tissue. In the case of MS, the cells that make myelin, the myelin itself, and/or the axons are attacked. Although 90% of those diagnosed are between the ages of 16 and 60, MS has been known to make its first appearance in early childhood or long after age 60 [5]. People presenting with multiple sclerosis after the age of 50 are typically classified as having late-onset multiple sclerosis In this age group, men are overrepresented and a progressive onset is more than the others. Most doctors believe that MS is an autoimmune disease because the plaques or scars in the myelin caused by MS appear to be the result of the person's immune system mistakenly attacking tissue in his or her own body [6]. The MS symptoms may occur and disappear completely where the permanent neurological problems happen when the disease timely advances [7].

The mechanism responsible for MS to appear can be summarized as two reasons: the immune system has destroyed the myelin sheath, and failure of the myelin-producing cells to produce new sheaths [6]. The two above mentioned reasons include numerous genetics and environmental factors e.g. heredity, pollution, microbial and viral infections [8]. The pathological hallmark of MS is the formation of large confluent plaques of primary demyelination in the white matter with variable axonal degeneration. Up to 5% of patients with multiple sclerosis develop their first symptoms in childhood, and these are almost always those of relapsing–remitting multiple sclerosis. In younger children (<12 years of age) multiple sclerosis can present differently in adolescents and adults; encephalopathy, multifocal neurological deficits (often with prominent brainstem or cerebellar involvement), and seizures are more common [9]. Understanding the pathophysiologic mechanisms underlying the course and prognosis of MS is important because these changes may impact therapeutic deductions. Neuropathologically, MS is characterized by circumscribed lesions located in the white matter of both cerebral hemispheres, cerebellum, and brain-stem. Lesions are more commonly found in periventricular white matter, basal ganglia, thalamus, and other subcortical areas, but may also be located in the gray–white matter junction [10]. It has long been established that demyelination alone is not the only pathological process at play in MS. Inflammation and axonal degeneration also contribute to neurological damage, leading to clinical disability. This has been evidenced by temporal discordance between indicators of tissue damage on neuroimaging versus acquisition of clinical disability later in life. It is speculated that early on, patients have only limited disability due to functional compensation in the presence of demyelination, and that much of the long term disability is due to axonal damage and subsequent neuronal death by retrograde degeneration [11]. MS is one of a broad category of *demyelinating* diseases that affect the CNS—the brain and spinal cord. Certain specific features on brain magnetic resonance images make the diagnosis of MS more likely. MS lesions often have an irregular and confluent shape and are located in the periventricular region, especially around the frontal, occipital, and temporal horn. Involvement of the corpus callosum, including subcallosal lesions and corpus callosum atrophy, is a common feature. Further, cortical and subcortical lesions can also be found in addition to lesions scattered in periventricular white matter. With improvements of MRI techniques, MR imaging of the spinal cord has become common practice showing focal and diffuse abnormalities [6, 12] (figure 5.1). Atrophy of both brain and spinal cord can be detected in MS patients, including relapsing patients with minimal neurologic deficits. Both axon and myelin loss contribute to tissue atrophy. The pathological hallmark of MS is the formation of large confluent plaques of primary demyelination in the white matter with variable axonal degeneration and astrocytic gliosis. The pathological hallmark of MS is the formation of large confluent plaques of primary demyelination in the white matter with variable axonal degeneration and astrocytic gliosis [13]. Degeneration is also likely to be a key mechanism in MS, particularly in progressive phases of the disease. A degenerative disease is a disease in which the function or structure of the affected tissues or organs progressively worsens over time, due to normal bodily wear and tear or lifestyle choices such as exercise or diet. Some examples include Alzheimer's disease, motor neuron disease, cancer, diabetes, heart disease, inflammatory bowel disease, Parkinson's disease and osteoarthritis. The growing evidence of a degenerative component to MS means that many lifestyle interventions such as diet and exercise which are known to be helpful in other degenerative diseases will also be of benefit to people with MS, and provides further rationale for why they are effective in MS [14].

MRI has become an extremely valuable tool in the diagnostic work-up of MS. T2-weighted imaging, using the spin echo, fast spin echo, or fast fluid-attenuated

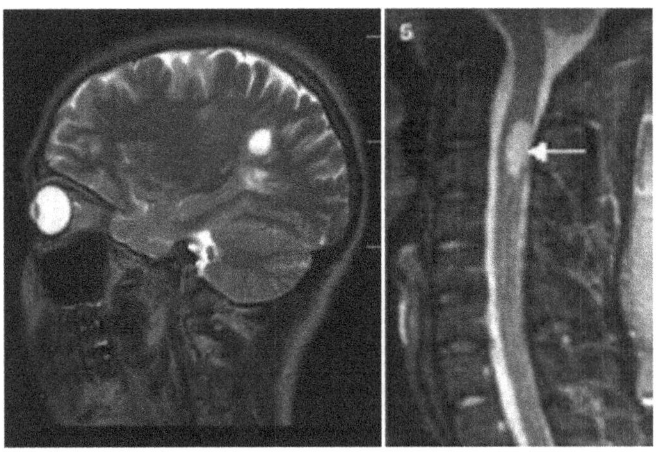

(a) (b)

Figure 5.1. An MRI image showing MS lesions in the brain (a) and spinal cord (b).

inversion recovery (FLAIR) technique, is highly sensitive in detecting MS plaques, the majority of which are clinically silent. Brain MRI is abnormal in 95% of patients with clinically definite MS and spinal cord MRI reveals lesions in about 75%. Together, one region or the other will reveal abnormalities in all but a very small number of patients assisting the diagnosis by demonstrating disseminated white matter lesions in space and also by showing a pattern of abnormalities that are characteristic of demyelination.

Typical features include:

- predominantly periventricular lesions with asymmetrical and irregular involvement;
- oval or round-shaped lesions;
- corpus callosum involvement;
- lesions abutting the corticomedullary junction;
- brain stem lesions, especially in the floor of the fourth ventricle or abutting the subarachnoid surface;
- gadolinium enhancement for the first few weeks after a lesion appears but not thereafter;
- nodular or ring-shaped enhancement, sometimes with an open (incomplete) ring; and
- spinal cord lesions of less than one vertebral segment in length, with partial cross-sectional involvement and often wedge-shaped and extending to the subarachnoid surface on axial images.

5.1.1 Neurodegenerative mechanisms of multiple sclerosis

In MS, the attack involves ***inflammation*** directed against the ***myelin*** and the cells that make myelin, the ***oligodendrocytes*** of the CNS, in a process called ***demyelination.*** Demyelination, although less obvious on gross inspection of the brain, is also present in the gray matter, in particular in the cerebral and cerebellar cortex but also in the brainstem and the spinal cord. Although the disease primarily affects myelin, axons too are injured in and lost from the lesions. While the functional consequences of inflammation and demyelination are at least in part reversible, the deficit due to axonal loss is irreversible. Thus axonal destruction in MS is a major correlate of permanent neurological deficit in patients. MS lesions can also in part be repaired spontaneously by remyelination. This can be quite extensive at early stages of the disease, where large plaques become completely remyelinated and remain in the CNS as so-called shadow plaques. At late stages of the disease and in particular in patients with progressive disease, the remyelinating capacity is low and remyelination is mostly restricted to small rims at the lesion edges [15]. Following activation of autoreactive T cells through some infectious agents that are molecular mimicking from proteins of myelin sheath, they pass through the blood brain barrier (BBB) and enter the CNS. These cells demyelinate the neurons through the neuro-inflammatory responses which finally lead to the destruction of myelin and axons of nervous cells and plaque formation in the brain white matter and spinal cord [16].

Neurons, or nerve cells, in the CNS are made up of the cell body, ***axons*** (the processes or extensions of nerve cells that conduct nervous impulses away from the cell body), and dendrites. Myelin is the insulation or coating that surrounds the axons and speeds nerve conduction. Demyelination results in ***plaques*** (also called *lesions* or *scars*) along the myelin sheath that interfere with nerve conduction (figure 5.2). The symptoms that occur in MS result from this inflammatory process, as well as from damage to the axons themselves. These symptoms can include loss of vision, double vision, stiffness, weakness, imbalance, numbness, pain, problems with bladder and bowel control, fatigue, sexual changes, speech and swallowing difficulties, emotional changes, and intellectual impairment. The type and number of symptoms vary from one individual to the next, depending on where in the CNS the myelin and ***axonal damage*** occurs [6].

Myelin is a fatty material that insulates nerves, acting like the covering of an electrical wire and allowing the nerve to transmit its impulses rapidly. It is the speed and efficiency with which these impulses are conducted that permits smooth, rapid,

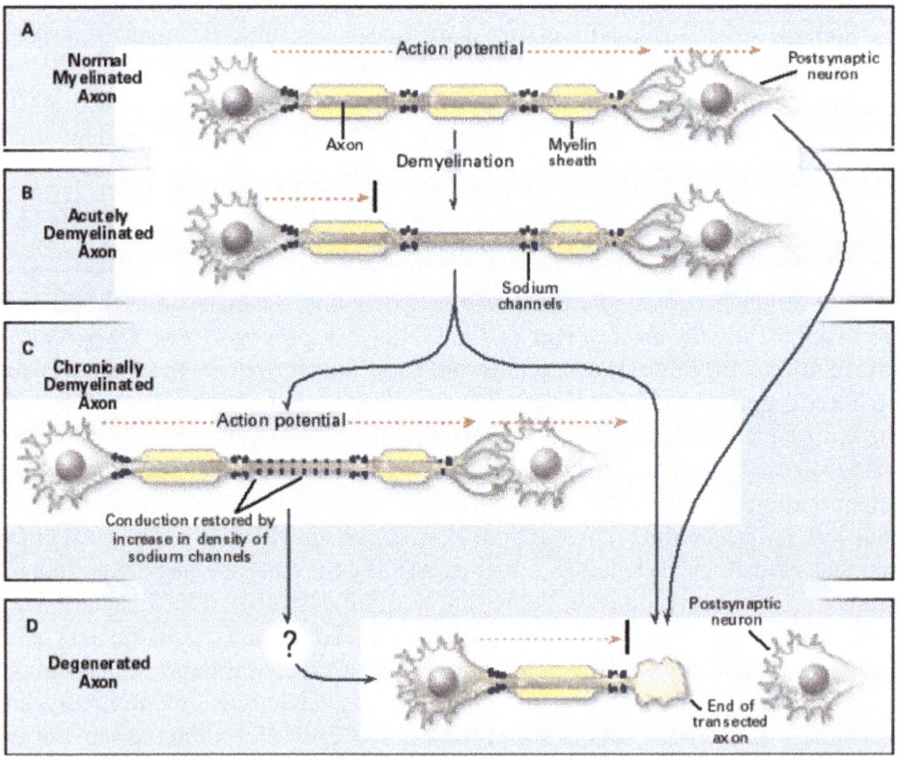

Figure 5.2. Demyelination and axonal degeneration in multiple sclerosis. (A) In a normal myelinated axon, the action potential (dashed arrow) travels, with high velocity and reliability, to the postsynaptic neuron. (B) In acutely demyelinated axons, conduction is blocked (black bar). (C) In some chronically demyelinated axons that acquire a higher-than-normal density of sodium channels, conduction is restored. (D) Axonal degeneration, by contrast, interrupts action potential propagation in a permanent manner. *Source*: Waxman, S G, 1998. Copyright 1998 Massachusetts Medical Society. All rights reserved. Reprinted with permission.

and coordinated movements that are performed with little conscious effort (figure 5.3). In MS the loss of myelin is accompanied by a loss of the ability to perform these movements. Without the myelin sheath, nerve cells lose their ability to conduct nerve impulses. As the number of damaged nerve cells increases, the body loses its ability to perform the functions controlled by these cells. The sites where myelin is lost appear as hardened *sclerotic* (scarred) areas, and because there tend to be many such areas within the CNS, the term *multiple sclerosis* (literally, many scars) is appropriate [17]. Active demyelination is associated with inflammation and blood–brain barrier leakage. In the progressive stage of the disease additional pathologies become prominent consisting of gradual expansion of pre-existing white matter

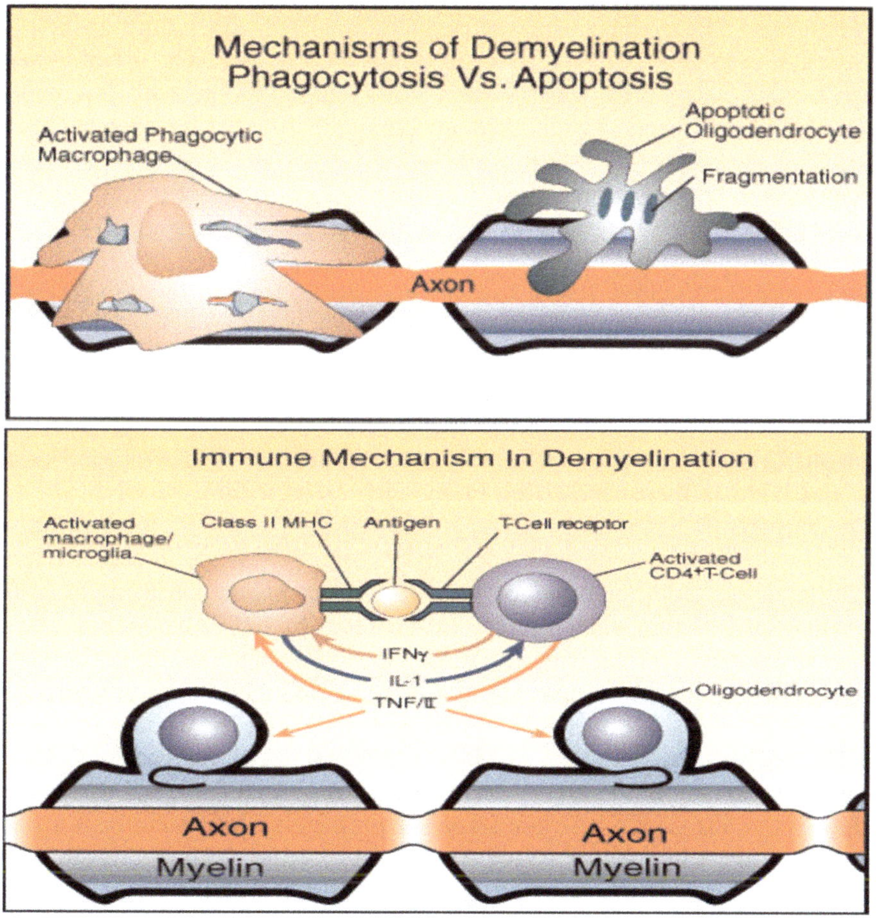

Figure 5.3. Possible mechanisms of demyelination. The mechanisms causing myelin damage are not completely known. Possible mechanisms include a direct toxic effect of tumor necrosis factor (TNF) on myelin (upper panel) or macrophage-mediated damage through either phagocytosis, in which the cell is engulfed and destroyed, or apoptosis, in which cells are induced to self-destruct (lower panel). *Note*: IL = interleukin; MHC = major histocompatibility antigen. *Source*: Adapted from New Directions in the Management of Multiple Sclerosis [1].

lesions in the absence of blood–brain barrier damage, widespread cortical demyelination and diffuse injury of the entire normal appearing white and gray matter. Altogether, these different modes of tissue injury finally result in extensive brain tissue loss and atrophy [18]. Irrespective of the stage of the disease, active tissue injury in MS is associated with inflammation, although the extent of inflammation is higher during early relapsing disease and declines with duration of the disease at late stages of progressive MS inflammation in the normal appearing white matter (NAWM) and the lesions may decline to levels seen in age-matched controls. In these patients, neurodegeneration also declines to levels seen in the respective controls [19].

There is no cure for MS to date. All the MS treatments try to attempt to improve the neuronal function following MS occurances and stop any progress of the disease [20]. The use of MS treatments in the early stage of MS can induce adverse side effects or can even be ineffective. The treatments with good results are observed in teenage women where MS appears early with relapsing type with few neurons damaged [21, 23]. MS decreases life with an average 5–10 years less than for healthy people [22].

Irrespective of the stage of the disease, active tissue injury in MS is associated with inflammation, although the extent of inflammation is higher during early relapsing disease and declines with duration of the disease [22].

Myelin is a fatty material that insulates nerves, acting like the covering of an electrical wire and allowing the nerve to transmit its impulses rapidly. It is the speed and efficiency with which these impulses are conducted that permits smooth, rapid, and coordinated movements that are performed with little conscious effort. In MS the loss of myelin is accompanied by a loss of the ability to perform these movements. The sites where myelin is lost appear as hardened *sclerotic* (scarred) areas, and because there tend to be many such areas within the CNS, the term *multiple sclerosis* (literally, many scars) is appropriate [7]. Active demyelination is associated with inflammation and blood–brain barrier leakage. In the progressive stage of the disease additional pathologies become prominent consisting of gradual expansion of pre-existing white matter lesions in the absence of blood–brain barrier damage, widespread cortical demyelination and diffuse injury of the entire normal appearing white and gray matter. Altogether, these different modes of tissue injury finally result in extensive brain tissue loss and atrophy [24]. Irrespective of the stage of the disease, active tissue injury in MS is associated with inflammation, although the extent of inflammation is higher during early relapsing disease and declines with duration of the disease [25]. At late stages of progressive MS inflammation in the normal appearing white matter (NAWM), the lesions may decline to levels seen in age-matched controls. In these patients, also neurodegeneration declines to levels seen in the respective controls [21]. Although a specific cause of MS has not yet been determined, several theories are plausible. MS generally is considered to be an autoimmune disease in which—for unknown reasons—the body's own immune system begins to attack normal body tissue. In the case of MS, the cells that make myelin, the myelin itself, and/or the axons are attacked. The body's actions and reactions to outside stimuli involve a lightning-quick and complicated process in which the body receives those stimuli through the various senses. This ongoing process depends on the coordinated transmission of nerve impulses from one nerve cell to the next. Nerve impulses pass along nerve fibers that connect at synapses. Although MS is generally considered to be a demyelinating disease, the importance of axonal and neuronal pathology cannot be overestimated. Although inflammation and demyelination lead to clinical deficit, which is at least in principle reversible, the consequences of axonal and neuronal loss can be compensated only by reorganization of CNS function, but not by repair. Axonal and neuronal pathology is undoubtedly an important feature of MS pathology and may already occur at early stages of the disease. Therapeutic strategies to prevent axonal and neuronal degeneration are thus urgently warranted. The extent and importance of axonal and neuronal destruction and loss in patients with MS have only recently been acknowledged. Since current immunological therapies of MS have little effect on disease progression and the development of axonal loss and atrophy in patients' brains, it has been suggested that the basic problem in MS may even be a neurodegenerative process, which may be superimposed and aggravated in its consequences by the inflammatory reaction. Although such a scenario cannot be ruled out at the present time, the data discussed in this chapter are more consistent with the notion that all aspects of MS pathology, including axonal and neuronal injury, are driven by an immune-mediated inflammatory response [11].

5.1.2 A word about anatomy

The anatomy of the nerves and muscles is intended to provide a quick reference for the reader. More specific information is included with each topic as needed. The integrative activity of the nervous system, which underlies motor, sensory, cognitive, and psychological behavior, depends on electrical signaling between neurons. Each neuron encodes its message in the form of action potentials (small all-or-none electrical impulses) that are carried to other neurons via axons, the cable-like fibers that extend from neuron cell bodies. Many axons within the brain and spinal cord are myelinated the *central nervous system*, which is somewhat analogous to the main processing unit of a computer; the *peripheral nervous system* (PNS), which links the CNS to the muscles; and the *sympathetic nervous system*, which links the CNS to the internal organs. The CNS has two major parts, the brain and spinal cord, which in turn have several subdivisions, each of which plays a unique role in regulating the functions of the body (figure 5.4). The portion of the brain referred to as the *cerebrum* acts as a master control system and is responsible for initiating all thought and movement. Memory, personality, vision, hearing, touch, and muscle tone all are housed within the cerebrum. Behind the cerebrum is the cerebellum, which coordinates movement and 'smoothes' muscle activity. The proper functioning of this region of the brain controls balance during walking and the smooth use of your hands and arms. Beneath the cerebrum and cerebellum is the *brain stem*, which contains the nerves that control eye movements and the vital centers that are involved in functions such as breathing and heart rate. Extending downward from the brain stem is the *spinal cord*, which functions very much like a large electrical

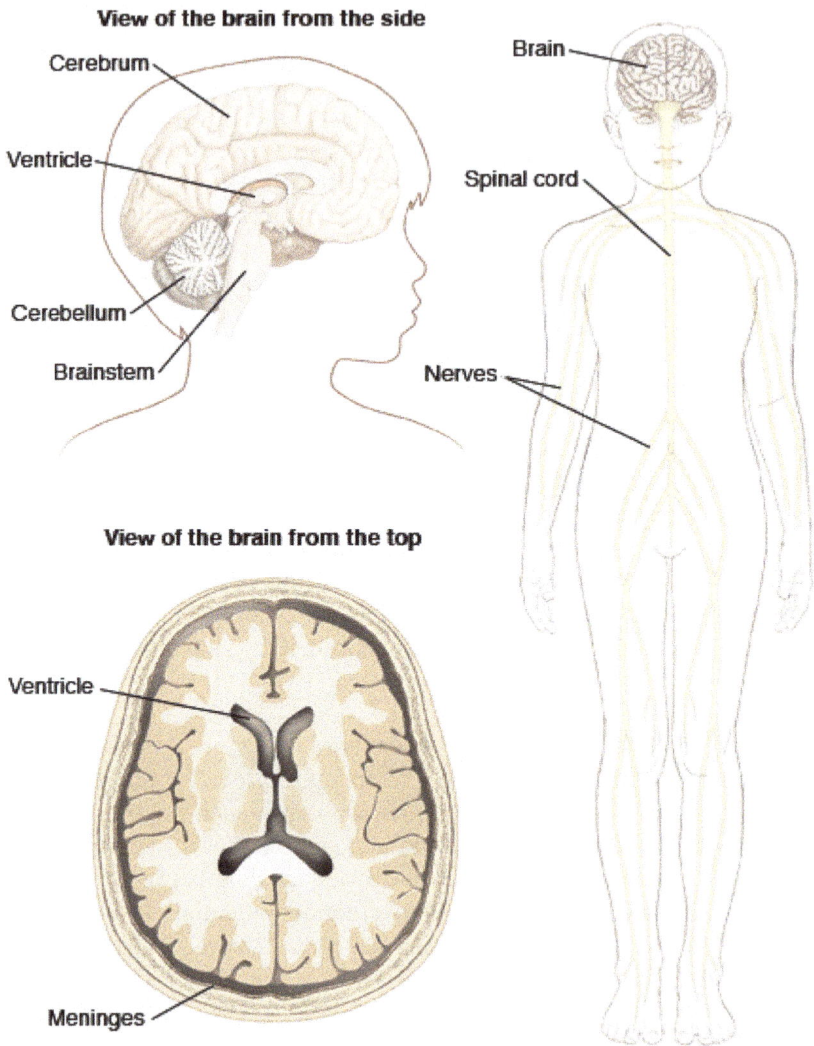

Figure 5.4. The nervous system.

cord that carries messages between the brain centers and all other parts of the body [26]. Although numerous biochemical reactions occur in the brain and spinal cord, their major role is to produce electrical activity that stimulates and regulates various bodily activities. These are delivered to the target structures very efficiently and effectively because the entire system is well insulated and shielded by the myelin that surrounds the conducting systems and allows the electrical nervous impulses to move through the pathways with little loss of information. The myelin in the brain and spinal cord is produced by a specific type of cell called an *oligodendrocyte* (oligo). Both oligos and myelin appear to be injured in MS. When they are injured, the nerve beneath the myelin is also sometimes injured (axonal damage). Oligos disappear as the affected myelin becomes hardened and scarred, forming what is called a *plaque* and causing a short-circuiting of electrical transmission. MS directly affects only the CNS, the disease has indirect effects on other systems and their functions because all components of the nervous system communicate with each other [18, 27].

5.1.3 The immune system

The immune system is made up of a complex mixture of cells that together protect the body against foreign invaders and toxins as well as stopping the development of internal cancers. The cells have individual functions like secreting antibodies, engulfing foreign viruses, or making and secreting chemicals that either promote inflammation or suppress it. The cells are all derived from the bone marrow. B cells come directly from the bone marrow to the bloodstream, where they secrete antibodies that attach themselves to foreign proteins or toxins to neutralise them. T cells are first processed by the thymus gland and differentiate into a number of sub-types. To oversimplify things, essentially their job is to initiate or turn off the immune response and to secrete chemicals (cytokines, eicosanoids and leukotrienes) which either whip up (T helper 1 or Th1 response) or dampen down (T helper 2 or Th2 response) the immune response. The Th2 cells are also known as suppressor cells. There is usually a balance between these responses, so that the immune system can set up an inflammatory response when it needs to get rid of a foreign invader, but also switch it off or suppress it so that it doesn't continue unabated when no longer needed. The Th1/Th2 hypothesis revolves around the patterns of chemicals released by these two cell types, and how they modulate immune responses. Mossman and Coffman initially proposed that mouse T-helper cells could be classified based on the chemicals they secreted. Th1 cells rely on interferon-gamma, interleukin-2 and interleukin-12. Th2 cells rely on interleukin-4 and sometimes interleukin-5. The immune system is designed to protect us from outside challenges to our bodies, whether from bacteria or viruses, foreign substances, poisons and so on. MS appears to be at least triggered by auto-immunity. The term auto-immune is used to describe a range of diseases where the immune system is fooled into recognising its own body's substances as foreign and starts attacking them. Examples of auto-immune diseases include systemic lupus erythematosus (SLE) and rheumatoid arthritis. In MS the immune system seems to recognise part of the myelin (fatty) sheath of nerves as foreign, and starts attacking it. It is now recognised that MS is typified by the balance between Th1 and Th2 responses shifting to a predominantly Th1 [18, 28].

This is a critical concept in MS. It fits nicely with the central thrust of this book, that balance is the key, and that there is a range of things we can do to shift that balance. In MS, we need to re-balance the immune system more towards a Th2 type response. Researchers have found that a number of lifestyle changes in the 20th and 21st centuries, particularly surrounding diet and exercise, have tended to shift people in Western societies to a predominantly Th1 response, making them more susceptible to auto-immune disease. For instance, infection with intestinal worms was once very common, and is still quite common in developing countries. Investigators have shown that such infestations, probably because of their continual challenge to the immune system, result in a chronic state of Th2 predominance. People with such infestations seem to be protected against the auto-immune diseases MS, diabetes and rheumatoid arthritis [26]. Despite many years of intensive research, however, MS still defies complete understanding and treatment remains suboptimal. The prevailing theory is that MS is immune mediated and that experimental autoimmune encephalomyelitis (EAE) is a suitable model. EAE as a model for MS. EAE is a complex condition in which the interaction between a variety of immunopathological and neuropathological mechanisms leads to an approximation of the key pathological features of MS: inflammation, demyelination, axonal loss and gliosis. EAE, however, may not be an adequate model as it represents more a model of acute CNS inflammation than the counterpart of MS. Researchers are currently reconsidering the utilisation of EAE, especially when this model is used to define therapy. This may in fact be helpful as it will also force us to examine MS without the restraints imposed by EAE, examining what it actually is rather than what it looks like.

5.2 Diagnosis of multiple sclerosis

The diagnosis of MS is based on both clinical parameters, such as medical history and neurological examination, and paraclinical parameters such as MRI, CSF oligoclonal banding, and evoked potentials. There is no MS-specific diagnostic test, and the intermittent nature of the disease and high variability in presenting symptoms make diagnosis difficult. The presentation of MS can be monosymptomatic or have multifocal signs and symptoms, and many neurodegenerative disorders are similar to MS in their presentation. The increasing use (and overuse) of MRI has led to renewed interest in the concept of 'preclinical' MS—the incidental identification of imagine abnormalities indicative of MS in patients who have never had a clinical attack. This clinical scenario has been called the 'radiologically isolated syndrome'. About one-third of patients with preclinical MS identified incidentally on MRI will experience a clinical attack within five years [30].

Traditionally, MS cannot be diagnosed until the patient has suffered clinical attacks involving different neuroanatomical sites at different times. However, a recent consensus statement allows the diagnosis of MS after only one clinical attack, if MRI of the brain or spinal cord 3 months later shows new disease activity (at least one lesion enhancing with the MRI contrast agent gadolinium). The incentive for changing the diagnostic criteria is to enable earlier treatment with disease-modifying agents. Patients with MS may present with a wide range of clinical symptoms (figure 5.5). Most of the symptoms experienced by patients, such as bladder and bowel dysfunction, sexual dysfunction, easy fatigability, optic nerve disease, and sensory complaints, are not associated with profound physical disability and are relatively responsive to symptomatic interventions. However, some symptom complexes that involve severe cognitive dysfunction, spastic paraplegia, and cerebellar dysfunction are poorly responsive to treatment and are profoundly disabling. Prognostic biomarkers that would predict the future occurrence of these symptoms would

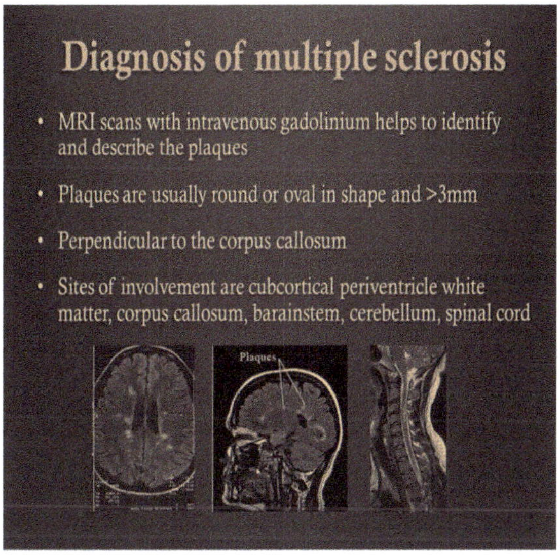

Figure 5.5. Diagnosis of MS.

Table 5.1. Clinical pathological correlations in common syndromes of MS.

Visual deficits	Often related to the involvement of the optic nerve as occurs in optic neuritis
Eye movement abnormalities	Frequently associated with plaques involving connections between the brainstem nuclei sub serving eye movements
Weakness and spasticity	One of the consequences of lesions involving the spinal cord or descending motor tracts in the white matter of internal capsule or brainstem
Ataxia	Usually the result of lesions in cerebellum or its input-output pathways
Dysarthria	Impairment of motor control of speech production. The current definition goes beyond its etymological 'disturbed articulation' to also include deficits in respiratory support, phonation and prosody
Cerebellum	Unsteady gait and slurred speech. Gait and limb ataxia, dysarthria, nystagmus
Optic nerve	Unilateral visual loss and painful eye movements. Relative afferent pupillary defect, lost colour vision/acuity, optic atrophy (late sign)
Cerebrum	Poor memory, personality change, epilepsy. Disinhibition dementia. The pattern of symptoms of MS is complex, variable and unpredictable. Symptoms in MS may be divided into those that are caused directly by demyelination within the brain and spinal cord and those that are not.

enable physicians to commence aggressive disease therapies. This in turn may abort future development of the symptom complexes associated with disability [1]. Predictably, they are presumably related to the location of the lesions, although clinically 'silent' demyelinating lesions also occur. These predominantly white matter lesions occur in multiple brain regions and appear at different times throughout the disease. Common syndromes correlated with lesions in specific areas include visual deficits, weakness and spasticity, eye movement abnormalities, and ataxia (table 5.1).

The initial presentation of multiple sclerosis varies according to both the location of lesions and the type of symptom onset (relapsing or progressive). Patients can present to a broad range of doctors depending on the neurological symptoms that could indicate an earlier unrecognised attack and thus help to establish the diagnosis and disease course (relapsing or progressive onset). Neurological examination is important to localize the site of involvement in the CNS and can provide evidence of other lesions—e.g. pathologically brisk reflexes or an extensor plantar response in a patient with optic neuritis.

5.3 Current classification includes

These four classes of measurement describe the types of measures, and provide a framework for assessment. The course of MS may be usefully characterized as the expression of two separate clinical phenomena, clinical relapses and disease progression these two phenomena correspond to distinct physiopathologic processes within the central nervous system (CNS). The interaction that takes place between relapses and progression during the course of MS has led to the separation of the disease into two phases and three types of evolution [1, 27].

- *Relapsing-remitting* (RR)

  This form of MS is characterized by clearly defined acute attacks, with either full recovery or some remaining neurologic signs/symptoms and residual deficit upon recovery. The early phase of the disease is marked by acute attacks characterized by unifocal (two-thirds of patients) or multifocal white matter lesions, gray matter lesions are not frequent in the early phase of the disease. The periods between relapses are characterized by a lack of disease progression. In the so-called relapsing–remitting (RR) phase of the illness, patients often resume their normal activity with minimal interference [33]. Relapses (also referred to as 'exacerbations,' 'attacks,' or 'bouts') are the clinical expression of the acute, self-limited, focal inflammatory events that occur episodically within the CNS of MS patients. It is thought that about 80% of MS begins in this manner. Over time the course may change and then the person moves into a different category.

- *Secondary progressive* (SP)

  This form of the disease begins with an initial RR course, followed by progression at a variable rate that also may include occasional relapses and minor remissions. many patients show progressive decline in neurological status, despite a decrease in the frequency of relapses. This secondary progressive (SP) phase of the illness is far more disabling and presents a greater barrier to high quality of life. About 10% of MS worsens right from the start and is called primary progressive.

- *Primary progressive*

  The disease shows progression of disability from its onset, without plateaus or remissions or with occasional plateaus and temporary minor improvements. It more commonly is seen in people who develop the disease after 40 years of age. About 5% of MS starts with a progressive course and becomes more fluctuating. It is called progressive-relapsing.
- *Progressive-relapsing*

  This pattern of MS shows progression from the onset but without clear acute relapses that may or may not have some recovery or remissions. This type is the lowest common type of MS types.

5.4 Clinical symptomatology

The clinical course of MS presents challenges because the disease has strikingly heterogeneous clinical manifestations that evolve over decades in most patients. MS is the most common inflammatory disease of the CNS affecting young adults. It is characterized by a huge interindividual variability of clinical symptoms and an unpredictable course ranging from asymptomatic sequelae to severe disability. Early initiation of treatment has proved effective in delaying the second neurological episode and reducing long-term disability [36]. It is therefore mandatory to identify as early as possible patients who may develop the disease. First attacks of MS, also called clinically isolated syndrome (CIS), usually consist of optic neuritis, brainstem involvement, or partial myelitis. Signs and symptoms of demyelinating lesions in multiple sclerosis include (figure 5.5):

Spinal cord: Limb weakness, Lhermitte's symptom[1], stiff legs, spasticity, pyramidal weakness, hyper-reflexia, sensory impairment (sometimes painful), erectile lost abdominal reflexes, extensor plantars, dysfunction, urinary frequency and retention, spinal sensory level constipation, flexor spasms.

Brain stem: Ataxia, diplopia, dysarthria, dysphagia, Internuclear ophthalmoplegia, nystagmus, gaze palsies, facial numbness/weakness facial sensory loss, 'rubral tremor'.

5.4.1 The brainstem

The brainstem is commonly affected in MS. The clinical syndromes produced by brainstem involvement in MS include: double vision (cranial nerves III, IV, VI), internuclear ophthalmoplegia (medial longitudinal fasciculus), facial weakness or myokymia (cranial nerve VII), vertigo (cranial nerve VIII), or bulbar (medullary) symptoms such as dysphagia, dysarthria, and tongue weakness (cranial nerves IX, X, XII). Facial sensory impairment (cranial nerve V) may arise from multiple localizations, including the brainstem, cervical cord (due to the fact that afferent trigeminal pathways descend from their entry at the pontomedullary junction to the level of the upper cervical spine), subcortical and cortical sensory pathways. Less

[1] ***Lhermitte's symptom*** is characteristic (neck flexion induces an 'electric shock' sensation running down the back, caused by a plaque in the cervical cord).

common brainstem symptoms in MS include hearing loss and severe bulbar signs. Involvement of cerebellar networks that connect [27].

5.4.2 Optic neuritis

Optic neuritis (inflammation of the optic nerve) is the most common visual disturbance in MS. In 17% of people with MS, optic neuritis was the first evidence of disease, but it can also occur subsequent to other symptoms. MRI is the most powerful predictor of whether MS will develop following optic neuritis, as evidenced by the presence and number of lesions in the brain. Loss of central vision is the major symptom reported in more than 90% of patients who have acute optic neuritis [31]. Others who have normal visual acuity may complain of a loss of peripheral vision to one side in the superior or inferior fields. The patient usually experiences mild orbital pain above or behind the eye, but the pain is mild even with severe visual loss. This dull retrobulbar pain may precede or occur concurrently with the visual loss. It may also be aggravated by upward eye movement and may occasionally last for as long as several weeks. The optic nerve inflammation may stimulate the trigeminal innervation of the optic nerve sheath to cause this orbital pain (figure 5.6). As visual acuity decreases over the next several days, the pain usually subsides when visual loss is maximal. Loss of color vision or dullness of vision is also more commonly noticed by patients than photophobia. Other less common symptoms are perception of phosphenes (flashing lights with noise or eye movement) and decreased depth perception in optic neuritis; patients experience pain in one eye, particularly on eye movement, and dimming of vision in that eye, often described as like looking through a dirty window or water. Color vision, especially red desaturation, and low-contrast vision are most prominently affected. Patients may complain of a 'blind spot' or 'blurry spot' within the visual field corresponding with a scotoma on formal visual field testing [32]. Acute demyelinating optic neuritis is the presenting symptom in about 20% of MS patients and affects about half of MS patients at some point in

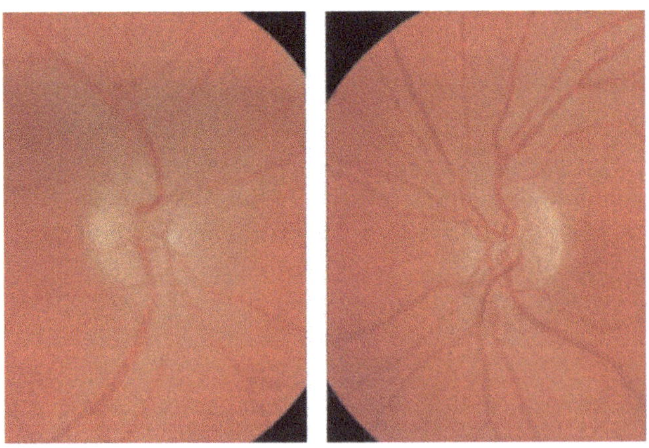

Figure 5.6. The left optic disc is normal, while the right optic disc is mildly swollen, as seen in anterior optic neuritis.

the disease course [31] and 20% of them have it as their presenting sign. The basic defect in optic neuritis/MS involves demyelination of the optic nerve, which blocks or slows the conduction of axonal transmission or decreases the amplitude of the nerve action potential. The perivenular demyelinating plaques from optic nerves of patients who have acute MS reveal similar pathology to the periventricular plaques found elsewhere in the brain. These plaques show a perivascular cuffing of T and B cells, edema in the myelin nerve sheaths, and subsequent myelin breakdown. In optic neuritis, the axons of the optic nerve are usually spared, resulting in good clinical recovery. More advanced lesions elsewhere in the CNS white matter often involve axonal degeneration, resulting in physical or mental disability. On histopathology, macrophages engulf the degraded myelin products and glial cells proliferate to cause permanent conduction block with no clinical recovery [33].

5.4.3 Myelitis

Acute partial transverse myelitis (APTM) may be the first clinical symptom of multiple sclerosis (MS) or may remain a monophasic event. Transverse myelitis is defined as impairment of motor, sensory, and bowel or bladder tracts in the spinal cord secondary to inflammatory-mediated injury. Partial myelitis is defined as involvement of one or more, but not all, of these functional spinal tracts. The myelitis that occurs in MS is typically partial and usually presents sub acutely [34, 35].

5.4.4 Sensory symptoms

Distortions of sensation on one side of the body are common in MS and can lead to many diagnostic errors and therapeutic misadventures. Nearly 15% or more of patients diagnosed with MS have had inappropriate surgery for their MS symptoms in the decade before diagnosis. Perhaps most common among these is podiatric surgery on toes and feet. These sensation impairments often lead to distortions of normal sensation or phantom sensations, which present diagnostic challenges. Some patients will present with a hand that has no position sense (the useless hand of Oppenheim). With this severe deficit, motor performance is impaired as well and probably results from the inability to organize a movement in the absence of appropriate sensation. The most common example of this occurs when one goes to the dentist and receives local anesthesia that numbs the tongue and lip on one side. No motor nerves have been blocked, but for 1 or 2 h after this procedure, one is often modestly dysarthric. Movement requires some degree of sensation to proceed normally. Patients with lesions in the dorsal columns of the spinal cord usually have proprioceptive defects on both sides [35, 36].

Numbness and paresthesias are common symptoms experienced by MS patients. When these symptoms are transient, lasting only seconds to minutes, they are unlikely to be due to an acute relapse in MS. Conversely, when they last many hours to days they may well reflect an acute inflammatory-demyelinating injury. Pain and other unpleasant sensations were reported as troubling symptoms by 54% of MS patients in a large survey. Pain in MS usually has neuropathic features such as burning, electrical or sharp sensations. Sensory symptoms may take the form of numbness, or may be more florid (e.g. a sensation that 'cold water is running down my leg'). Weakness in MS may develop gradually in one or more limbs, increasing with use and often described as a feeling of heaviness and clumsiness. Depending on the site of the lesion, signs of an upper motor neuron lesion may be present while involvement of the cerebellum and its connections produces ataxic symptoms which usually occur in combination with corticospinal damage. Spinal demyelination causes progressive weakness in both legs. In individuals where there is extensive demyelination adjacent to the dorsal root entry zones, lower motor neuron signs may be present. People with MS who suffer from *loss of muscle activation and control* often have difficulty when participating in activities of daily living and leisure activities. This, in turn, results in a gradual decrease in physical activity. It has been shown that physical limitations are positively correlated with physiological changes in people with MS, which have been shown to be similar to those that occur in healthy people who have experienced prolonged physical inactivity [37].

5.4.5 Heat sensitivity

Heat characteristically aggravates MS symptoms and can transiently bring out old symptoms that had previously remitted. This can occur in the context of a hot day, a hot shower, or with vigorous exercise. The physiologic basis for heat sensitivity in MS—Uhthoff's phenomenon—is less efficient conduction of demyelinated nerves at higher temperatures [35].

5.4.6 Motor symptoms

The motor problems in MS are, again, various and complicated. The most common motor manifestation is a paraparesis or quadriparesis primarily resulting from cord lesions. This often begins with a slowing of gait, a tendency for one of the legs to give way, and, when coupled with spasticity, may produce calf discomfort after walking some distance, closely resembling claudication. If the anterior tibial muscles are weak, tripping will be the predominant presentation. When spasticity is present, extensor spasms and spontaneous ankle clonus are often present. With a severe paraparesis, there may be flexor spasms that represent a form of the triple flexion response [35].

Focal weakness in the limbs in MS is usually due to involvement of the corticospinal tract and, thus, it is often accompanied by other signs of the upper motor neuron syndrome, such as hyperreflexia, spasticity, and an extensor plantar response on Babinski or Chaddock testing [35].

5.4.7 Spasticity

Spinal cord lesions, may lead to stiffness, flexor spasms, cramps or spontaneous clonus. Spasticity, a velocity-dependent increase in resistance to passive muscle stretch, is associated with stiffness, spasms, cramping, and gait impairment, and can occur in the absence of weakness. Spasticity is a very common symptom in patients with MS and represents one main cause of disability, even more than strength loss, contractures and sensory evoked muscle spasms being the most debilitating aspects of spasticity in MS [35].

Spasticity tends to occur most frequently in a specific group of muscles that are responsible for maintaining upright posture. These muscles are called *antigravity* or *postural* muscles. They include the muscles of the calf (gastrocnemius), thigh (quadriceps), buttock (gluteus maximus), groin (adductor), and occasionally the back (erector spinae). When spasticity is present, the increased stiffness in the muscles means that a great deal of energy is required to perform daily activities. Reducing spasticity produces greater freedom of movement and strength, and frequently also lessens fatigue and increases coordination. The major ways in which spasticity is reduced include stretching exercises, physical therapy, and the use of medication. If spasticity does not respond to these measures and causes discomfort, a surgical procedure may be necessary. Paroxysmal tonic 'seizures' are involuntary contractions of the limbs, which are sometimes rhythmic. Tonic seizures are often seen in association with spinal cord and brainstem lesions [37].

As with spasticity, the muscle weakness seen in chronic spinal MS probably results from changes in motoneurons and interneuron electrophysiology that are comparable to those observed in incomplete spinal cord injury. These changes result in disruptions of interneuron and motoneuron pathways and in monoaminergic input to spinal motoneurons. Other peripheral changes that may contribute to muscle weakness include muscle wasting, fiber loss, muscle contracture, and joint contractures [35]

Tonic spasms should be distinguished from muscle spasms, which are often associated with spasticity, as the treatments are different. Tonic spasms are probably related to other paroxysmal syndromes that occur in MS, such as paroxysmal dysarthria–ataxia [37].

More than 80% of patients with multiple sclerosis (MS) experience deficits of balance and/or coordination during the course of their disease. Impaired balance is often one of their earliest complaints. Intention tremor is also an ataxic symptom. In MS it may be absent, mild, or indeed devastating. Paroxy small attacks of dysarthria and ataxia, characterized by sudden onset and frequent repetition, have been previously described in MS patients. ***Ataxia of the limbs*** may be caused by a lesion of the cerebellum or its connections, or by de-afferentation from a dorsal column spinal plaque, however, the pathophysiology of this neurological dysfunction remains unclear. Some authors have proposed that a transversely spreading, ephaptic activation of axons within a partially demyelinated lesion may cause the paroxysmal phenomena in MS. A lesion affecting a fiber tract involved in central motor control, such as the brachium conjunctivum, can produce ataxia [27]. Paroxysmal dysarthria and ataxia appeared during the recovery phase of an MS relapse so we can hypothesize that the remyelination process may have induced the ephaptic transmission and the interruption of the cerebello-thalamo-cortical pathway. Carbamazepine may have reduced the ephaptic transmission by blocking the sodium channels, thus repristinating the physiological conduction through the cerebello-thalamo-cortical pathway [35].

Patients with ataxia usually complain of balance deficits and/or intentional tremor and dysmetria, which impair mostly manual activities.

Balance is necessary to perform coordinated movements, whether one is standing, sitting, or lying down. It involves the function of many neurologic centers. The *cerebellum* is the main center for balance, but the eyes, ears, and nerves to the arms and legs also contribute to balance not working properly [21]. Balance problems and falls are common in people with multiple sclerosis (MS). It is known that MS affects many areas of the central nervous system that can impact postural responses to maintain balance, including the cerebellum and the spinal cord. Cerebellar balance disorders are associated with normal latencies but reduced scaling of postural responses. Impaired balance can result in falls and injury, and reduced activity participation. Given the wide distribution of CNS lesions in people with MS, poor balance control in this population may be caused by impairments in cognitive, visual, vestibular, motor, sensory, and/or coordination functions, and the contributions of each of these factors may vary among individuals [23]. A number of medications may aid in decreasing tremor. The most common tremor seen in MS, and the most difficult to treat, occurs as a result of demyelination in the cerebellum. This area of the brain is responsible for balance and has connections throughout the brain stem (the back of the brain) and the spinal cord. Demyelination in this area often results in a gross tremor that is relatively slow and occurs during purposeful movements of the arm or leg [21].

5.4.8 Speech, vocal

Speech, vocal quality, and other communication disorders are found in 40% of people with multiple sclerosis (MS) [35]. Autoimmune disease in which demyelination of the nerve cells in the central nervous system leads to weaknesses in speech musculature. The weakness of the speech musculature in the degenerative neurological diseases affects all the speech subsystems to varying degrees. This consequently decreases the speech intelligibility and verbal communication skills [21]. Any changes in the speech subsystems caused by neurological disorders can be detected by applying acoustic analyses with prevalence around 45%. Dysarthria (abnormal speech production) is the most common expressive communication deficit presenting in patients with MS. MS ***plaques*** (also called *lesions*) in the brain can interfere with muscle control in the lips, tongue, soft palate (the soft muscle tissue extending back from the roof of the mouth), vocal cords, and diaphragm (the dome-like muscle under the lungs that plays an important role in breathing). These muscles control speech production and voice quality as well as the process of swallowing. A person who develops problems with speech or swallowing is usually referred by his or her physician to a ***speechllanguage pathologist***, who specializes in the diagnosis and treatment of speech and swallowing disorders. Existing evidence suggests that dysarthria in people with MS (PwMS) is typically mild in nature, with patients rarely becoming unintelligible. Nevertheless, impaired speech is known to have a negative impact on employment status, social participation and overall quality of life in this population [38].

5.4.9 Bladder and bowel dysfunction

Many people with MS experience difficulties with bladder control and urination at some point during the course of the disease. Bladder symptoms are more common in women than men. Impotence may be prevalent in males. Sphincter control may be lost or impaired. Disinhibition causes urgency and frequency which lead to incontinence [39]. Bowel incontinence may also be present. Bladder symptoms usually can be controlled with medication or other approaches that minimize any changes in daily activities and life-style. Bladder dysfunction affects up to 90% of people with MS at some time during their illness. Bladder dysfunction is the presenting feature in approximately 5% of patients, but the incidence increases as the disease progresses. The level of dysfunction relates to the stage of disease, and more than half of patients who cannot walk have bladder complaints (personal communication). The symptoms of bladder dysfunction are disruptive to social, vocational, and sexual activities, but they are generally treatable and can be successfully managed. Bowel dysfunction is less prevalent than bladder dysfunction in MS, affecting up to 68% of patients [29], but it might be related to bladder dysfunction since people with bladder problems are sometimes reluctant to consume enough fluids, which leads to constipation. Chia *et al* [29] found that 52% of patients with urinary symptoms also had some degree of bowel dysfunction. The neurological basis for bowel dysfunction in MS is not as clearly defined as it is for the bladder, and treatment options are limited. Probably the most common type of bladder problem in MS results from a *small spastic bladder*, sometimes referred to as a 'failure to store' bladder, which results from demyelination of the spinal cord pathways between the voiding reflex center and the brain (figure 5.7). Because the pathways to the brain are blocked, bladder emptying is no longer under voluntary control. Voiding then becomes a reflex activity, with messages to 'empty' coming only from the spinal center. A small spastic bladder may produce symptoms of increased frequency, urgency, dribbling, and/or incontinence [38]. Bladder dysfunction in MS results from interruption of the neural control systems, most often in the sacral nerves [16]. As a result, the loss of bladder control is likely to coincide with lower limb spasticity and the diminished ability to respond to urinary urgency by moving to a toilet [21].

5.4.10 Sexual problems

Sexuality has both psychological and physiological components, and both aspects contribute to the level of a person's sexual functioning. MS can affect the experience of sexuality in a variety of ways. People sometimes report feeling less sexually interested or aroused, either as a direct result of neurologic changes or because of their efforts to cope with the impact of these changes on their lives [40]. Partners often misinterpret the sexual changes they observe in the person with MS, and may also experience their own changes in sexual responsiveness in the face of the illness. Both members of the couple often find it difficult to communicate with one another about their changing sexual and intimacy needs. The few studies on the ***prevalence*** of sexual problems in MS have relied primarily on the survey or questionnaire method.

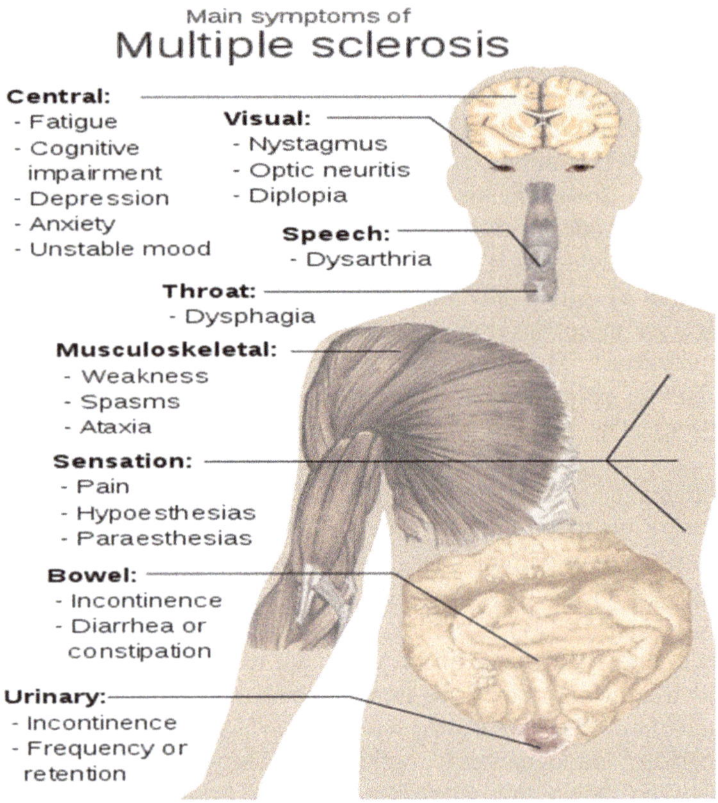

Figure 5.7. Most of the symptoms experienced by patients, such as visual, bladder and bowel dysfunction, sexual dysfunction, easy fatigability, optic nerve disease, and sensory complaint.

In these studies—most of which were conducted in Europe or Australia—up to 85% of men with MS reported at least occasional sexual problems, with erectile difficulties being the most commonly reported symptom. The proportion of women reporting sexual problems ranged from 56% to 74%, with loss of libido (sexual desire) and changes in vaginal sensation and lubrication being the most commonly cited problems. Although these statistics may seem disturbing, it is important to keep in mind that the prevalence of at least occasional sexual dysfunction in the general US population ranges between 34% for men and 41% for women. MS can interfere directly or indirectly with orgasm. *Primary orgasmic dysfunction* stems from MS ***plaques*** (also called lesions) in the spinal cord or brain that directly interfere with orgasm. Orgasm depends on ***nervous system*** pathways originating in the brain (the center of emotion and fantasy during masturbation or intercourse) and pathways in the upper, middle, and lower parts of the spinal cord (which control sensations from erogenous zones such as lips, nipples, clitoris, and so on). Sensation and orgasmic response can be diminished or absent if these pathways are disrupted by plaques. Orgasm can also be inhibited by secondary or indirect symptoms, such as sensory ***paresthesias***, cognitive problems, and other MS-related changes. In addition, anxiety, depression, and loss of sexual self-confidence or sexual self-esteem represent tertiary symptoms that can interfere with one's ability to enjoy the sexual experience and thus inhibit orgasm [21].

5.4.11 Dysarthria

Clinically evident dysarthria often presents in more advanced stages of the disease thus being significantly correlated with overall disease severity as rated in EDSS. Accordingly, overt dysarthria is more frequently described in primary and secondary progressive subtypes of MS. However, it should be noted that MS-related disability is inconsistently reported in the published literature. There are also several less common speech presentations reported within the literature. At least forty-nine patients with paroxysmal episodes of dysarthria have been described. The case reports describe acute onset of frank dysarthria lasting only for a few seconds per episode, and recurring often and daily, frequently associated with other cerebellar/ brain-stem symptoms (e.g. generalized ataxia). They occurred approximately 6–10 weeks after a classic relapsing episode. Six (more recent) cases were investigated at the time of the primary relapse with magnetic resonance imaging (MRI), reporting new enhancing lesions including one or more at or below the red nucleus.

5.5 The incidence and prevalence of psychiatric disorders in multiple sclerosis

Psychiatric comorbidity is associated with lower quality of life, greater levels of fatigue, and reduced adherence to disease-modifying therapy in MS. Patients frequently experience depression, stress and anxiety, anger, fatigue, and cognitive dysfunction, known as the hidden symptoms of MS. Symptoms appear as overlapping comorbidities that are directly associated with markers of inflammation or neurodegeneration. The impact of MS on neuropsychological (NP) function is well recognized [41].

5.5.1 Quality of life

MS has a major and widespread effect on the patient. It tends to affect young adults at a crucial stage in their lives when they are establishing their careers, setting up home and having a family [10, 41]. The variable and unpredictable manifestations of MS tend to result in progressive disability over time without significantly affecting longevity. After an MS diagnosis, individuals change their entire functional dynamics; their behaviour changes, both personally and within the family. They try to adapt to a new reality, leading to changes in quality of life. The disease thus affects people in their most active years: young adults readying themselves to leave home in pursuit of academic, vocational, or social goals; men and women in the process of launching careers and families of their own; and those in middle age who are enjoying their productive years and planning for their retirement. In each of these age groups, the diagnosis of a chronic and unpredictable disease has significant impact, not only on the individual who receives the diagnosis of MS, but also on the family members and loved ones whose lives are interwoven with that person. All parts of the CNS can be affected by MS, and it commonly results in difficulty with mobility and upper limb function, bladder, bowel and sexual dysfunction. speech and swallowing, vision and cognition. In addition, there may be severe fatigue and acute and chronic pain. Many of these disabilities interact. In relation to loss of mobility, it is estimated that at 15 years, 50% of patients require assistance to walk 100 m. MS places major strain on relationships and is associated with a high level of divorce. It is also associated with high levels of unemployment, depression and an increased suicide rate. As in MS, all neurological diseases cause biopsychosocial consequences. The deterioration of the symptoms and the lack of a cure make MS a very stressful condition and adjustment problems are more prevalent [27].

5.5.2 Fatigue

Fatigue is a phenomenon that most people experience in their daily life and has been described as an inability to sustain cognitive or physical effort required to achieve a specific goal.

The nature of fatigue in MS has yet to be fully characterized, but it is interrelated with physical activity and social engagement. Plausible mechanisms related to impaired motor function include slowing or alteration of neurotransmitter release and increased nerve conduction times. Physical fatigue is higher in MS patients with pyramidal tract signs and during relapses [21].

Although controversial, at least two forms of fatigue can be distinguished: peripheral fatigue, characterized as a failure to maintain specific muscular pressure, and central fatigue that is described as an inability to sustain cognitive performance (feeling fatigued after a long day at work) due to mental exhaustion [42]. MS can lead to depression and depression can lead to fatigue. This is especially important to understand because there are treatments for depression that are efficient and effective. Demyelination in the brain typically leads to changes in the neurochemistry in the brain This may manifest as the signs of depression, with sleep disturbances, eating disturbances, and fatigue. The specific serotonin release inhibiting medications, of which there are many, can be of significant value because they not only treat depression, but also can energize in the process. Thus, these medications should accompany counseling for this specific type of fatigue.

Definitions

1. A feeling of physical tiredness of lack of energy that many people experience (general fatigue).
2. A subjective lack of physical or mental energy, or both, that is perceived by the individual or care partner, or both, to interfere with usual and desired activities (MS fatigue). It appears early in the disease and is not related to the amount of disability a person might have and may affect both motor and cognitive dysfunction. Fatigue can severely affect the ability to perform activities of daily life and is a major reason for unemployment. Therefore, fatigue is related to disability and poor quality of life [27].

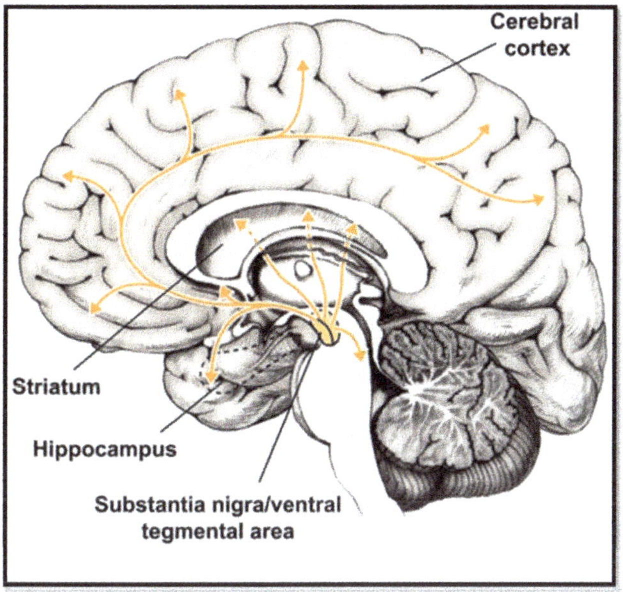

Figure 5.8. Representation of dopaminergic projections throughout the brain.

Fatigue is a common symptom in MS, with up to 90% of individuals with MS reporting fatigue. Moreover, more than half of individuals with MS report fatigue to be their worst symptom. The actual cause of MS fatigue is not clear but is felt to be a combination of immune system irregularities, CNS damage, and heat that affects conduction of messages related to physical activity. Although fatigue has been studied extensively, in part because it affects such a wide range of clinical populations, there has been no unifying framework within which to understand fatigue. Dopamine imbalance can be caused by changes in brain structure, particularly when structures critical for dopaminergic projections are damaged (figure 5.8). Recent structural neuroimaging studies implicate regions of the mesocorticolimbic pathway [43].

Although MS fatigue might be associated with frontal cortex and basal ganglia dysfunction resulting from demyelination of frontal white matter, other neuroimaging studies have failed to find a significant correlation between fatigue and neuropathology in MS patients. Neuroimaging of chronic fatigue syndrome, which has been much more widely studied in this regard than MS, has likewise yielded conflicting results. At this stage, reports of fatigue-associated neuropathology in MS should be interpreted cautiously.

5.5.3 Cognitive

Cognitive disorders (CDs) are common, described in 30%–70% of patients according to published studies. CDs can occur at an early stage of the disease regardless of the form of MS affecting information processing speed. episodic memory and executive function. No drug therapy to date has been shown to be effective in MS [44].

Cognitive dysfunction is characterized by decline in such specific domains as processing speed, attention, memory, executive functions, and learning. Alterations in these are may be detected by means of sophisticated neuropsychological test batteries even in early stages of MS [27]. Cognitive dysfunction seems to be most closely correlated with increased numbers of lesions in the brain in general and with involvement of the corpus callosum. The corpus callosum is a collection of fibers that allow the right and left sections of your brain to communicate, which is important to accomplish complex tasks. Cognitive dysfunction is also found when there is increased atrophy (tissue loss due to lesions) of the brain. The total number of lesions in the brain seems to be more related to problems with recent memory and abstract or conceptual reasoning. Lesions in the corpus callosum are more related to problems with the speed of information processing, sustained attention, problem solving, and mental arithmetic. MS caused cognitive dysfunction affects the following domains: MS features gray and white matter damage in the brain, as well as progressive physical disability. Cognitive dysfunction is moderately related to traditional magnetic resonance (MR) measures like lesion load and whole-brain volume. A process called 'functional reorganization' is hypothesized to change regional brain function to delay functional decline [45, 46].

The functional consequences of MS-related cognitive impairment can be devastating. Cognitive impairment has a direct impact on the ability to maintain employment, driving skills and safety, involvement in social activities, personal and community independence, and the likelihood of benefiting from in-patient rehabilitation. Not surprisingly, it is a major source of strain for caregivers. Cognitive changes can affect anyone with MS, whether they have had the disease for 30 years or 30 days and whether they are confined to a wheelchair or running a marathon. In other words, there is little or no relationship between duration of the disease, or severity of physical symptoms, and cognitive changes. Although people who have had MS for a long time, or have a progressive course, are at slightly greater risk for cognitive changes, even those who are recently diagnosed and/or have a relapsing–remitting disease course, can have such deficits. Cognitive deficits can worsen during an exacerbation and lessen as a remission sets in, although the fluctuations in these symptoms appear to be less dramatic than the changes seen in physical symptoms such as walking and vision. Cognitive changes can and do progress like other MS symptoms, but the progression appears to be very slow in most cases. Cognitive impairment is directly related to cerebral abnormalities produced by MS. All other cognitive functions depend on good powers of concentration. Attention and/or concentration problems may be manifested as the inability to focus for long periods of time or as extreme distractibility during a task. In MS, it is the more complex forms of attention that seem to be affected (e.g. divided attention tasks, which require a person to pay attention to more than one thing at a time). Because fatigue and stress can also affect these functions, the person with MS may be at very high risk for attention and/or concentration problems [33].

5.5.4 Memory

Memory is probably the function that is most frequently cited as being affected by MS. This may be true for a couple of reasons: memory is crucial to almost everything we do; and memory lapses are easy to spot because they involve discrete bits of information and minor disasters (e.g. missed appointments). Memory is a catch-all term that encompasses many processes such as learning information (e.g. studying for an exam) and retrieving information (e.g. taking an exam). In recent years, increasing attention has been focused on 'working memory,' which refers to the short-term storage of information that is required, for example, to hold a phone number in memory for a few seconds. MS can affect almost any part of the memory process. People with MS related memory loss may need to spend more time learning new material if they want to retain and eventually recall it when needed [27].

5.5.5 Emotional disturbances

Emotional disturbances are common in MS; they consist of disturbances of affect, in which emotional expression may be blunted, flat, inappropriate, or labile and disturbances of mood, such as depression, mania, stress and anxiety. The terms 'affect' and 'mood' are often used interchangeably, but the differences between them are important and have etiological, diagnostic, and treatment implications. Mood refers to a sustained and pervasive emotion that influences perception of self, others, and the world. Affect refers to more fluctuating changes in the outward expression of inner feeling states. The disorders of affect, euphoria, pathological laughing and weeping, and other frontal lobe syndromes are direct consequences of the pathological process in MS, are highly characteristic features of the disease, and follow the same course as the other signs and symptoms of MS. There are effective treatments for pathological laughing and weeping and, to some extent, for the apathy associated with frontal lobe and subcortical syndromes. By contrast, the relationship between MS and the disorders of mood—major depressive disorder, dysthymic disorder, bipolar disorder, panic disorder, and generalized anxiety disorder—is multifactorial and complex, and the extent to which mood disorders are direct consequences of the disease process or psychological reactions to it remains unclear. Whatever their cause, however, mood disorders in MS are phenomenologically no different from mood disorders more generally and respond similarly to standard treatment [26].

MS is a complex and unpredictable disease. Because no two people are psychologically identical, or experience MS in exactly the same way, each person's reaction to the disease will be unique. Uncertainty and anxiety set in as soon as the first symptoms appear. MS can begin in a variety of ways, perhaps with a strange tingling sensation or numbness, sudden loss of vision, or unexplained weakness. Uncertainty surrounds these upsetting and unexplained symptoms. Because the disease is unpredictable, people with MS are called upon to adjust to a lifetime of uncertainty about their health. They often do not know how they are going to feel or function tomorrow or next week, let alone several years down the road. Because the disease is unpredictable, people with MS are called upon to adjust to a lifetime of uncertainty about their health. They often do not know how they are going to feel or function tomorrow or next week, let alone several years down the road. In addition, there is uncertainty associated with the disease-modifying therapies that are recommended for relapsing forms of MS. These medications have been shown to reduce the number and severity of attacks and may slow disease progression; They are not, however, designed to reduce symptoms or make people feel better. Because of the way these medications function in the body, it is virtually impossible for any one individual to know the degree to which the disease-modifying medication is 'working' at any given time. This much uncertainty can lead to a constant state of anxiety. The effects of uncertainty and its attendant anxiety can include anger and irritability, indecision, difficulty in planning, feelings of helplessness, and pessimism about the future [33].

Mood disorders are common in patients with MS and depression is the most frequent one. Moreover, in everyday neurological practice MS patients often describe a psychological stressor as a trigger for their disease relapse. Untreated depression may be one of the most disabling aspects of MS. Indeed, the World Health Organization (WHO) estimated that, over the next 20 years, disability due to depression will be exceeded only by ischemic heart disease [11]. With highly effective and well-tolerated treatments now available, we can dramatically reduce the personal suffering, disrupted relationships, occupational impairment, and the number of deaths by suicide that result from depression. General healthcare providers have a particular opportunity to decrease depression related morbidity and mortality since the majority of depressed patients are seen first in medical settings, but unfortunately they too often fail to identify, diagnose, and treat mood disorders appropriately [19]. Approximately 48% of MS patients experience anxiety, stress and depression within the first year of diagnosing the disease. Research suggests that 56%–60% of MS patients suffer from depression and 37%–40% from anxiety. These symptoms are associated with social dysfunction, suicidal thoughts and increasing number of relapses, which seriously degrade the patients' quality of life [47]. Depression is generally associated with an increased risk of suicide; about 15% of all people with major depression commit suicide. Recognition and treatment of depression thus is an important tool in suicide prevention. At the same time, patients and family members often have trouble acknowledging emotional difficulties, discussing them with healthcare providers, and following recommendations for psychiatric consultation and treatment.

As a multi-dimensional and multifactorial phenomenon, stress can be considered a complication of MS as well as a factor contributing to the aggravation or relapse of symptoms. Moreover, stress can be life threatening in MS patients and leads to divorce, job loss and family conflicts. Major depression affects about 30%–45% of MS patients depending on the screening methodology used. The cause is unclear, but in some patients it may relate to injury of frontotemporal networks from MS, whereas in others it may simply be a comorbid condition [27].

5.5.6 Pain

Nearly one-half of individuals with MS experience clinically significant pain at some time during the course of the disease. Significantly more women than men report pain. The longer the duration of the disease and the older the patient, the more likely it is that pain will be reported. The disconnect between the incidence and severity of the pain and the realization by physicians of its importance to the patient is a major problem for the management of MS. Pain is a frequent accompaniment of MS, and for a small group of MS patients, pain is the worst aspect of the disease. Despite treatment, many MS patients have ongoing pain. Pain may be due to inflammatory disease activity, in which case it is usually transient and may respond to glucocorticoids. In other cases, the accumulating burden of CNS damage may lead to irreversible lesions that cause neuropathic pain. The neuropathic pain syndromes are of two types: paroxysmal and constant. Paroxysmal phenomena (trigeminal neuralgia and painful tonic spasms) are recurrent and appear to respond well to anticonvulsant medications. Constant dysesthetic pains vary in intensity and appear to be resistant to currently available treatments. However, the committee did not find any satisfying data on this point. Another set of pain types are musculoskeletal [27, 48, 50].

5.6 Conclusion

Although MS is postulated to have an underlying immune-mediated pathogenesis, there is as yet no biologic marker that is disease specific and can be used for diagnostic purposes. Similarly, there is insufficient evidence to allow detection of any putative disease-related infectious agent as a basis for defining the disease. MS may well be heterogeneous when viewed from the perspective of genetics, pathogenic mechanisms, clinical phenotypes, and immunopathology. To be considered a truly distinctive variant of MS, any putative distinct disease subtypes defined in one of these categories would have to be correlated with the distinctive features identified in each of the other categories. Symptomatic management of patients with MS is a complex and varied problem that must take into consideration the many dimensions of quality of life. Pain and paresthesias can be disabling to patients with MS. Many physicians underestimate the importance of these symptoms and are challenged to devise a rational treatment plan. Improving the lives of people with MS rests on better understanding of both their needs and their successes, specifically research into the conditions of life with MS, which requires objective, reliable research tools. The most essential tools are the various survey instruments that measure abilities to function and quality of life. These tools not only provide for objective assessment of the needs of people with MS, but also are an essential element of measuring the effectiveness of any sort of therapeutic intervention be it a rehabilitation process, a self-help program, or a disease-modifying therapy. Quality-of-life measures can also reveal aspects of the disease process that are not readily captured in standard clinical measures and can often provide more sensitive outcome measures of the clinical efficacy of new therapies. Given the chronicity and uncertain course of MS, tracking its impact over time can assist with care of individual patients, suggesting near-term prognoses and the need for various interventions. Tabulating these findings across individuals offers insight into the burden of MS related disability within populations, information increasingly used to set research, health, and social policy priorities. Longitudinal studies of the trajectory of functioning and quality of life should help to define the natural history of the disease and expand understanding of its clinical epidemiology and patterns of progression. Finally, functional status and quality of life are critical end points in measuring the effectiveness of therapy, both for clinical trials and for routine patient care. Clinical neurology should move toward adopting as a standard of care a concise measurement of health status that includes quality-of-life measures, as well as impairment and disability measures. This could serve as the basis for communication between physicians and other caregivers and for increasing the efficiency and thoroughness of consultations between patients and physicians, particularly if filled out by the patient. Although MS is not commonly thought of as a painful disease, when MS patients are asked, a surprisingly high proportion report significant pain problems.

The management of MS in the current millennium clearly has emphasized stabilization of the disease itself. The past decade has seen the common use of disease modifying therapies and the future is bright for more treatments that can alter the course of MS. However, from a very practical point of view, the management of the symptoms caused by the destructive process of MS remains of major importance.

References

[1] Joy J E and Johnston R B 2001 *Multiple Sclerosis Current Status and Strategies for the Future* (Washington DC: National Academies Press)

[2] Kappos L, Freedman M S and Polman C H *et al* BENEFIT Study Group 2007 Effect of early versus delayed interferon beta-1b treatment on disability after a first clinical event suggestive of multiple sclerosis: a 3-year follow-up analysis of the BENEFIT study *Lancet* **370** 389–97

[3] Zimmermann H, Oberwahrenbrock T, Brandt A U, Paul F and Dörr J-M 2014 Optical coherence tomography for retinal imaging in multiple sclerosis *Degener. Neurol. Neuromuscul. Dis.* **4** 153–62

[4] Tolley K, Hutchinson M and You X *et al* 2015 A network meta-analysis of efficacy and evaluation of safety of subcutaneous pegylated interferon beta-1a versus other injectable therapies for the treatment of relapsing–remitting multiple sclerosis *PLoS One* **10** e0127960

[5] Calabrese M, Bernardi V and Atzori M *et al* 2012 Effect of disease-modifying drugs on cortical lesions and atrophy in relapsing–remitting multiple sclerosis *Mult. Scler.* **18** 418–24

[6] Soufi G, Aitbenhaddou E, Hajji Z, Tazrout S, Benomar A, Soufi M, Boulanouar A, Abouqal R and Yahyaoui M 2015 Evaluation of retinal nerve fiber layer thickness measured by optical coherence tomography in Moroccan patients with multiple sclerosis *J. Fr. Ophtalmol.* **38** 497–503

[7] Cioncoloni D, Innocenti I, Bartalini S, Santarnecchi E, Rossi S and Rossi A 2014 Individual factors enhance poor health-related quality of life outcome in multiple sclerosis patients. Significance of predictive determinants *J. Neurol. Sci.* **345** 213–9

[8] Loma I and Heyman R 2011 Multiple sclerosis: pathogenesis and treatment *Curr. Neuropharmacol.* **9** 409–16

[9] Chan C-L 2018 The neural encoding of reward in the striatal-pallidal circuitry *Dissertation Abstracts International: section B: The Sciences and Engineering* 78

[10] Feinstein A, Freeman J L and Albert C 2015 Treatment of progressive multiple sclerosis: What works, what does not, and what is needed *Lancet Neurol.* **14** 194–207

[11] Miller D M and Allen R 2010 Quality of life in multiple sclerosis: determinants, measurement, and use in clinical practice *Curr. Neurol. Neurosci. Rep.* **10** 397–406

[12] Frischer J M, Bramow S, Dal-Bianco A, Lucchinetti C F, Rauschka H, Schmidbauer M, Laursen H, Sorensen P S and Lassmann H 2009 The relation between inflammation and neurodegeneration in multiple sclerosis brains *Brain* **32** 1175–89

[13] Khayati R, Vafadust M, Towhidkhah F and Nabavi M 2008 Fully automatic segmentation of multiple sclerosis lesions in brain MR FLAIR images using adaptive mixtures method and markov random field model *Comput. Biol. Med.* **38** 379–90

[14] Gioia M C, Cerasa A, Valentino P, Fera F, Nisticò R and Liguori M 2009 Neurofunctional correlates of personality traits in relapsing-remitting multiple sclerosis: An fMRI study *Brain Cogn.* **71** 320–7

[15] De Sa J C, Airas L, Bartholome E, Grigoriadis N, Mattle H and Oreja-Guevara C *et al* 2011 Symptomatic therapy in multiple sclerosis:a review for a multimodal approach in clinical practice *Ther. Adv. Neurol. Disord.* **24** 139–68

[16] Gharibi T, Ahmadi M, Seyfizadeh N, Jadidi-Niaragh F and Yousefi M 2015 Immunomodulatory characteristics of mesenchymal stem cells and their role in the treatment of multiple sclerosis *Cell. Immunol.* **293** 113–21

[17] Feuillet L, Reuter F, Audoin B, Malikova I, Barrau K and Cherif A A *et al* 2007 Early cognitive impairment in patients with clinically isolated syndrome suggestive of multiple sclerosis *Mult. Scler.* **13** 124–7

[18] Harris V K and Sadiq S A 2009 Disease biomarkers in multiple sclerosis *Mol. Diagn. Ther.* **13** 225–44

[19] Chua A S, Egorova S, Anderson M C, Polgar-Turcsanyi M, Chitnis T, Weiner H L, Guttmann C R, Bakshi R and Healy B C 2015 Using multiple imputation to efficiently correct cerebral MRI whole brain lesion and atrophy data in patients with multiple sclerosis *NeuroImage* **119** 81–8

[20] Martinez-Lapiscina E H *et al* 2016 Retinal thickness measured with optical coherence tomography and risk of disability worsening in multiple sclerosis: A cohort study *Lancet Neurol.* **15** 574–84

[21] Phillips J T *et al* 2011 Sustained improvement in Expanded Disability Status Scale as a new efficacy measure of neurological change in multiple sclerosis: Treatment effects with natalizumab in patients with relapsing multiple sclerosis *Mult. Scler. J.* **17** 970–9

[22] Tanović E, Vrabac D, Aldijana K, Rama A and Tanović H 2014 Evaluation of the treatment efficacy of patients with multiple sclerosis using Barthel index and expanded disability status scale *J. Health Sci.* **4** 110–3

[23] Schapiro R T 2003 *Managing the Symptoms of Multiple Sclerosis* 4th edn (New York: Demos Medical)

[24] Kuhlmann T, Lassmann H and Bruck W 2008 Diagnosis of inflammatory demyelination in biopsy specimens: A practical approach *Acta Neuropathol.* **115** 275–87

[25] Tabansky I *et al* 2015 Advancing drug delivery systems for the treatment of multiple sclerosis *Immunol. Res.* **63** 58–69
[26] Lin W, Zhang Y, Zhou F, Gao L, He L, Zeng X and Gong H 2016 Altered intra- and interregional synchronization in relapsing–remitting multiple sclerosis: A resting-state fMRI study *Neuropsychiatr. Dis. Treat.* **12** 853–62
[27] Selkirk S M and Shi J 2005 Relapsing-remitting tumefactive multiple sclerosis *Mult. Scler.* **11** 731–4
[28] Gelfand J M 2014 Multiple sclerosis: diagnosis, differential diagnosis, and clinical presentation *Mult. Scler. Relat. Disord.* **124** 269–90
[29] Kalb R 2008 *Multiple Sclerosis: The Questions You Have—The Answers You Need* (New York: Demos Medical)
[30] Olek M J and Weiner H L 2005 *Multiple Sclerosis Etiology, Diagnosis, and New Treatment Strategies* (New York: Humana)
[31] Johnston B, Richard J and Janet E 2001 *Multiple Sclerosis: Current Status and Strategies for the Future Institute of Medicine* (Washington DC: The National Academies Press)
[32] Dobryakova E, DeLuca J, Genova H M and Wylie G R 2013 Neural correlates of cognitive fatigue: cortico-striatal circuitry and effort–reward imbalance *J. Int. Neuropsychol. Soc.* **19** 849–53
[33] Jelinek G 2009 *Overcoming Multiple Sclerosis: An Evidence-Based Guide to Recovery* (Sydney: Allen & Unwin) p 394
[34] Kappos L, Freedman M S and Polman C H *et al* BENEFIT Study Group 2007 Effect of early versus delayed interferon beta-1b treatment on disability after a first clinical event suggestive of multiple sclerosis: a 3-year follow-up analysis of the BENEFIT study *Lancet* **370** 389–97
[35] Kalb C and Kalb R 2006 *Multiple Sclerosis: A Guide for Families* 3rd edn (New York: Demos Medical) p 305
[36] Strober L, Englert J, Munschauer F, Weinstock-Guttman B, Rao S and Benedict R H 2009 Sensitivity of conventional memory tests in multiple sclerosis: comparing the Rao brief repeatable neuropsychological battery and the minimal assessment of cognitive function in MS *Mult. Scler.* **15** 1077–84
[37] Huppke P and Gärtner J 2010 A practical guide to pediatric multiple sclerosis *Neuropediatrics* **41** 157–62
[38] Opdenakker G 2005 Immunohistopathology to guide multiple sclerosis treatment *Lancet* **366** 526–7
[39] Hoang P 2010 *Multiple Sclerosis* https://researchgate.net/publication/230554483
[40] Schairer L C, Foley F W, Zemon V, Tyry T, Campagnolo D, Marrie R A, Gromisch E S and Schairer D 2014 The impact of sexual dysfunction on health-related quality of life in people with multiple sclerosis *Mult. Scler. J.* **20** 610–6
[41] Albuquerque C, Geraldo A M and Rosa Ribeiro O 2015 Quality of life of people with multiple sclerosis: clinical and psychosocial determinants *Procedia—Soc. Behav. Sci.* **171** 359–65
[42] Filippi M, Rocca M A and Benedict R H *et al* 2010 The contribution of MRI in assessing cognitive impairment in multiple sclerosis *Neurology* **75** 2121–8
[43] Benedict R H, Wahlig E, Bakshi R, Fishman I, Munschauer F, Zivadinov R and Weinstock-Guttman B 2005 Predicting quality of life in multiple sclerosis: Accounting for physical

disability, fatigue, cognition, mood disorder, personality, and behavior change *J. Neurol. Sci.* **231** 29–34
[44] Krupp B L 2004 *Fatigue in Multiple Sclerosis: A Guide to Diagnosis and Management* (New York: Demos)
[45] Tabrizi F M and Radfar M 2015 Fatigue, sleep quality, and disability in relation to quality of life in multiple sclerosis *Int. J. MS Care* **17** 268–74
[46] Martin S T and Mario Suttner N 2015 *Multiple Sclerosis: Recovery of Function and Neurorehabilitation* (Cambridge: Cambridge University Press) pp 1507–11
[47] Langdon D W, Amato M P, Boringa J, Brochet B, Foley F and Fredrikson S *et al* 2012 Recommendations for a Brief International Cognitive Assessment for Multiple Sclerosis (BICAMS) *Mult. Scler.* **18** 891–8
[48] Amato M P, Portaccio E, Goretti B, Zipolli V, Hakiki B and Giannini M *et al* 2010 Cognitive impairment in early stages of multiple sclerosis *Neurol. Sci.* **31** S211
[49] Janalipour K, Kafi M, Hatamian H and Rezapour P 2017 The effectiveness of yoga therapy in reducing anxiety, stress and depression in women with multiple sclerosis *Caspian J. Neurol. Sci.* **3** 151–8
[50] Latov N 2006 *Peripheral Neuropathy: When the Numbness, Weakness, and Pain Won't Stop* (New York: Demos) p 151

IOP Publishing

Neurological Disorders and Imaging Physics, Volume 2
Engineering and clinical perspectives of multiple sclerosis
Ayman El-Baz and Jasjit S Suri

Chapter 6

Using transcranial direct current stimulation to manage symptoms of multiple sclerosis

Michael Shaw, Giuseppina Pilloni and Leigh Charvet

This chapter reviews the use of noninvasive brain stimulation with transcranial direct current stimulation (tDCS) to help manage the symptoms of multiple sclerosis (MS). Technical considerations are discussed for use of tDCS in treatment and imaging research. Emphasis is placed on the use of the remotely supervised tDCS (RS-tDCS) protocol and how it can enable at-home delivery of tDCS to patients with MS and broad participation across the MS population.

6.1 Introduction

6.1.1 Symptom management in MS

MS is associated with episodes of acute neuronal damage and varying presentation of neurological symptoms. As the autoimmune disease processes destroy nervous tissue in the central nervous system (CNS) and lesions form, normal neurological processes are disrupted. In the short term, these lesions typically result in weakness, numbness, or degradation of tissue specific functions. Over a lifetime of MS, deficits or problems may accumulate that individuals do not recover from, leading to significant symptom burden. Among the most common symptoms associated with MS are feelings of fatigue, motor disability, pain, visual disturbances, cognitive impairment, and a loss of tactile sensation or paresthesia (table 6.1) [1, 2].

As an autoimmune disease, MS is primarily managed with disease modifying therapies (DMTs) that target and restrain the immunological capabilities of the body to prevent accumulation of neuronal damage. However, while DMTs may prevent the frequency of autoimmune relapses, they do not resolve and can even worsen symptoms across the disease course [3]. Most common symptoms associated with MS lack effective and reliable treatment options. Effective near-term treatment options are needed to manage this high symptom burden for individuals with MS.

doi:10.1088/978-0-7503-1762-7ch6

Table 6.1. Common symptoms of MS. Individuals with MS can present with highly variable symptoms that can interfere with daily living.

Fatigue	Spasticity and tremors
Motor weakness or difficulties	Mood changes (i.e. pseudobulbar affect)
Pain (including neuropathic and mixed)	Vertigo
Cognitive changes or impairment	Numbness (hypoesthetic)
Vision changes or problems	Swallowing (dysphagia)

Noninvasive brain stimulation is an emerging approach with potential therapeutic uses across a range of neurological disorders. This chapter will review the use of transcranial direct current stimulation (tDCS), one of the more common brain stimulation methods, for use in the management of MS-related symptoms.

6.1.2 Neuromodulation in MS

There is a growing focus on harnessing the plasticity mechanisms in the brain to mediate the damage of the MS disease process. A recent study demonstrated the possibility for functional plastic recovery from relapses, despite lack of resolution of myelin and axonal injuries associated with the disease course [4]. Some MS patients can respond to demyelinating processes with the same rapid adaptive plasticity responsible for clinical recovery in healthy individuals [5]. Functional magnetic resonance imaging (fMRI) studies suggest that adaptive cortical reorganization occurs in MS patients through activation of parallel existing pathways, local synaptic reorganization, or expansion of functional cortex reorganization at distant sites [6]. This functional reorganization mechanism may help to prevent functional loss of cognitive and motor functions and maintain the ability to learn adaptive strategies [7], despite the extent and type of neuroplastic changes that vary across phases and stages of the disease course [8].

Neuromodulation techniques are an emerging group of treatment options that encompass a broad range of electrical and pharmaceutical techniques that affect nerve functioning at the cellular level. Noninvasive approaches to brain stimulation use external devices to alter the activity of neural networks to achieve specific behavioral effects. For example, transcranial stimulation techniques use externally placed electrodes or magnets or other treatment delivery devices to stimulate and alter electrical activity within the brain through the stimulation of cortical and/or cranial neurons.

Transcranial magnetic stimulation (TMS) and transcranial electrical stimulation (TES) remain the two most popular techniques studied to treat hundreds of different conditions ranging from cognitive and physical impairments, to managing addictive tendencies and obesity, as well as other problems including depression, anxiety, and pain [9–12]. Both TMS and TES apply or induct an electrical field in the brain to modulate the dynamics of cortical networks.

TMS operates on Faraday's principle of electromagnetic induction by which the transmission of a large, brief pulse of current through loops of copper wire generates a fluctuating magnetic field perpendicular to the plane of the coil that subsequently induces an electric field predominantly parallel to the inner surface of the volume conductor adjacent to the coil [12–14]. In this way, the electric field generates secondary currents that flow through the targeted region of the brain. Upon delivery of sufficiently intense TMS to the targeted area, the cortical neurons depolarize, and action potentials are generated. Thus, TMS pulses can induce massive depolarization of a group of neurons and trigger action potentials or motor evoked potentials.

In contrast to TMS, TES refers to techniques that apply weak electrical currents by means of multiple electrodes placed on the body, of which at least one is placed over a targeted brain area. TES effects on brain function are slight and induce a mild polarizing effect on the resting membrane potential of neurons thereby modulating their spontaneous firing rates, but TES paradigms are generally unable to elicit neuron action potentials.

6.1.3 Introduction to tDCS

The most common form of TES, and the focus of this chapter, is tDCS. tDCS typically uses a small battery-operated device to pass a low intensity direct electrical current through electrodes, of which, at least one is placed on the scalp. This electrical stimulation technique affords many different treatment permutations as the cortical targets and intensity of the stimulation can be adjusted to manage the specific symptom or problem. There is rapidly expanding interest in the field of noninvasive brain stimulation, and tDCS in particular (figure 6.1).

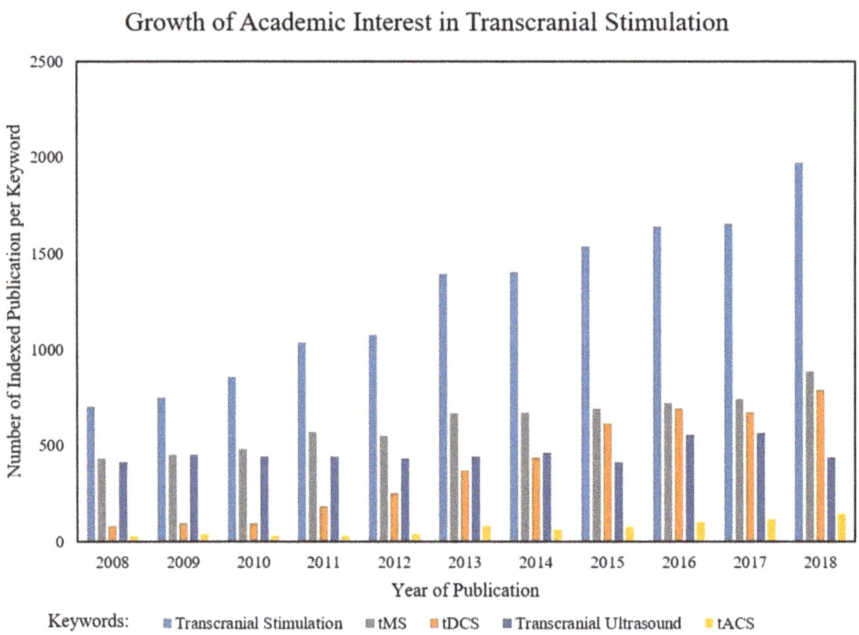

Figure 6.1. Growth of academic interest in transcranial stimulation. As neuromodulation, noninvasive brain stimulation, and transcranial stimulation techniques all gain more popularity and interest throughout the scientific community, the number of studies and publications grow steadily each year. tDCS publications, in particular, have more than tripled over the last ten years.

tDCS has many advantages compared to other approaches, including the relative inexpensiveness of the stimulation device and strong safety profile (figure 6.3). tDCS can be delivered with minimal hardware such as handheld stimulator devices that can be sent home with research participants, while transcranial magnetic stimulation (TMS) requires a large magnet and device to harness the magnetic stimulation.

6.1.3.1 The effect of tDCS on cortical excitability

tDCS modulates cortical excitability in a polarity-specific manner, facilitating or inhibiting neuronal processes. Generally, anodal stimulation is able to facilitate the depolarization of neurons, while cathodal stimulation hyperpolarizes the resting membrane potential, reducing the spontaneous neuronal firing [15].

It is important to recognize that tDCS does not target individual neurons, but, instead, broadly bathes target and adjacent cortical regions with electrical current. Electrical current flow and application is affected by the positioning of electrodes upon the scalp and electrodes can be positioned to target specific brain regions of interest (figure 6.2).

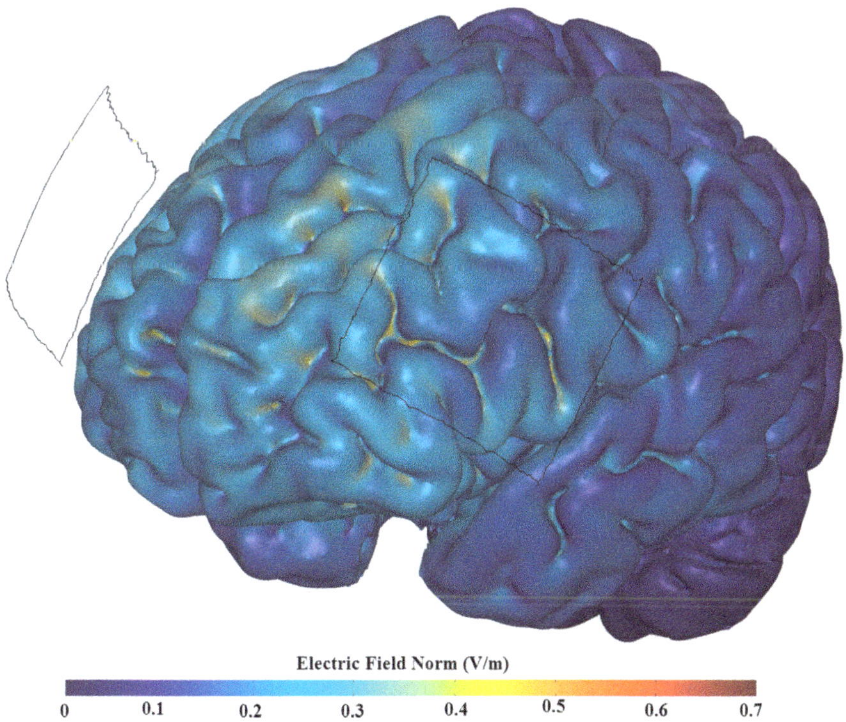

Figure 6.2. Modeling of the electric field intensity of left dorsolateral prefrontal cortex (DLPFC) electrode placement. Theoretical model of electric field distribution generated using the DLPFC montage with anodal electrode over the left prefrontal lobe (F3) and cathodal electrode on supraorbital region (FP3).

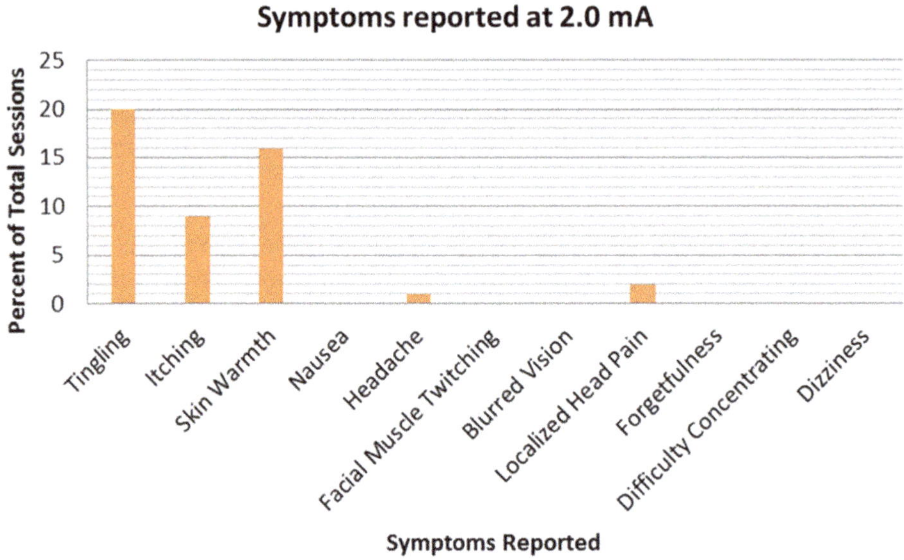

Figure 6.3. Adverse events experienced with RS-tDCS (current intensity set to 2 mA). Across all RS-tDCS studies with MS patients to date, incident rates of adverse events have been on a par with the overall tDCS field. It is important to note that no individual experienced a burn or skin lesion from the tDCS and instead remarked that they felt a mild sensation of skin burning or warmth from the scalp electrodes.

6.1.3.2 tDCS Delivery

tDCS can be delivered from small handheld equipment, which has allowed development of innovative protocols and studies to investigate clinical problems. For example, protocols have been developed for MS patients that use active tDCS paired simultaneously with motor exercises to improve motor functioning [16]. Such a protocol is more difficult to achieve with TMS, which requires use of a large magnetic stimulation device that the participant is effectively tethered to for the duration of a stimulation session. Consider the RS-tDCS protocol, which allows MS participants to complete stimulation at home while simultaneously completing cognitive remediation exercises. Specifically, RS-tDCS uses equipment designed by Soterix Medical (www.soterixmedical.com) including the mini-CT devices, SPAPpads, and specially designed headstraps for fixed electrode positioning. Since the RS-tDCS protocol enables effective electrode placement via use of a headband that holds the anode and cathode in place for each session and remote supervision, MS participants are able to participate from home, which has facilitated study recruitment and retention [17–19].

6.1.3.3 tDCS safety

An additional advantage of tDCS is its strong safety profile (figure 6.3). In Bikson *et al*'s 2016 review of safety [9] in tDCS, no serious adverse events have been reported in clinical trials to date tDCS sessions with MS participants treatment of varying stimulation intensities has been very well tolerated [9, 17].

6.2 Techincal considerations for tDCS

6.2.1 Technical standards for tDCS

6.2.1.1 Dosing

Many facets of tDCS constitute the overall treatment dose such as duration, stimulation intensity, stimulation targets, and number of treatments. These parameters of dose have been manipulated across tDCS studies to achieve different clinical effect with specific optimal guidelines yet to be defined.

- Current intensity has ranged across studies and is typically between 1 and 2.5 mA [20]. Although the safety intensity threshold is set at 2 mA [21], there are several studies that have been testing greater stimulation intensities (up to 4 mA) [22]. Specific to studies within the MS literature, stimulation intensities have varied between 1.0–2.0 mA.
- The duration of stimulation is directly proportional to the electrical energy that is transmitted and conducted through the brain over the course of a session. Duration of stimulation also influences the length of time of after effects and time needed for cortical excitability to return to baseline levels (i.e. tDCS applied between the range of 5 and 13 min leads to proportionate increases in the duration of after effects [23]). Several studies have investigated whether there are diminishing returns with regard to the upper limits of stimulation duration, and some have shown that the relationship between tDCS duration and effect is not necessarily linear. For example, the application of 26 min of anodal tDCS finally resulted in inhibitory effects [24] and cathodal tDCS continuously applied for 20 min resulted in excitatory changes (but conventional practice holds that cathodal tDCS leads to inhibitory effects) [25]. Conventional stimulation duration across the MS literature is 20 min.
- tDCS should be completed across multiple daily sessions for cumulative benefit. Promoting long-term potentiation and plastic changes are believed to be the mediating effect for improved rehabilitative outcomes in tDCS treatment trials. However, multiple sessions are needed to produce robust and lasting effects in the neural networks and thus multiple consecutive treatment sessions are needed [26]. This need for multiple, consecutive treatments may constitute the largest barrier to achieving clinical benefit with tDCS and many studies in both the MS tDCS literature and tDCS literature are limited by small numbers of treatment sessions administered.
- Electrode size and placement has varied greatly across the MS literature as the targeted problems and symptoms have respectively varied. For example, some motor functioning studies have used stimulation targeted at the motor cortex of the brain that corresponds to the limb or side with more significant motor problems.

Table 6.2 below reviews tDCS studies published in MS to date along with the specific dose, electrode montage, and cortical target.

6.2.1.2 Electrode placement

Conventional tDCS uses two sponge electrodes, an anode and a cathode, placed over regions of the scalp to deliver low-level direct current directly to the brain. Small deviations during electrode placement procedures can lead to distinct changes in the distribution of current across cortical regions [27]. To ensure that both electrodes are reliably placed on an individual's scalp one can consult the international 10/20 EEG coordinate system [28] to find an approximation of certain brain regions to target or one can institute localization methods that use EEG or TMS to guide the placement of the tDCS electrodes [28]. Additionally, placement aids such as predesigned headbands that hold electrodes in place that incorporate tactile and visual aids can improve the reliability of electrode placement between tDCS sessions [29].

The location of the electrodes generally depends on the pathology treated and/or on the behavioral task studied, as neurons are expected to be recruited and utilized within the target area and stimulation is then broadly aimed at them. Due to the critical role of electrode montage, there are different alternatives for electrode placement depending on the clinical target or behavioral response desired. For example, to improve cognitive functioning, the anodal electrode is most commonly placed on the scalp in correspondence of the left dorsolateral prefrontal cortex (DLPFC), which typically corresponds to F3/F4 on the 10–20 EEG system, and the cathode over the right supraorbital area or Fp2 on the 10–20 EEG system (figure 6.4). This electrode montage promotes broad stimulation of the frontal brain regions that are implicated in cognitive processes. When tDCS is used to improve motor function, the most common configuration of the electrodes places the anode on the primary motor cortex (M1 and C3/C4) and the cathode on the supraorbital area (Fp2/Fp3) [30] (figure 6.4). Electrode size is yet another dimension of tDCS to be considered as it affects the distribution and density of the current that flows between the electrodes. For this reason, electrode size (i.e. a sponge with the dimensions 5 cm × 5 cm or 5 cm × 7 cm) should be considered when targeting specific cortical regions.

Some investigators use sophisticated electrode montages to guide the injected electrical current flow in a given cerebral region. High definition tDCS or HD-tDCS uses multiple anodes and cathodes to direct current flow more focally than conventional tDCS. Electrode placement is arguably more sensitive when employing this tDCS method. To date, there have been no publications using HD-tDCS for individuals with MS. However, personalized electrodes have been used in MS that specifically target cortical regions based on high-resolution magnetic resonance imaging [31, 32].

In summary, further study is needed to identify the most effective stimulation paradigms for tDCS, especially for treatment of MS symptoms.

Table 6.2. tDCS Studies Used in MS. The asterisks denote a study completed by the authors and using the RS-tDCS methodology. All studies were found using pubmed and the search terms: 'tdcs', 'multiple sclerosis', 'transcranial direct current stimulation'.

Reference and year	Targeted symptom or outcome	Cortical target	Electrode characteristics	Duration and intensity (min mA^{-1})	n	Number of sessions	Notes
			Treatment of motor symptoms				
Rumpf *et al* 2018 [36]	Motor consolidation	Anode: Left Primary Motor Cortex Cathode: Right supraorbital (SO) region	Sponge electrodes: Anode: 25 cm^2 Cathode: 25 cm^2	15/1.0	$n = 14$	2 (1 active session)	Double-blind, sham-controlled, crossover study design
Cosentino *et al* 2018 [37]	Swallowing problems/ Dysphagia	Anode: Right swallowing motor cortex	Sponge electrodes: Anode: 25 cm^2 Cathode: 25 cm^2	20/2.0	$n = 6$	5	TMS guided electrode placement. Open-label pilot study design
Iodice *et al* 2015 [38]	Lower limb spasticity	Anode: Primary motor cortex contralateral to spastic limb Cathode: SO ipsilateral to spastic limb	Sponge electrodes: Anode: 35 cm^2 Cathode: 35 cm^2	20/2.0	$n = 20$	10	TMS guided electrode placement. Randomized, double-blind, sham-controlled study design
Meesen *et al* 2014 [16]	Hand motor performance	Anode First Dorsal Interosseous (FDI) contralateral to intervention hand, cathode on contralateral SO	Sponge electrodes: Anode: 25 cm^2 Cathode: 50 cm^2	20/1.0	$n = 31$	2 (1 active session)	TMS guided electrode placement. Randomized, double-blind, sham-controlled, crossover study design

Cuypers *et al* 2013 [39]	Corticospinal Output	Anode: M1 contralateral to impaired hand Cathode: SO Ipsilateral impaired hand	Sponge electrodes: Anode: 25 cm^2 Cathode: 50 cm^2	20/1.0	$n = 10$	2 (1 active session)	TMS guided electrode placement. Randomized, double-blind, sham-controlled, crossover study design
Treatment of cognitive symptoms							
Fiene *et al* 2018 [40]	Cognitive fatigue	Anode: Left DLPFC Cathode: Right shoulder	Sponge electrodes: Anode: 25 cm^2 Cathode:35 cm^2	30/1.5	$n = 15$	2 (1 active session)	Randomized, double-blind, sham-controlled, crossover study design
*Charvet *et al* 2018 [18]	Cognitive functioning	Anode: Left DLPFC Cathode: Contralateral SO	Sponge electrodes: Anode: 35 cm^2 Cathode: 35 cm^2	20/1.5	$n = 26$	10	Remotely delivered. Open-label pilot study design
Mattioli *et al* 2015 [41]	Cognitive Functioning	Anode: Left DLPFC Cathode: Right shoulder	Sponge electrodes: Anode: 25 cm^2 Cathode: 60 cm^2	20/2.0	$n = 20$	10	Randomized, double-blind, sham controlled study design
Fatigue							
*Charvet *et al* 2017 [19]	MS fatigue	Anode Left DLPFC Cathode: Contralateral SO	Sponge electrodes: Anode: 25 cm^2 Cathode: 25 cm^2	20/1.5 and 2.0 for studies 1 and 2	$n = 15$ and $n = 27$	10 and 20	Two different studies, the second of which was randomized, double-blinded, and sham controlled. Both studies were remotely delivered.

(*Continued*)

Table 6.2. *(Continued)*

Reference and year	Targeted symptom or outcome	Cortical target	Electrode characteristics	Duration and intensity (min mA^{-1})	n	Number of sessions	Notes
Cancelli *et al* 2017 [32]	MS fatigue	Anode: Somatosensory cortex Cathode: occipital	Personalized electrode: Anode: 35 cm^2 Cathode: 70 cm^2	15/1.5	$n = 10$	10 (5 active sessions)	Randomized, double-blind, sham-controlled, crossover study design. MRI guided electrode placement
Chalah *et al* 2016 [42]	MS fatigue	Electrode targets: Left DLPFC and contralateral SO or Right Posterior Parietal Cortex (P4) and Cz	Sponge electrodes: Anode: 25 cm^2 Cathode: 25 cm^2	20/2.0	$n = 10$	15 (5 active sessions target DLPFC and 5 active sessions target PPC)	Randomized, double-blind, sham-controlled, crossover study design with three different treatment blocks
Hanken *et al* 2016 [43]	MS fatigue	Anode: Right parietal cortex Cathode: Contralateral SO	Sponge electrodes: Anode: 35 cm^2 Cathode: 35 cm^2	20/1.5	$n = 46$	1	Randomized, double-blind, sham-controlled study design
Tecchio *et al* 2015 [31]	MS fatigue	Anode: Central sulcus trace/ somatosensory cortex Cathode: Occipital	Personalized electrode: Anode: 35 cm^2 Cathode: 84 cm^2	15/1.5	$n = 21$	10 (5 active sessions)	Randomized, double-blind, sham controlled, crossover study design. MRI guided electrode placement

Tecchio *et al* 2014 [44]	MS fatigue	Anode: Central Sulcus Trace/somatosensory cortex. Cathode: Occipital	Personalized electrode: Anode: 35 cm^2 Cathode: 70 cm^2	20/1.5	n = 10	10 (5 active sessions)	Randomized, double-blind, sham controlled, crossover study design. MRI guided electrode placement
Saiote *et al* 2014 [45]	MS fatigue	Anode: Left DLPFC Cathode: Contralateral SO	Sponge electrodes: Anode: 35 cm^2 Cathode: 90 cm^2	20/1.0	$n = 13$	10 (5 active sessions)	Randomized, double-blind, sham-controlled, crossover study design
Ferrucci *et al* 2014 [46]	MS fatigue	Anodal targets: Both motor cortices with two anodes Anode: M1 bilaterally (two electrodes: C3-C4) Cathode: Right deltoid muscle	Sponge electrodes: Anode: 25 cm^2 Cathode: 25 cm^2	15/1.5	$n = 25$	10 (5 active sessions)	Randomized, sham-controlled, double-blind, crossover study design
Treatment of sensorimotor deficits							
Ayache *et al* 2016 [47]	Neuropathic pain	Anode: Left DLPFC Cathode: Contralateral SO	Sponge electrodes: Anode: 25 cm^2 Cathode: 25 cm^2	20/2.0	$n = 16$	6 (3 active sessions)	Randomized, double-blind, sham-controlled, crossover study design
Mori *et al* 2013 [48]	Tactile sensory deficits	Anode: 2 cm posterior to C3/4 of affected hypoesthetic limb Cathode: Contralateral SO	Sponge electrodes: Anode: 25 cm^2 Cathode: 25 cm^2	20/2.0	$n = 20$	5	Randomized, double-blind, sham-controlled study design

(*Continued*)

Table 6.2. (*Continued*)

Reference and year	Targeted symptom or outcome	Cortical target	Electrode characteristics	Duration and intensity (min mA^{-1})	n	Number of sessions	Notes
Mori *et al* 2010 [49]	Neuropathic pain	Anode: C3 or C4 position contralateral to painful somatic area Cathode: Contralateral SO	Sponge electrodes: Anode: 35 cm^2 Cathode: 35 cm^2	20/2.0	$n = 19$	5	Randomized, double-blind, sham-controlled study design

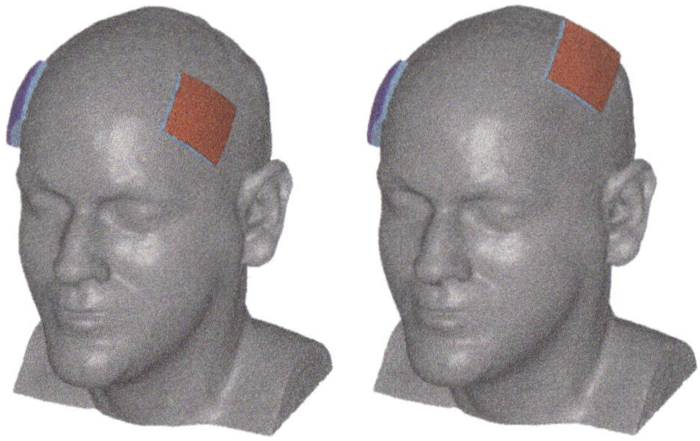

Figure 6.4. Commonly used electrode montages. The left model represents the motor montage, where the anode is placed over primary motor cortex (C3) and the cathode over the right supra-orbital area (FP3). The right model represents the left dorsolateral prefrontal cortex (DLPFC) montage that is used to target the left pre-frontal lobe. Specifically, the anode (red) is positioned over F3 and the cathode (blue) over FP3 based on 10–20 EEG system.

6.2.2 Using at-home protocols to reach MS patients

Additionally, for strong and lasting clinical tDCS efficacy, consecutive tDCS treatments are needed [26]. The need to visit the clinic for treatment has limited sample sizes and treatment session number in MS research in the past [33]. This treatment need for multiple in-person clinical visits can present obstacles for MS patients, especially those living with higher burden of disability. Remotely supervised treatment delivery options and protocols have been developed to enable this population to participate.

RS-tDCS was developed for clinical populations that cannot attend the clinic multiple times each week in order to enable participation of the individuals and populations that most stand to benefit from tDCS. RS-tDCS uses real time monitoring and a stop-go series of quality checks as enabled through videoconferencing and remote desktop software to deliver reliable and reproducible treatments to patients.

The RS-tDCS methodology has been piloted in and verified for use with MS populations over multiple successful studies. RS-tDCS has a deliberate series of steps to ensure that clinical standards are maintained even while patients complete their treatment from their own home [29, 34]. RS-tDCS requires an internet connection and tDCS device and associated equipment (i.e. sponge electrodes, saline solution, etc) to allow for treatment delivery.

Prior to beginning all tDCS treatments, an initial clinical visit is required to distribute study equipment, establish a baseline of performance or symptom severity, and finally to train the participant on the use of the tDCS equipment. The first tDCS session is completed in clinic with the help of a staff tDCS technician to confirm the tolerability of the treatment and aptitude of the participant to prepare the treatment. Following the first successful clinical visit, the participant takes all equipment home and proceeds to complete the remainder of their study participation and tDCS treatments in a quiet and distraction-free setting at home. tDCS technicians call patients on their computer and begin videoconferencing to guide patients with self-placement of a specifically designed headstrap that holds tDCS electrodes in place on the head. Once technicians have determined correct headset placement, the impedance of the device is measured to assure that a safe current can be conducted through the scalp and if impedance is measured to be too great to continue then the technician troubleshoots the problem with the patient. Once sufficient contact quality between the electrodes is established, the patient needs a device unlock code to release stimulation for treatment, which is given by the technician once all clinical standards are met. Treatment begins once the device unlock code is entered and technicians monitor patients for the duration of the session to immediately address or troubleshoot any problems that should arise during a given tDCS treatment.

Multiple studies are currently underway or have been completed that use this RS-tDCS protocol. It has powered robust study designs that overcome the limitations, sample size and limited number of treatments, typically observed in the tDCS field [18, 19]. Additionally, RS-tDCS has been found to be highly feasible with for those with MS. RS-tDCS has been successfully piloted and found to be feasible in a large range of MS patients from ages 18–71 and EDSS range 0.0–8.5. Compliance rates have been found to be high [17] and patients were able to successfully follow all study direction while completing treatment remotely.

tDCS treatment has a good tolerability profile and adverse event rates (most commonly including tingling, itching, and warmth sensations) for those with MS have been consistent with those published in the tDCS literature and have been, on average, mild in severity. tDCS in the stimulation range of 1.5–2.5 mA is well tolerated by individuals with MS.

6.3 Potential clinical applications in MS

Use of tDCS to treat and manage specific symptoms of MS has been relatively limited compared to other neurological conditions. Clinical use remains limited to date, as tDCS lacks a formal FDA indication in the US and generally remains an experimental treatment tDCS research has been diverse in scope and grown in quantity significantly over the last decade. Research efforts are underway to establish its use for the treatment of MS problems and specific symptoms [18, 19, 29, 35].

6.3.1 Fatigue

The majority of individuals with MS experience fatigue, either sporadically or persistently during their disease course, which has serious effects on daily functioning and quality of life [50]. Estimates of the incidence of fatigue in the MS population is typically high, at 75% or more [50, 51]. Furthermore, the majority of those who experience fatigue tend to rate fatigue as one of their worst symptoms with 14% rating as the single worst symptom [52].

MS fatigue is defined by the subjective sense of overwhelming tiredness and exhaustion that does not resolve with sleep. Fatigue can affect MS patients significantly and lead to exit from the work force, increased healthcare utilization, and depression [53]. Multiple pathological factors contribute to fatigue, including CNS demyelination and axonal loss [54], immunological changes, other MS-related problems (trigeminal neuralgia, spasms), psychological and chronic illness factors (depression, pain, poor sleep), and medications [55, 56].

Despite the scope of this problem and its impact on individuals with MS there remains no accepted or standardized treatment for fatigue [57]. There is little evidence of consistent benefit for fatigue with disease modifying therapies [58, 59], while some therapies have been associated with depreciations in quality of life and worsening of fatigue symptoms [3].

Over the last two decades, MS fatigue has been a common target for clinical tDCS research. tDCS has shown promise for the treatment of MS fatigue [19], potentially through a non-specific activating effect in the brain that leads to broad excitation of neurons at the electrode target sites and neighboring cortical regions. This diffuse excitation of cortical regions is believed to lead to direct improvement of fatigue symptomology [44]. Importantly, recent studies have demonstrated that tDCS leads to clinically significant improvements in fatigue following an extended treatment paradigm delivered remotely in patients' homes by investigators [19].

6.3.2 Cognition

Cognitive impairment presents in many individuals with MS (estimates between 40%–70% of the population [64]) and can seriously affect their employment opportunities, familial obligations, and overall quality of life [65, 66]. Cognitive deficits may present at the earlier stages of the disease course and may accumulate over a short time to hinder the familial and professional duties of young and working-age individuals [67, 68]. In order to prevent cognitive decline, investigators have worked hard to identify possible cognitively protective and restorative treatments and therapies.

Functionally significant deficits can present across many cognitive domains in those with MS. Among the most commonly affected cognitive domains are memory, information processing speed, attention, executive function, and visual perceptual function [69].

To manage these cognitive problems, many treatment approaches, both pharmacological and behavioral, have been studied.

Brain stimulation techniques like tDCS stand to benefit cognitive symptoms via simultaneous administration of stimulation and cognitive remediation techniques. Additionally, tDCS applied alone has cognitively enhancing effects including increased vigilance and attentiveness [71] and perceptual sensitivity [72] for healthy adults. Thus, the improved cognitive functioning observed with cognitive training in MS patients [70] may be increased when paired with tDCS, and specifically for complex attention [19]. Studies focused on remediating cognitive symptoms in persons with MS have typically paired anodal stimulation (targeting the dorsolateral prefrontal cortex) with cognitive remediation techniques such as computerized training platforms [18, 41]. Improvements in attention, executive functioning, and cognitive response variability have been reproduced across the literature for those with MS that complete multiple sessions of tDCS paired with cognitive training.

Previous positive effects and outcomes for tDCS and cognitive remediation warrant further clinical research and use of tDCS for cognitive impairment. However, it is important to recognize that the efficacy of the tDCS may rely upon the therapeutic activity of the cognitive remediation treatment. For this reason, one should consider carefully what cognitive deficit or domain is affected by the MS disease course and what remediation technique may best be paired with tDCS to achieve optimal clinical benefit.

6.3.3 Upper limb motor functioning

Motor impairments are very common and highly disabling for individuals with MS: 80% of people with MS experience gait and mobility impairments, 75% report balance disorders [73] and 76% report some manual dexterity problems [74]. However, motor disabilities cannot fully be controlled by drug treatment. Currently, physical rehabilitation has been identified as the most useful and effective approach to improve some of the typical motor impairments associated with MS. In the last decade or so, several sham-controlled studies conducted across neurological diseases have published encouraging results for improvement of motor symptoms using tDCS alone or in conjunction with rehabilitative therapy. Studies in the literature generally concentrate on primary motor cortex (M1) as the target area in an attempt to modulate cortical excitability.

In a randomized double-blind cross-over study, Cuypers *et al* [39] demonstrated that, after one single session of anodal tDCS with current intensity of 1 mA for 20 min over the M1 contralateral to the most impaired hand, a significant increase in corticospinal excitability was detected. Conversely, no facilitation of motor improvements was observed in another sham controlled double-blind crossover study [16] of one session of anodal tDCS (1 mA for 20 min) on M1 area contralateral to the most impaired hand. Recently, Proessl *et al* [75] showed that one single session of anodal tDCS (2 mA for 20 min) combined with an endurance task is not able to significantly quantitative increase of the time to task failure and muscles activation strategy. Effect of tDCS in motor consolidation was explored in the study of Rumpf *et al* [36]. One single session of anodal tDCS (2 mA for 20 min), applied immediately after a training session of a sequential finger-tapping task, did not produce significant improvement in the functional motor tests.

As these studies do not conclusively demonstrate clinical improvements after one single session of tDCS, further studies are needed to explore the effects of extended treatment schedules (i.e. multiple consecutive treatment sessions) combined with physical rehabilitation.

6.3.4 Pain and sensory deficits

Sensory problems such as neuropathic pain [47, 49, 76] and tactile deficits [48] can be serious symptoms of MS that stand to benefit from therapeutic application of tDCS [77]. While the pathophysiological causes of neuropathic MS pain and tactile sensory deficits are different, they can be similarly modulated and ameliorated by tDCS. Incident rates for these types of symptomatic problems are high, with estimates above 60% of the MS population [2] and, similar to other common MS symptoms, treatment options are lacking [78].

At this point, the hypothetical basis for the improvement of both neuropathic pain and tactile deficits is that multiple sessions of tDCS induce long-lasting, functional, plastic changes in interconnected [49, 79] and somatosensory cortical regions [48]. For pain, these plastic changes in the brain may directly modulate how individuals with MS experience neuropathic pain and for sensory deficits, somatosensory cortex of tactile regions may be stimulated, which may lead to plastic functional improvements in maladaptive neuronal processes incurred by the disease course.

6.3.5 Imaging and future directions

While there is clear potential for the clinical benefit of tDCS in MS, many questions remain regarding the mechanism of action of tDCS and its effects on the underlying brain tissue, both in regions local to the site of stimulation and those more anatomically distant [80, 81]. Among the neuroimaging techniques available, magnetic resonance imaging (MRI) may advance the understanding of underlying mechanisms and ultimately determine biomarkers of efficacy for tDCS.

Methodologically, tDCS can be combined with MRI either sequentially or simultaneously:

- In the sequential approach, the participant is scanned before and after stimulation in order to detect any neurological brain changes. This approach has also been used to determine whether functional brain changes occur after long periods of tDCS treatment.
- Recently, methods to deliver the stimulation within the bore of the scanner (simultaneous approach) have been developed. This approach allows delivery of tDCS during MRI data collection sequences or even during a resting period. While there are advantages to scanning during active delivery of treatment, the integration of tDCS within an MRI requires specific preparation including a customize stimulation kit, MRI compatible equipment to prevent imaging artifacts, and forethought to address adverse events that may arise from treatment the MRI sequences (figure 6.5).

The simultaneous approach can also be used to determine whether tDCS induces acute neuronal activation in both healthy and MS participants. Recent work has shown that the cerebral oxygen metabolism of both MS patients and healthy participants, as assessed via TRUST imaging, increases during application of tDCS. This indicates a higher level of neuronal reactivity during direct current stimulation

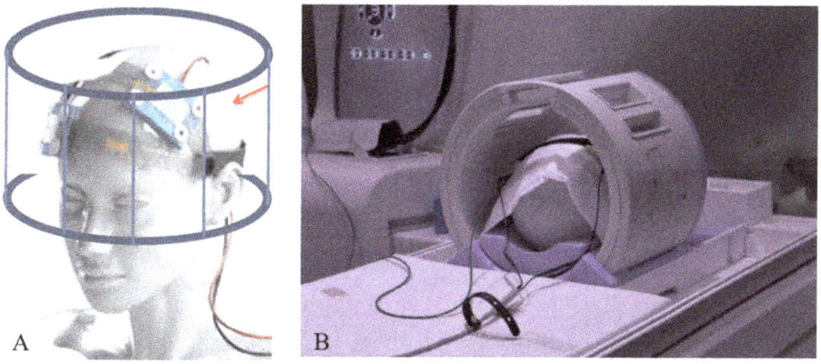

Figure 6.5. Demonstration of simultaneous tDCS MRI configuration. (A) The headset can be inserted within and around the locking coil as long as the cables have been specially designed to prevent imaging artifacts. (B) Example of prepared tDCS MRI configuration.

[82]. Incorporating imaging assessment may play a pivotal role in determining the specific mechanism of action and predictor of the treatment's efficacy

6.4 Conclusions

tDCS holds promise for use in the clinical managment of MS. However, the optimal parameters for clinical benefit remain to be identified and include factors such as electrode placement or montage, stimulation duration, and number of treatments needed for benefit. Beyond parameters, reliable predictors of response to tDCS are needed to determine who will benefit most from treatment with tDCS.

Adequately powered clinical trials that build off the successes of the initial pilot studies in MS are needed to demonstrate whether tDCS can be used to manage comorbid symptoms and problems. The long-term effects of tDCS have been sparingly studied in general tDCS research, and even less so in the MS population, with the longest treatment schedule of 20 sessions over 4 weeks with MS participants [9]. Protocols that enable participation of individuals with MS, such as RS-tDCS, may best promote success [18, 19, 29, 34, 35, 83–86].

Imaging assessment may play a pivotal role in determining how tDCS can be used to rehabilitate and manage symptoms of individuals with MS.

References

[1] Amtmann D, Bamer A M, Kim J, Chung H and Salem R 2018 People with multiple sclerosis report significantly worse symptoms and health related quality of life than the US general population as measured by PROMIS and NeuroQoL outcome measures *Disabil. Health J.* **11** 99–107

[2] Rae-Grant A D, Eckert N J, Bartz S and Reed J F 1999 Sensory symptoms of multiple sclerosis: a hidden reservoir of morbidity *Mult. Scler.* **5** 179–83

[3] Simone I L, Ceccarelli A, Tortorella C, Bellacosa A, Pellegrini F, Plasmati I, De Caro M F, Lopez M, Girolamo F and Livrea P 2006 Influence of Interferon beta treatment on quality of life in multiple sclerosis patients *Health Qual. Life Outcomes* **4** 96

[4] Hirst C, Ingram G, Pearson O, Pickersgill T, Scolding N and Robertson N 2008 Contribution of relapses to disability in multiple sclerosis *J. Neurol.* **255** 280–7
[5] Zeller D *et al* 2010 Rapid-onset central motor plasticity in multiple sclerosis *Neurology* **74** 728–35
[6] Filippi M and Rocca M A 2004 Cortical reorganisation in patients with MS *J. Neurol. Neurosurg. Psychiatry* **75** 1087–9
[7] Tomassini V, Johansen-Berg H, Leonardi L, Paixao L, Jbabdi S, Palace J, Pozzilli C and Matthews P M 2011 Preservation of motor skill learning in patients with multiple sclerosis *Mult. Scler.* **17** 103–15
[8] Rocca M A, Colombo B, Falini A, Ghezzi A, Martinelli V, Scotti G, Comi G and Filippi M 2005 Cortical adaptation in patients with MS: a cross-sectional functional MRI study of disease phenotypes *Lancet Neurol.* **4** 618–26
[9] Bikson M *et al* 2016 Safety of transcranial direct current stimulation: evidence based update 2016 *Brain Stimul.* **9** 641–61
[10] Brunoni A R *et al* 2012 Clinical research with transcranial direct current stimulation (tDCS): challenges and future directions *Brain Stimul.* **5** 175–95
[11] Palm U, Ayache S S, Padberg F and Lefaucheur J P 2014 Non-invasive brain stimulation therapy in multiple sclerosis: a review of tDCS, rTMS and ECT results *Brain Stimul.* **7** 849–54
[12] Hallett M 2007 Transcranial magnetic stimulation: a primer *Neuron* **55** 187–99
[13] Cohen L G, Roth B J, Wassermann E M, Topka H, Fuhr P, Schultz J and Hallett M 1991 Magnetic stimulation of the human cerebral cortex, an indicator of reorganization in motor pathways in certain pathological conditions *J. Clin. Neurophysiol.* **8** 56–65
[14] Roth B J and Basser P J 1990 A model of the stimulation of a nerve fiber by electromagnetic induction *IEEE Trans. Biomed. Eng.* **37** 588–97
[15] Stagg C J and Nitsche M A 2011 Physiological basis of transcranial direct current stimulation *Neuroscientist* **17** 37–53
[16] Meesen R L, Thijs H, Leenus D J and Cuypers K 2014 A single session of 1 mA anodal tDCS-supported motor training does not improve motor performance in patients with multiple sclerosis *Restor. Neurol. Neurosci.* **32** 293–300
[17] Kasschau M *et al* 2016 Transcranial direct current stimulation is feasible for remotely supervised home delivery in multiple sclerosis *Neuromodulation* **19** 824–31
[18] Charvet L, Shaw M, Dobbs B, Frontario A, Sherman K, Bikson M, Datta A, Krupp L, Zeinapour E and Kasschau M 2018 Remotely supervised transcranial direct current stimulation increases the benefit of at-home cognitive training in multiple sclerosis *Neuromodulation* **21** 383–9
[19] Charvet L E, Dobbs B, Shaw M T, Bikson M, Datta A and Krupp L B 2018 Remotely supervised transcranial direct current stimulation for the treatment of fatigue in multiple sclerosis: Results from a randomized, sham-controlled trial *Mult. Scler.* **24** 1760–9
[20] Bikson M, Datta A and Elwassif M 2009 Establishing safety limits for transcranial direct current stimulation *Clin. Neurophysiol.* **120** 1033–4
[21] Iyer M B, Mattu U, Grafman J, Lomarev M, Sato S and Wassermann E M 2005 Safety and cognitive effect of frontal DC brain polarization in healthy individuals *Neurology* **64** 872–5
[22] Chhatbar P Y, Chen R, Deardorff R, Dellenbach B, Kautz S A, George M S and Feng W 2017 Safety and tolerability of transcranial direct current stimulation to stroke patients—A phase I current escalation study *Brain Stimul.* **10** 553–9

[23] Nitsche M A and Paulus W 2001 Sustained excitability elevations induced by transcranial DC motor cortex stimulation in humans *Neurology* **57** 1899–901
[24] Monte-Silva K, Kuo M F, Hessenthaler S, Fresnoza S, Liebetanz D, Paulus W and Nitsche M A 2013 Induction of late LTP-like plasticity in the human motor cortex by repeated non-invasive brain stimulation *Brain Stimul.* **6** 424–32
[25] Batsikadze G, Moliadze V, Paulus W, Kuo M F and Nitsche M A 2013 Partially non-linear stimulation intensity-dependent effects of direct current stimulation on motor cortex excitability in humans *J. Physiol.* **591** 1987–2000
[26] Loo C K, Alonzo A, Martin D, Mitchell P B, Galvez V and Sachdev P 2012 Transcranial direct current stimulation for depression: 3-week, randomised, sham-controlled trial *Br. J. Psychiatry* **200** 52–9
[27] Ramaraju S, Roula M A and McCarthy P W 2018 Modelling the effect of electrode displacement on transcranial direct current stimulation (tDCS) *J. Neural Eng.* **15** 016019
[28] Rich T L, Menk J S, Rudser K D, Chen M, Meekins G D, Pena E, Feyma T, Bawroski K, Bush C and Gillick B T 2017 Determining electrode placement for transcranial direct current stimulation: a comparison of EEG- versus TMS-guided methods *Clin. EEG Neurosci.* **48** 367–75
[29] Kasschau M, Sherman K, Haider L, Frontario A, Shaw M, Datta A, Bikson M and Charvet L 2015 A protocol for the use of remotely-supervised transcranial direct current stimulation (tDCS) in multiple sclerosis (MS) *J. Vis. Exp.* e53542
[30] DaSilva A F, Volz M S, Bikson M and Fregni F 2011 Electrode positioning and montage in transcranial direct current stimulation *J. Vis. Exp.* 2744
[31] Tecchio F *et al* 2015 Brain plasticity effects of neuromodulation against multiple sclerosis fatigue *Front. Neurol.* **6** 141
[32] Cancelli A, Cottone C, Giordani A, Migliore S, Lupoi D, Porcaro C, Mirabella M, Rossini P M, Filippi M M and Tecchio F 2018 Personalized, bilateral whole-body somatosensory cortex stimulation to relieve fatigue in multiple sclerosis *Mult. Scler.* **24** 1366–74
[33] Chiaravalloti N D, Moore N B, Nikelshpur O M and DeLuca J 2013 An RCT to treat learning impairment in multiple sclerosis: The MEMREHAB trial *Neurology* **81** 2066–72
[34] Shaw M T, Kasschau M, Dobbs B, Pawlak N, Pau W, Sherman K, Bikson M, Datta A and Charvet L E 2017 Remotely supervised transcranial direct current stimulation: an update on safety and tolerability *J. Vis. Exp.*
[35] Kasschau M, Reisner J, Sherman K, Bikson M, Datta A and Charvet L E 2016 Transcranial direct current stimulation is feasible for remotely supervised home delivery in multiple sclerosis *Neuromodulation* **19** 824–31
[36] Rumpf J J, Dietrich S, Stoppe M, Fricke C, Weise D, Then Bergh F and Classen J 2018 Compromised tDCS-induced facilitation of motor consolidation in patients with multiple sclerosis *J. Neurol.* **265** 2302–11
[37] Cosentino G *et al* 2018 Anodal tDCS of the swallowing motor cortex for treatment of dysphagia in multiple sclerosis: a pilot open-label study *Neurol. Sci.* **39** 1471–3
[38] Iodice R, Dubbioso R, Ruggiero L, Santoro L and Manganelli F 2015 Anodal transcranial direct current stimulation of motor cortex does not ameliorate spasticity in multiple sclerosis *Restor. Neurol. Neurosci.* **33** 487–92
[39] Cuypers K, Leenus D J, Van Wijmeersch B, Thijs H, Levin O, Swinnen S P and Meesen R L 2013 Anodal tDCS increases corticospinal output and projection strength in multiple sclerosis *Neurosci. Lett.* **554** 151–5

[40] Fiene M, Rufener K S, Kuehne M, Matzke M, Heinze H J and Zaehle T 2018 Electrophysiological and behavioral effects of frontal transcranial direct current stimulation on cognitive fatigue in multiple sclerosis *J. Neurol.* **265** 607–17

[41] Mattioli F, Bellomi F, Stampatori C, Capra R and Miniussi C 2015 Neuroenhancement through cognitive training and anodal tDCS in multiple sclerosis *Mult. Scler.* **22** 222–30

[42] Chalah M A, Riachi N, Ahdab R, Mhalla A, Abdellaoui M, Creange A, Lefaucheur J P and Ayache S S 2017 Effects of left DLPFC versus right PPC tDCS on multiple sclerosis fatigue *J. Neurol. Sci.* **372** 131–7

[43] Hanken K, Bosse M, Mohrke K, Eling P, Kastrup A, Antal A and Hildebrandt H 2016 Counteracting fatigue in multiple sclerosis with right parietal anodal transcranial direct current stimulation *Front. Neurol.* **7** 154

[44] Tecchio F, Cancelli A, Cottone C, Zito G, Pasqualetti P, Ghazaryan A, Rossini P M and Filippi M M 2014 Multiple sclerosis fatigue relief by bilateral somatosensory cortex neuromodulation *J. Neurol.* **261** 1552–8

[45] Saiote C, Goldschmidt T, Timaus C, Steenwijk M D, Opitz A, Antal A, Paulus W and Nitsche M A 2014 Impact of transcranial direct current stimulation on fatigue in multiple sclerosis *Restor. Neurol. Neurosci.* **32** 423–36

[46] Ferrucci R, Vergari M, Cogiamanian F, Bocci T, Ciocca M, Tomasini E, De Riz M, Scarpini E and Priori A 2014 Transcranial direct current stimulation (tDCS) for fatigue in multiple sclerosis *NeuroRehabilitation* **34** 121–7

[47] Ayache S S, Palm U, Chalah M A, Al-Ani T, Brignol A, Abdellaoui M, Dimitri D, Sorel M, Creange A and Lefaucheur J P 2016 Prefrontal tDCS decreases pain in patients with multiple sclerosis *Front. Neurosci.* **10** 147

[48] Mori F, Nicoletti C G, Kusayanagi H, Foti C, Restivo D A, Marciani M G and Centonze D 2013 Transcranial direct current stimulation ameliorates tactile sensory deficit in multiple sclerosis *Brain Stimul.* **6** 654–9

[49] Mori F, Codeca C, Kusayanagi H, Monteleone F, Buttari F, Fiore S, Bernardi G, Koch G and Centonze D 2010 Effects of anodal transcranial direct current stimulation on chronic neuropathic pain in patients with multiple sclerosis *J. Pain* **11** 436–42

[50] Lerdal A, Celius E G, Krupp L and Dahl A A 2007 A prospective study of patterns of fatigue in multiple sclerosis *Eur. J. Neurol.* **14** 1338–43

[51] Khan F, Amatya B and Galea M 2014 Management of fatigue in persons with multiple sclerosis *Front. Neurol.* **5** 177

[52] Fisk J D, Pontefract A, Ritvo P G, Archibald C J and Murray T J 1994 The impact of fatigue on patients with multiple sclerosis *Can. J. Neurol. Sci.* **21** 9–14

[53] Fernandez-Munoz J J, Moron-Verdasco A, Cigaran-Mendez M, Munoz-Hellin E, Perez-de-Heredia-Torres M and Fernandez-de-Las-Penas C 2015 Disability, quality of life, personality, cognitive and psychological variables associated with fatigue in patients with multiple sclerosis *Acta Neurol. Scand.* **132** 118–24

[54] Genova H M, Rajagopalan V, Deluca J, Das A, Binder A, Arjunan A, Chiaravalloti N and Wylie G 2013 Examination of cognitive fatigue in multiple sclerosis using functional magnetic resonance imaging and diffusion tensor imaging *PLoS One* **8** e78811

[55] Kos D, Kerckhofs E, Nagels G, D'Hooghe M B and Ilsbroukx S 2008 Origin of fatigue in multiple sclerosis: review of the literature *Neurorehabil. Neural Repair* **22** 91–100

[56] Braley T J and Chervin R D 2010 Fatigue in multiple sclerosis: mechanisms, evaluation, and treatment *Sleep* **33** 1061–7

[57] Charvet L E, Serafin D and Krupp L B 2014 Fatigue in multiple sclerosis *Fatigue* **2** 3–13
[58] Svenningsson A, Falk E, Celius E G, Fuchs S, Schreiber K, Berko S, Sun J, Penner I K and Tynergy Trial Investigators 2013 Natalizumab treatment reduces fatigue in multiple sclerosis. Results from the TYNERGY trial; a study in the real life setting *PLoS One* **8** e58643
[59] Kraft G, Bamer A, McMullen K and Amtmann D 2012 Multiple sclerosis patients taking disease modifying treatments endorse less severe symptoms and improved quality of life compared with patients not on treatment *Neurology* **78** P07.094
[60] Lange R, Volkmer M, Heesen C and Liepert J 2009 Modafinil effects in multiple sclerosis patients with fatigue *J. Neurol.* **256** 645–50
[61] Krupp L B, Coyle P K, Doscher C, Miller A, Cross A H, Jandorf L, Halper J, Johnson B, Morgante L and Grimson R 1995 Fatigue therapy in multiple sclerosis: results of a double-blind, randomized, parallel trial of amantadine, pemoline, and placebo *Neurology* **45** 1956–61
[62] Asano M and Finlayson M L 2014 Meta-analysis of three different types of fatigue management interventions for people with multiple sclerosis: exercise, education, and medication *Mult. Scler. Int.* **2014** 798285
[63] Hugos C L, Copperman L F, Fuller B E, Yadav V, Lovera J and Bourdette D N 2016 Clinical trial of a formal group fatigue program in multiple sclerosis *Mult. Scler.* **16** 724–32
[64] Chiaravalloti N D and DeLuca J 2008 Cognitive impairment in multiple sclerosis *Lancet Neurol.* **7** 1139–51
[65] Hankomaki E, Multanen J, Kinnunen E and Hamalainen P 2014 The progress of cognitive decline in newly diagnosed MS patients *Acta Neurol. Scand.* **129** 184–91
[66] Strober L, Chiaravalloti N, Moore N and DeLuca J 2014 Unemployment in multiple sclerosis (MS): utility of the MS Functional Composite and cognitive testing *Mult. Scler.* **20** 112–5
[67] Glanz B I, Healy B C, Hviid L E, Chitnis T and Weiner H L 2012 Cognitive deterioration in patients with early multiple sclerosis: a 5-year study *J. Neurol. Neurosurg. Psychiatry* **83** 38–43
[68] Jonsson A, Andresen J, Storr L, Tscherning T, Soelberg Sorensen P and Ravnborg M 2006 Cognitive impairment in newly diagnosed multiple sclerosis patients: a 4-year follow-up study *J. Neurol. Sci.* **245** 77–85
[69] Grzegorski T and Losy J 2017 Cognitive impairment in multiple sclerosis—a review of current knowledge and recent research *Rev. Neurosci.* **28** 845–60
[70] Charvet L E, Yang J, Shaw M T, Sherman K, Haider L, Xu J and Krupp L B 2017 Cognitive function in multiple sclerosis improves with telerehabilitation: Results from a randomized controlled trial *PLoS One* **12** e0177177
[71] Clark V P, Coffman B A, Mayer A R, Weisend M P, Lane T D, Calhoun V D, Raybourn E M, Garcia C M and Wassermann E M 2012 TDCS guided using fMRI significantly accelerates learning to identify concealed objects *Neuroimage* **59** 117–28
[72] Falcone B, Coffman B A, Clark V P and Parasuraman R 2012 Transcranial direct current stimulation augments perceptual sensitivity and 24-hour retention in a complex threat detection task *PLoS One* **7** e34993
[73] Feinstein A, Freeman J and Lo A C 2015 Treatment of progressive multiple sclerosis: what works, what does not, and what is needed *Lancet Neurol.* **14** 194–207
[74] Johansson S, Ytterberg C, Claesson I M, Lindberg J, Hillert J, Andersson M, Widen Holmqvist L and von Koch L 2007 High concurrent presence of disability in multiple sclerosis. Associations with perceived health *J. Neurol.* **254** 767–73
[75] Proessl F, Ketelhut N B and Rudroff T 2018 No association of leg strength asymmetry with walking ability, fatigability, and fatigue in multiple sclerosis *Int. J. Rehabil. Res.* **41** 267–9

[76] Kenner M, Menon U and Elliott D G 2007 Multiple sclerosis as a painful disease *Int. Rev. Neurobiol.* **79** 303–21

[77] Amatya B, Young J and Khan F 2018 Non-pharmacological interventions for chronic pain in multiple sclerosis *Cochrane Database Syst. Rev.* **12** CD012622

[78] Moulin D *et al* 2014 Pharmacological management of chronic neuropathic pain: revised consensus statement from the Canadian Pain Society *Pain Res. Manag.* **19** 328–35

[79] Dostrovsky J O 2000 Role of thalamus in pain *Prog. Brain Res.* **129** 245–57

[80] Polania R, Paulus W and Nitsche M A 2012 Modulating cortico-striatal and thalamo-cortical functional connectivity with transcranial direct current stimulation *Hum. Brain Mapp.* **33** 2499–508

[81] Turi Z, Paulus W and Antal A 2012 Functional neuroimaging and transcranial electrical stimulation *Clin. EEG Neurosci.* **43** 200–8

[82] Ge Y, Datta A, Dobbs B, Shaw M, Clayton A, Gonen O and Charvet L 2018 Simultaneous assessment of tDCS-induced neuronal responses with oxygen metabolic MRI *Int. Society for Margnetic Resonance in Medicine (Paris, France)*

[83] Clayton A M, Howard J, Dobbs B, Shaw M T and Charvet L E 2018 Remotely supervised transcranial direct current stimulation after ECT improves mood and cognition in a patient with multiple sclerosis: a case study *J. ECT* **34** e15

[84] Agarwal S, Pawlak N, Cucca A, Sharma K, Dobbs B, Shaw M, Charvet L and Biagioni M 2018 Remotely-supervised transcranial direct current stimulation paired with cognitive training in Parkinson's disease: an open-label study *J. Clin. Neurosci.* **57** 51–7

[85] Dobbs B, Pawlak N, Biagioni M, Agarwal S, Shaw M, Pilloni G, Bikson M, Datta A and Charvet L 2018 Generalizing remotely supervised transcranial direct current stimulation (tDCS): feasibility and benefit in Parkinson's disease *J. Neuroeng. Rehabil.* **15** 114

[86] Pilloni G, Shaw M, Feinberg C, Clayton A, Palmeri M, Datta A and Charvet L E 2019 Long term at-home treatment with transcranial direct current stimulation (tDCS) improves symptoms of cerebellar ataxia: a case report *J. Neuroeng. Rehabil.* **16** 41

IOP Publishing

Neurological Disorders and Imaging Physics, Volume 2
Engineering and clinical perspectives of multiple sclerosis
Ayman El-Baz and Jasjit S Suri

Chapter 7

Oxidative stress and sterile inflammation in multiple sclerosis

Necat Yilmaz and Esin Eren

Time has shown us change is inevitable. In evolution, due to the restricted availability of resources, the sole purpose of organisms was to survive long enough to transmit their genes to the next generation.

During their short lifetime, living organisms used pathogen-associated and damage-associated molecular pathways as an inflammatory response against pathogens (exogenous factors) and tissue damage (endogenous factors), respectively. Now, despite advances in human life-time, it appears that an increasing number of diseases such as multiple sclerosis (MS) are associated with inflammation. Excessive glucose, lipid and protein intake leads to the formation of endogenous crystals, i.e., mono sodium urate (MSU) and cholesterol crystals, which can induce a sterile inflammatory immune response that manifests as a vicious cycle. Moreover, MS is the most common neurological disorder in young adults. With an initial age of 20 to 40 years, it affects more than 3 million people worldwide. In this chapter, we evaluate the possible relationship between a crystal-based sterile inflammatory response and oxidative stress (OS) response in MS. In addition, the chapter will focus on the causes of OS and its relationship with MS.

7.1 Introduction to the disease

MS is a chronic multifactorial and polygenic autoimmune disease of the central nervous system (CNS), affecting predominantly young females. It affects women more often than men (3:1 ratio), but its incidence also varies according to ethnicity and geographical location, with Northern Europeans and their descendants being more susceptible to develop the disease. The etiology of MS is yet uncertain, but the most updated working model for disease pathogenesis proposes the interplay between genetic and environmental factors as necessary for MS manifestation [1–6].

doi:10.1088/978-0-7503-1762-7ch7

Escalating evidence has shown that MS is the outcome of inappropriate immune response, characterized by auto-inflammation, making it a highly unpredictable neurologic disease. MS is a chronic inflammatory disease of the CNS, in which the body's own immune cells attack the lipids, insulating myelin sheath surrounding nerve fibers [7, 8]. Moreover, evidence shows that OS plays a role in demyelination. Nowadays it is well known that OS poses a high risk to human health [9, 10]. Many studies have highlighted the role of diverse environmental and genetic factors in MS etiopathogenesis, each adding a new puzzle to MS and therefore making it a multifactorial and polygenic disease [11]. In spite of being of unknown etiology, the pathological hallmarks of MS lesions are well-defined. Generally lesions implicate focal as well as diffuse demyelination, oligodendrocyte damage, and activation of brain immune cells such as microglia and astrocytes, and injury of the neuro-axonal unit [11–14].

In conclusion, MS is a multiphase disease of the CNS, characterized by inflammation, demyelination, and axonal loss. The clinical process of MS is incalculable and recognized by relapses and remissions. Indeed, most patients show relapsing–remitting MS (RRMS) displaying typical symptoms that maintain for days followed by spontaneous amelioration or in response to treatment with steroids. A few patients develop continuous CNS disorders increasing disability; this type of MS is familiar as secondary progressive MS (SPMS). The last MS patient group has primary progressive MS (PPMS), which is characterized by relapses at the onset of the disease and a gradual progressive clinical course. But more research is still needed to find a cure for this chronic, unpredictable disease [15, 16].

7.1.1 History of MS

The abundance of knowledge available about MS in the 21st century has accumulated exponentially since the 19th century. Towards the end of the 19th century, Jean-Martin Charcot set a relationship between plaques in an autopsy and trembling, speech disorder and irregular eye movements that the deceased woman had suffered. Later, Walter Moxon and Dr Edward Seguin observed many neurological symptoms in MS patients. They found that MS disease affected females more often than males. Doctors also determined that MS wasn't strictly genetic, because parents didn't necessarily pass the disease down to their children [17].

Then 20th century researchers have observed a revival of medical breakthroughs that helped the study the progression and portray the symptoms of MS disease [18]. This came about because it was now possible to view cells under a microscope. Moreover, it was also possible to detect abnormalities in spinal cord fluid and record electrical activity of the nerves. In 1935, the pieces of the MS puzzle started to come together, revealing that MS was not just a simple viral disease of the immune system. One theory from many researchers in the 1960s suggested the immune system attacked the myelin coating of the nerves and acted like an autoimmune disease. Fortunately, there were major technological advances in magnetic resonance imaging (MRI) in the late 1970s, and it was very helpful as a diagnostic tool for

MS patients. For the first time, in 1981, MRI was used in the diagnosis of a patient with MS [18, 19].

Genetic researches in the second half of the 19th century had shed light on the genetic component of the disease for the first time. Hereby, the potent genetic evocation signal in MS is set in the major tissue adherence complex (MHC) in the chromosome 6p21.3. So, compared with a lifetime risk of 0.2% in the general population, siblings of individuals affected by MHC are 10–20 times more likely to develop disease [20, 21].

However, a critical point should not be overlooked, which is the fact that the relative risk does not reach 100% even in identical twins, indicating that other factors beyond the identity of the DNA sequence must be involved in the creation of conditions that cause irregularity of the MS-associated immune response. Clearly, no single gene or environmental factor has been identified as a causal agent for MS. There is a broad range of determinants in the formation of MS. These include toxin-filled environmental exposures, smoking, viral infections, overfeeding and microbiome, and also include epigenetic interaction, DNA methylation patterns, histone modifications, and non-coding RNAs [20, 21].

Really, the 20th century could be named the 'MS drug explosion' century for MS treatments. In 1951, steroids were first used to treat MS relapses. Also, steroids were found to abbreviate the severity of the MS relapse and to reduce MS duration; on the other hand steroids had no long-term effects on the MS treatment. Thus, the first drug trial to be effective in the long-term treatment of MS received approval only 25 years ago [18]. Presently, about 20 different drugs are now approved for MS treatment, with many more on the way. However, these are described as disease-modifying therapies (DMTs). While these medications do not cure MS, they do work to slow disease activity as well as reduce the severity and frequency of flare-ups. Additionally, these DMTs may delay disease progression, delay disability, and increase longevity [22, 23]. The use of interferon for immunosuppressive therapy in MS patients was also first introduced in 1990. Interferon, an injectable drug, was approved for a relapsing–remitting MS treatment in the early 1990s. Now, many sophisticated drugs used for the treatment of MS can change the way the immune system attacks healthy tissues in MS disease. But, it is still unknown what exactly causes demyelinating lesions in MS [18, 19].

Generally, it is believed that there is a strange autoimmune mechanism in MS. Nowadays, many different theories about the factors leading to MS are being proposed. For example, in many studies published in the medical literature over the last decade, it has been reported that vitamin D can protect against MS. In addition, many different studies in the literature suggest that oxygen may be able to help prevent myelin damage. Until now, the etiology of MS remains extremely enigmatic, with no sufficient evidence of the exact cause of the disease [20].

Interestingly, the hygiene hypothesis was proposed as a causative agent of MS, suggesting that exposure to microbes in childhood may assistant in building up and preserving the immune system [24]. Evidence suggests that these neuro-inflammatory diseases are much more common in the developed world where antibiotics are frequently used to reduce children's exposure to microbes [24, 25].

Our living journey in the world is a very short period of time in the evolutionary processes of living beings that has lasted 2.3 million years. As a result, although the world is becoming more hygienic, such a sterile environment is becoming dangerous for more people [1]. Also, it can be said that cumulative effects of OS-incorporated environmental factors as well as many genes cause the formation of MS [26].

Many new hypotheses are suggested along with the hygiene hypothesis about the cause of MS. There is no doubt that the role of OS in MS has begun to be broadly discussed more recently. So, it is thought that the development of MS may be affected by OS. Furthermore, in the acute phase of the disease, OS is responsible for initiating inflammation and continues the neurodegenerative process in to the chronic phase. Redox mechanisms in MS may be related to the irregularity of crystal-based sterile inflammation, axonal bioenergetics, cerebral iron accumulation, mitochondrial dysfunction, impaired oxidant/antioxidant balance, and OS damage [1, 27].

It is possible that MS may have been triggered by a 'chemical silent killer' that is perhaps caused by free radicals (FRs). So, OS is now thought to make a significant contribution to all inflammatory-related diseases. Because new researches point towards all oxidative/inflammatory cascades being the effect that leads to the damage, this offers new thoughts on ways to prevent the myelin damage in MS patients. In fact, all evidence suggests a combination of anti-crystal, anti-inflammatory, anti-oxidative and anti-neurodegenerative strategies for treatment in MS [1].

Nowadays, FRs, ROS, OS and antioxidants have become commonly used terms in current discussions of disease mechanisms. A good understanding of the terms associated with the redox mechanism is necessary. Let us try to explain these terms a little more deeply.

7.2 Redox system

7.2.1 Redox term

Reduction–oxidation (redox) reactions at the base of life are at the center of cell metabolic machines. With the simplest definition, redox reactions involve the transfer of electrons or hydrogen atoms from one reactant to another. The process of taking away electrons is called 'oxidation,' because molecular oxygen does it so well. The molecules receiving electrons attain a 'reduced' state. Unfortunately, the redox process may sometimes damage the live cell. Frequently, the reason that overproduction of FRs is a feature of such a wide spectrum of diseases emerges from the fact that the oxidative metabolism is an essential part of every cell's metabolism [28, 29].

7.2.2 History of oxidative stress

A world-famous scientist, Myron Wentz, said: 'We live too short and die too long'; truly, increased OS is killing us slowly [30]. How can this be? Let us begin by considering a machine—the perfect machine. Although perfect, the human body compared to such a design is gradually disrupted by the increased OS. Now, let us try to answer the question of what is OS? Reactive oxygen species (ROS) should be well defined primarily as disrupted redox balance leading to OS.

Superoxide radicals ($O_2^{\bullet-}$), hydrogen peroxide (H_2O_2), hydroxyl radicals ($^{\bullet}OH$), and singlet oxygen ($1O_2$) are commonly defined as ROS (figure 7.1). All ROS are generated as natural metabolic by-products by biological systems, whilst an imbalance between the production of ROS and the detoxification of their reactive intermediates causes OS in an oxygen dependent organism. A living organism must respond effectively and fast to this imbalance before the ROS damages cellular structures, particularly DNA. The definition of OS is quite recent, having been made in the late 20th century. Simply, the term OS was defined as a disturbance in the balance between the production of ROS/RNS and antioxidant defenses, which may lead to cell injury [30, 31]. The origin of the basic principle of the biological stress term and stress responses dates back to Selye in 1936 [32, 33]. In a famous paper in 1954, Rebecca Gershman and Dan Gilbert put forward a relationship between the effects of O_2 and ionizing radiation and suggested that most of the damaging effects of O_2 are due to oxygen radicals [34]. In 1970, the original medical wording '*cells were subjected to oxidative stress*' was used to describe the addition of H_2O_2 to erythrocytes. In 1985, Barry Halliwell and John M C Gutteridge published the textbook *Free Radicals in Biology and Medicine*. In this book a comprehensive chapter describes OS [28, 34]. The notion of OS and OS responses was formulated in 1985 in the book entitled *Oxidative Stress* written by Helmut Sies [28, 31].

As seen, the definition and use of OS has been improved recently. However, it is the subject of a large number of studies because it can form the basic mechanism of diseases. Presently, an exponentially growing number of scientific articles and books are appearing that focus on OS.

OS as a concept in redox medicine has witnessed fulminant development over the past 30 odd years. As an example, there are 200 931 publications in PubMed as of December 2018. On the other hand, there were only 5 publications in PubMed in 1975 that included the words oxidative stress. In the last year alone, >30 books appeared dealing with OS. The majority of these books handle OS in connection with a number of different specific diseases, for instance: MS, Alzheimer's or Parkinson's disease. In the last two decades, many international research journals

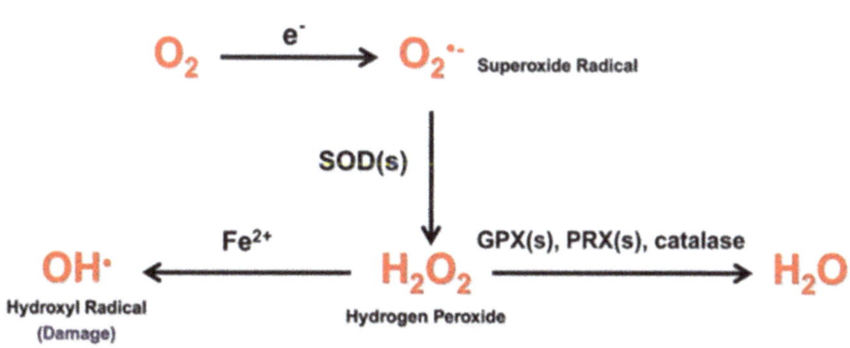

Figure 7.1. Reactive oxygen species.

(*Free Radical Research, Free Radicals in Biology and Medicine, Redox Reports, Antioxidant Redox Signaling, Redox Biology Oxidative Medicine and Cellular Longevity*) specialising in OS were launched. The higher number of OS-related studies in the medical literature nowadays shows a very important role in OS disease formation.

7.2.3 What is the concept of oxidative stress?

'*The dose makes the poison*' by Paracelsus is a 21st century toxicology paradigm, appropriately applicable to OS. Numerous diseases have a more-or-less OS component, including, neurodegenerative diseases such as MS.

Nowadays, how OS damages cells and organs is better understood. The new definition of OS is certainly essential: '*an imbalance between oxidants and antioxidants in favor of the oxidants, leading to a disruption of redox signaling and control and/or molecular damage*'. So an imbalance between the production of free radicals (FRs) and the antioxidative defense leads to OS and nitrosative stress (NS). To counter the possible noxious effects of oxygen, intracellular homeostasis is maintained by a balancing of redox reactions, the so-called '*intracellular redox equilibrium'*. In excessive cases, whenever metabolic processes or toxic degradation lead to a situation where pro-oxidants outbalance their anti-oxidative counterparts, a state of '*oxidative stress*' is achieved [31]. At a glance only from a chemical point of view, OS is a consequence of the imbalance between the production and consumption of oxidants in biological systems. However, FRs and ROS are a very important part of the normal functioning of the living organism.

For example processes, like protein phosphorylation, activation of several transcriptional factors, apoptosis, immunity, and differentiation, are all dependent on a proper FRs/ROS production. Its presence inside cells that need to be kept at a low level can be classified according to its density, with intensity scales ranging from physiological OS (*eustress*) to toxic OS which damages biomolecules (*distress*). When production of ROS rises (*distress*), they start showing harmful effects on important cellular structures like proteins, lipids, and nucleic acids. '*Distress*' activates disposal programs such as autophagy, mitophagy, apoptosis, necroptosis, ferroptosis in the cell. In neuro-inflammatory diseases such as MS, this '*distress*' process takes place in the myelin part of the neurons [31–36].

7.2.4 Redox code

Naturally, the oxidative molecules utilized in redox signaling directly or indirectly target transcription factors. The redox code of the metabolic and protein ingredient provides a supreme complement to the genetic code, the epigenetic code, and the histone code in the molecular logic of life. Unlike the genetic code and histone code, which underlie information storage and transfer for use, the epigenetic code and the redox code define the operations of the genetic and histone codes in the organizational structure, differentiation, and adaptation of an organism to the environment. In this way, the living organism can adapt to the environment better with its redox code and epigenetic code [28, 29, 31]. So, redox code and epigenetic code may have a superior adaptation advantage in the evolutionary process. That could be because the redox code covers specific, reversible oxidative changes in proteins that modulate protein tertiary structure, interactions, molecular signaling and activity. No doubt, 'chef regulators' of redox code are the Nrf2/Keap1 and the NF-κB/IkB systems in the upkeep of redox balance. These two main pathway molecules work in the opposite direction to provide the oxidative balance, because Nrf2, after translocation to the nucleus, activates a pattern of anti-oxidant defense enzymes. Contrariwise, NF-κB, after translocation to the nucleus activates the expression of genes involved in inflammatory, immune and acute phase responses [29, 34].

In fact, these contrary pathways are more essential in sustained low-dose OS in oxygen-dependent life balance. So, hormesis as a phenomenon of mounting defense patterns upon low-dose OS has received cautious attention in recent years. For the first time in 1943, Arndt-Schulz used the '*hormesis*' term. Thus, a brief simple definition of hormesis is: *'a process in which exposure to a low dose of a chemical agent or environmental factor that is damaging at higher doses induces an adaptive beneficial effect on the cell or organism'* [28, 36].

Many findings have elucidated the cellular signaling pathways and molecular mechanisms that mediate '*hormetic*' responses which typically involve enzymes such as kinases and deacetylases, and transcription factors such as Nrf-2 and NF-κB. During these helpful '*hormetic*' responses, cells increase their production of cytoprotective and restorative proteins including growth factors, phase 2 and antioxidant enzymes, and protein chaperones. The reaction to mild mitochondrial OS, named '*mitohormesis*', addresses such far-reaching questions such as how raised OS promotes longevity and metabolic health [28, 31, 36].

We have defined the terms related to OS and also briefly discussed the historical development. Now let us try to recognize dangerous molecules that are the cause of OS.

7.2.5 History of free radicals

In the last decade there has been increasing attention on analyzing the role of FRs in neurological disease, because of their principal role in physiological conditions as well as their involvement in a many kinds of diseases. As stated before, if in excess, FRs and oxidants give rise to a phenomenon known as distress; higher OS is a harmful process that can negatively affect several cellular structures, such as membranes, lipids, proteins, lipoproteins, and nucleic acids.

There is nothing more powerful than an idea whose time has come. V Hugo.

In the 1600s, scientists began to understand that there was an element in the air that was essential for life. They then essentially described a component termed 'eminently breathable air', subsequently termed 'oxygen' in the science world.

Could oxygen be harmful to a living organism? Although oxygen is obligatory for life in most organisms, some of oxygen's metabolic product can be harmful. Firstly, in 1954, Rebeca Gerschman proposed the 'free radical theory of oxygen toxicity', according to which, the toxicity of oxygen is because of its capability to form FRs. Subsequently, the presence of free radicals in biological materials was confirmed by

Commoner *et al.* And soon thereafter, Denham Harman, in 1956, proposed the 'free radical theory of aging', which states that FRs play a central role in the aging process. 'FR theory'was developed in 1969 by Mc Cord and Fridovich, who discovered superoxide dismutase, the first enzymatic defense system against superoxide anion. For the first time in 1971, Loschen indicated that the ROS are generated in normal cellular metabolic respiration. Later, in 1977, Mittal and Murad reported that the hydroxyl radical, $OH^{\bullet}$ induces the formation of the second messenger cyclic GMP by activating the enzyme guanylate cyclase. In 1989, Halliwell and Gutteridge reported that ROS include both free radical and non-radical derivatives of oxygen [28, 34, 37, 38].

7.3 Why is a free radical dangerous?

An atom consists of a nucleus with protons and neutrons, and pairs of electrons orbiting this electrically-charged space. The behavior of the atom depends on the number of electrically-charged particles. Dioxygen (O_2) is 'paramagnetic' and has two electrons with 'parallel spins'. This renders reactions with O_2 difficult, since the organic donor has to undergo a 'slow spin inversion' so that it can donate its electrons. To bypass this necessity, O_2 is either unified with a paramagnetic metal, for example, copper or iron, or electrons are added to oxygen in phases. This means that O_2 is reduced to H_2O by producing the superoxide anion radical ($^{\bullet}O_{2-}$), hydrogen peroxide (H_2O_2) and hydroxyl radical ($^{\bullet}OH$). These trash intermediates, called FRs, can pose a threat to cells [39, 40].

When, during a chemical reaction, an electron is pulled from one of the pairs of electrons of an oxygen molecule, that oxygen molecule with an unpaired electron becomes a FR. So, FRs are any atom with an unpaired electron. This is so because it must seek out another electron to make a new pair, and might cause damage by pulling an electron from an otherwise normal cell of your body. Now the newly damaged molecule is itself left with an unpaired electron and must scavenge an electron in what has now become a '*cascade*' of free-radical damage. Otherwise, the odd number of electrons of a free radical makes it unstable, short lived and highly reactive. Because of their high reactivity, they can extract electrons from other compounds to attain stability. Thus the attacked molecule loses its electron and becomes a FR itself, beginning a chain reaction cascade which finally damages the living cell. However, the FRs chain reaction may lead to broken cell membranes, which can alter what enters and exits the cell. OS occurs when there are too many FRs and too much cellular damage [36, 39, 40].

The FRs sources may be divided into an endogenous and exogenous base. For example, lifestyle factors (exposome) impinge on both these types of sources. In addition, ROS/RNS may be generated in the body in response to electromagnetic radiation from the environment and acquired directly as oxidizing pollutants such as ozone and nitrogen dioxide [36].

FRs can be produced by several different metabolic processes within the living organism including: reduction of molecular oxygen pending aerobic respiration yielding superoxide and hydroxyl radicals; by-products of chemistry such as oxidation of catecholamines and activation of the arachidonic acid cascade product electrons, which can reduce molecular oxygen to superoxide; production of superoxide and hypochlorous acid, a powerful oxidant, by activated phagocytes; nitric oxide production by vascular endothelium and other cells. FRs are inherently unstable molecules because of the presence of unpaired electrons. As a result, they can be highly reactive, although this varies from radical to radical, reacting locally to accept or donate electrons to other molecules to achieve a more stable state. In addition, FRs can be produced in response to external electromagnetic radiation, such as gamma rays, which can split water to produce hydroxyl radicals [36–41].

However, FRs are essential to life—the body's ability to turn air and food into chemical energy depends on a chain reaction of FRs. Eventually there are continuously produced antioxidant molecules and antioxidant defense mechanisms to combat OS in a cell. That is not all so simple, because FRs which are involved in the formation of OS, are the products of normal cellular metabolism. For example, FRs are a crucial part of the immune system, floating through the veins and attacking foreign invaders.

7.3.1 What is the difference between FRs and ROS?

Certainly oxygen is fundamental for multicellular life, because for aerobic organisms oxidation has become the major instrument of energy generation. At the same time it is one of the most reactive and life threatening elements known. As mentioned above, FRs are any atom with an unpaired electron. So, FRs are constituted by an atom or a molecule formed from more atoms that has an unpaired electron, but not always containing oxygen. However, ROS are the entire FRs that are commonly found in biology that involve oxygen. So ROS's are FRs that specifically involve oxygen [39].

Often, factors inducing OS are chemical compounds classed as ROS or reactive nitrogen species (RNS) in cells. ROS/RNS are both unstable, and mostly present in a radical form, which means that they contain unpaired electrons on the outer orbital. On the other hand, a helpful functional aspect of ROS/RNS has been less well studied: low levels of ROS/RNS can act as second messengers for signal transduction/amplification and fulfil specific intracellular functions. Key transcription factors regulated by ROS include, NF-κB, the Nrf2 and p53, AP-1 (c-Jun, c-Fos) [38–40].

7.3.2 Main endogenous oxidant sources

As previously mentioned, FRs are generated from both endogenous and exogenous sources. In contrast, ROS production basically relies on enzymatic and non-enzymatic reactions in an oxygen dependent living organism. Mostly enzymatic reactions able to generate ROS are those involved in respiratory chain, prostaglandin synthesis, phagocytosis, and cytochrome P450 system.

For instance, superoxide radical ($O_2^{\bullet -}$) is achieved by NADPH oxidase, xanthine oxidase, and peroxidases. A superoxide radical once created, is involved in several main reactions that in turn generate hydrogen peroxide, hydroxyl radical, peroxynitrite, hypochlorous acid, and so on. Also, hydrogen peroxide (a non-radical) is produced by multiple oxidase enzymes, that is, amino acid oxidase and xanthine oxidase. These ROS species formed in the cell are unfortunately extremely dangerous molecules. Thus, a hydroxyl radical ($OH^{\bullet}$), the most reactive among all the FR species *in vivo*, is generated by reaction of $O_2^{\bullet-}$ with H_2O_2, with Fe^{2+} or Cu^{+} as a reaction catalyst (Fenton reaction). Also, nitric oxide radical ($NO^{\bullet}$), which plays some important biochemical roles, is synthesized from arginine-to-citrulline oxidation by nitric oxide synthase (NOS). Moreover, NO synthases and cytochrome P-450 enzymes, when uncoupled, further contribute to endogenous oxidant production. Nowadays, more than thirty cellular (mitochondrial or non-mitochondrial) hydrogen peroxides-producing enzymes have been compiled in cells. As a result, also organic hydroperoxides composed of polyunsaturated fatty acids and radical attack contribute to the design of endogenous oxidants. This is because hydroperoxides are highly reactive functional groups, so they contain an oxidant (O–O bond) adjacent to a reductant (C–H bonds) [36–42].

Of course, higher immune cell activation, severe inflammation, ischemia, infection, cancer, excessive exercise, mental stress, and aging are all responsible for further endogenous ROS production. In addition, non-enzymatic ROS production can occur as well during mitochondrial respiration. Also, non-enzymatic reactions can be responsible for ROS production, that is, when oxygen reacts with organic compounds or when cells are exposed to ionizing radiation [36].

As now we well understand, living cells are constantly producing endogenous ROS. At the same time, ROS are a normal metabolic product and necessary to some degree.

7.3.3 Exogenous oxidant sources: exposome

The '*exposome*', conceptually and practically, ensures a holistic view of human health and disease. Success in mapping the human genome has supported the integral notion of the exposome. Also, the exposome can be defined as the measure of all the environmental exposures of an individual in a lifetime and how all those exposures relate to health.

So, exposome includes all exposures from our diets, our lifestyles, and our behaviors. It also includes how our bodies respond to these challenges. A person's FRs exposure begins before birth and also includes deformation from environmental and occupational sources. The whole of external FRs has been denoted as the 'exposome' [36, 42].

Another word, '*exposomics*' is the investigation of the exposome on the application of internal and external exposure evaluation methods. Internal exposure relies on fields of study such as 'genomics', 'metabonomics,' 'lipidomics', 'transcriptomics', and 'proteomics'. Exogenous FRs production can occur as a result of exposure to environmental pollutants, heavy metals, certain drugs, chemical solvents, cooking, cigarette smoke, alcohol, and radiations.

When these exogenous compounds penetrate the body, they are metabolized, and FRs are generated as by-products. The '*exposome memory*' might find biomarkers such as measurement of telomere length or '*metabolic memory*', a new emerging field in molecular expression of epigenetic changes. Consequently, redox processes, and therefore OS, provide a prominent contribution to the human disease network, newly termed as the '*diseasome*'. After this part we will explain the effect of FRs on neurological diseases and especially on the development of MS [36, 43].

7.4 Oxidative stress in multiple sclerosis

Unfortunately, to date MS is a neurological disease of still unresolved etiology. But neuroinflammation and OS are very important elements in the pathogenesis of MS. It is certain that OS related harmful processes cause demyelination, axonal damage, loss of neurons over years, and consequently lead to neurodegeneration (figure 7.2). Many studies in the last two decades have stressed that alterations in the oxidant/ antioxidant balance contribute to the pathophysiology of MS. Further, this degenerative OS harm, mitochondrial injury, and energy failure may be involved in plaque formation and neurodegeneration in white and grey matter lesions in MS. Also, the presence of rising ROS in the nervous tissue may be neurotoxic; for example, peroxynitrite increases neuroinflammation and in the chronic phase leads to such a high ROS concentration that it may lead to neurodegeneration [25, 26, 35, 38].

MS is a multifactorial disease of the CNS in which both inflammatory and neurodegenerative processes occur simultaneously. Various forms of MS exist: RRMS, SPMS, and PPMS. The most common form of MS is RRMS which may

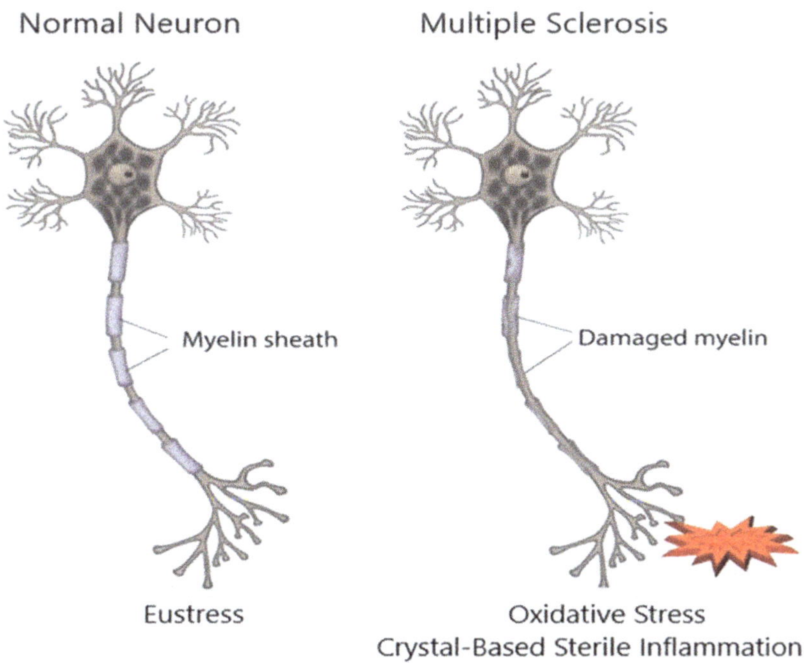

Figure 7.2. Oxidative stress and demyelination.

progress to SPMS after years of remission. However, in RRMS an inflammatory process dominates, while in SPMS and PPMS a neurodegenerative act is more strongly expressed. However, between the relapses patients fully or partially recover from the deficit. Interestingly, the examination of the cerebrospinal fluid (CSF) during exacerbation of MS has revealed a redox failure that was associated with an increased mitochondrial proton leak and an increased expression of genes involved in neurooxidative damage. Importantly, the neurodegenerative process is complicated and still poorly understood [25, 26, 44, 45].

7.4.1 General symptoms of oxidative stress

According to the medical literature, three primary factors initiate and propagate neuro-oxidative damage: the consumption of rancid fats, insufficient antioxidant levels, and strong ROS production. OS is most dangerous because it is the main precursor causing oxidative damage in a neuron. But interestingly, according to many scientific articles in medical literature, there are no officially recognized general symptoms of OS. However, some of the general symptoms of OS may include fatigue, headaches, noise sensitivity, memory loss and brain fog, muscle and joint pain, wrinkles and gray hair, decreased eyesight, and susceptibility to infections. As seen, most of the general symptoms attributed to OS concern neurons. However, OS has also been linked to several neurological diseases; such as MS. In MS, many experimental and clinical researches showed that neurooxidative damage plays a pivotal role in myelin loss and progression to MS. However, the relationship between neuroinflammation and OS is still poorly understood. Importantly, the CNS's cells are particularly vulnerable to oxidative damage since it has a very active mitochondrial metabolism, which leads to high levels of intracellular superoxide anions. So, cells of the CNS are very active in oxidative metabolism, as they are constantly exposed to low-to-moderate levels of ROS, and specifically these ROS are removed by antioxidants and antioxidant enzymes [43, 45, 46].

Of course, the CNS and neuronal tissue is very sensitive to the action of ROS owing to its very high demand for oxygen and a limited possibility of obtaining antioxidants. An imbalance between ROS production and antioxidative defense results in OS and nitrosative stress. Consequently, the more fat-containing neurons in their structures are more vulnerable to ROS attack. Researchers suggest that this disregulation of axonal bioenergetics plays a critical role in OS and subsequent axonal injury [35]. Two molecular mechanisms proposed to explain how ROS could specifically mediate neurologic diseases are the following:

(a) The lower levels of antioxidants in neuron can promote OS related neuronal damage, thereby raising the immune neuro-inflammatory processes in the neuron.
(b) In MS, the damage to myelin can be caused by non-quality activation of T cells which may be activated by ROS.

Undoubtedly, OS results with reduced activity of valuable neuronal antioxidant enzyme SOD and the increase in neuronal glutamine. This process is then followed by OH• and the production of hydroperoxides which ultimately has a negative affected on myelin. Thus increased ROS also reveal axonal damage. So, damage to axons is mediated by the following cascade; failure in mitochondrial energy metabolism due to inhibition of the respiratory chain by NO, which in turn causes a decrease in Na^{+}/K^{+} ATPase activity and alters Na^{+}-dependent glutamate transporters, over-expression of glutamate receptors, oligodendroglial excitotoxicity, massive influx of extracellular Ca^{++}, activation of proteases, and impaired axonal transport. In chronic inflammatory diseases, such as MS, antioxidant defenses are overcome, which leads to OS. Finally, chronic OS and ROS are involved in auto immune mediated tissue damage in MS also by inducing proliferation, inflammation and activation of astrocytes, microglia and T cells. The development of neurodegeneration in MS is a complex process that may be related to primary apoptosis, synaptopathy, and excitotoxicity associated with glutamate overload, ionic channel dysfunction, calcium overload, mitochondriopathy, proteolytic enzyme production, and activation of apoptotic pathways [20–26].

7.4.2 'OS memory' in MS

As mentioned before, MS is a neuroinflammatory disease of still unresolved etiology. An increasing number of studies on OS markers have been published on a number of neurologic diseases. However, the studies for MS disease are still quite few. Interestingly, persistent hyper activation of oxidative enzymes suggests an '*OS memory*' in such areas as chronic neuroinflammation. The brain tissue is very sensitive to the action of radicals due to its high demand for oxygen and a limited possibility of obtaining antioxidants.

The activation of microglia (specialized macrophages of the CNS) and mitochondrial dysfunction may play a particular role in CNS's OS memory processes. In particular, it is also important that mitochondrial dysfunction results in an increased production of ROS, which is harmful to neurons and glia in created OS memory [26].

Indeed, ROS are produced primarily by leakage of electrons in the mitochondrial respiratory chain in neurons. Increased ROS by activated microglia during the immune response gives a state of increased lipid peroxidation, and moreover, the oligodendrocyte cell is the cell most susceptible to damage by ROS. Then, microglia activated T-lymphocytes release proteolytic enzymes, cytokines, oxidative products, and free radicals. In addition, there is no doubt that macrophages have an important role in the creation of memory in OS in neurons. Also, the endogenous sources of ROS include mitochondria, peroxisomes, endoplasmic reticulum, and phagocytic cells. Indeed the inflammatory active MS lesion is characterized by the expression of ROS generating NADPH oxidase in microglia and infiltrating macrophages phagocytic cells. Macrophages constitute a major factor responsible for the production of ROS due to high oxygen consumption [20–26].

Meanwhile, the presence of markers associated with OS, such as lipid peroxidation, coincide with marked up regulation of antioxidant enzymes, such as SOD 1 and 2 in neurons. Overall, OS memory installed microglia has a number of antioxidative protective properties. On the other hand, increasing OS damages the mitochondria, which disrupts the transport of ATP along the axon, and consequently leads to neurodegeneration [2, 35].

Unfortunately, the ROS are generated by a number of cellular oxidative and metabolic processes including activity of the enzymes of the mitochondrial respiratory chain, xanthine oxidase, NADPH oxidase, monoamine oxidases, and metabolism of arachidonic acid mediated by the activity of lipoxygenases (LOX). Collectively, they all provide memory formation in OS; superoxide anion, hydrogen peroxide and hydroxyl radical. In addition, RNS are nitrogen-derived reactive species and include nitric oxide and peroxynitrite [47].

The ROS/RNS take electrons from proteins, lipids, carbohydrates, and nucleic acids, causing damage to neurons membranes, genetic material, and other macromolecules. Unsaturated fatty acids are the most vulnerable to ROS, and because myelin has a high lipid-to-protein ratio, it is a preferred target of ROS in MS. Recent observations confirm the fact OS became an important factor associated with the development of demyelination in MS. These processes cause demyelination, axonal damage, loss of neurons over years and consequently lead to neurodegeneration in MS. Despite all the considerable scientific information, the relationship between neuro-inflammation and OS memory is still poorly understood [26, 47, 48].

Unfortunately, oligodendrocytes have low levels of antioxidant enzymes and a high concentration of redox active iron. Redox active iron collection in the brain is of major importance in MS. This collection process leads to chronic OS, resulting in axonal and neuronal death. So, abnormal iron accumulation has frequently been reported in MS plaques.

Also, extracellular hemoglobin may harmfully lead to local OS through the globin radical which was responsible for myelin basic protein oxidative cross-linking and '*heme*' involved in lipid peroxidation. Also, myelin degradation may be the result of LOX mediated by peroxides. Ferrous iron may strengthen oxidative injury in the presence of FRs produced by the oxidative burst. A diffuse neurodegenerative process is related to the high iron content in the basal ganglia. In conclusion, the process of neurodegeneration depends on the liberation of iron from the myelin sheath during demyelination but the role of these specific toxic factors in the pathogenesis of MS remains partially elusive [47, 48].

Recent studies have suggested the importance of ceramides in the CSF as signaling molecules leading to impaired mitochondrial function. It was reported that the short-chain ceramides stimulated oxygen species production and led to neuronal death [49].

As OS has arisen among other culprits, anti-oxidative defense of the neurons has attracted more attention in the scientific area. For example, uric acid (UA), the most potent internal antioxidant is responsible for about 60% of total plasma antioxidant capacity. Two decades ago, the endogenous antioxidant UA was marked as a strong peroxynitrite scavenger. Previous data pointed out that peroxynitrite, as a marker of OS, also has a role in the MS evolution. Meanwhile, many studies in MS patients have shown an increase in the production of OS markers (such as cholesteryl ester hydroperoxides) and lower levels of UA [27].

However, the increase in ROS coupled with decreased antioxidant capacity is not enough to entirely explain the pathogenesis of MS. Many other scientific reports suggest that the loss of myelin nerve sheath is possible because the immune system participates in combination with defects in the mitochondria, and these defects cause the generation of ROS and RNS. Mechanisms of axonal damage are the consequence of the presence of TNF-α, matrix metalloproteinases, ROS, antibodies, increased glutamate, and aspartate, and these molecules cause excitotoxicity in MS patients. Under physiologic conditions, NO is produced from L-arginine by constitutive NO synthase (cNOS) and participates in a variety of important biological functions such as immunoregulation of inflammatory reactions, the downregulation of tumor necrosis factor (TNF)-α production, MHC II expression in macrophages, induction of apoptosis in CD4 cells, physiological regulation of the mitochondrial respiratory chain, inhibition of antigen presentation, and leukocyte adhesion and migration [10–15] (figure 7.3).

Chronic inflammation related macrophages and monocytes release ROS that degrade unsaturated fatty acids. However, during neuro-inflammatory reactions, exposure of macrophages to interferon (IFN)-γ and TNF-α results in the activation of the inducible isoenzyme of NOS, which increases up to 10 times the levels of NO. Releasing abundant RNS may have also been implicated as a mediator of demyelination of axonal damage in MS. interestingly, NO can produce a more damaging radical for neurons. The role of NO in MS is therefore complex, and in fact, peroxynitrite is definitely more toxic than NO [40, 48].

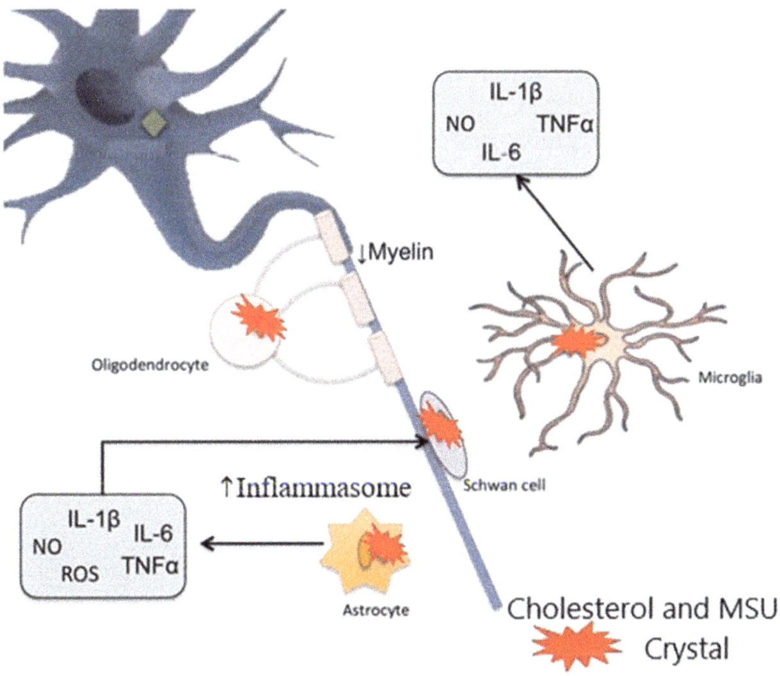

Figure 7.3. Crystal-based sterile inflammation.

Mature oligodendrocytes and astrocytes are highly sensitive to glutamate. Glutamate is increased in MS patients (active lesions), especially in white matter of normal appearance. Glutamate in turn may cause neurodegeneration through the different pathways and receptors in oligodendrocytes and astrocytes. It is possible to explain the role of mediators using an experimental model of autoimmune neuroinflammation in MS. These mechanisms produce glutamate excitotoxicity and increased generation of NO leading to '*nitrosative stress*' [50]. Only cells capable of generating a high flow of $NO^{\bullet}$ have the potential for causing nitrosative stress such as neurons. Finally, NO may be a highly toxic element that by itself blocks nerve conduction, especially in demyelinated axons, and stimulates apoptosis [48, 50, 51].

I would like to make a summary of the section. '*OS memory*', which plays an important role in the pathogenesis of MS, deserves further investigation in the coming years. In the evolutionary process of living things that has lasted for millions of years, human beings have been able to sustain their lives with success. Today, the penalty exacted by nature to humanity is an increase in chronic diseases for humans. Now people no longer suffer from plague or famine. Yet since the 20th century, humanity has had to struggle with nutritional abundance and environmental toxins. In the next section you will find that the abundance of nutrients can take place in the pathogenesis of MS.

7.5 Dangerous crystals

Neuroinflammation coexists sometimes with an immunological origin such as MS. Such chronic inflammatory response is generally referred to as sterile inflammation because microbial pathogens are not typically involved, but rather, the response is directed by damage-associated inflammatory inducers [1]. Sterile inflammation is linked to a plethora of inflammatory pathways within and outside of the CNS. Such triggering inflammatory pathways can be caused by endogenous molecules. Researchers have discovered a novel signaling pathway that plays a significant role in the pathogenesis of sterile neuroinflammation in MS [52].

Indeed, scientists have found cross-talk between cholesterol metabolism and inflammatory pathways and the immune system. This phenomenon is very important and may be relevant in relation to MS pathogenesis, as the immune system derangement is seen in MS. The best example of links between cholesterol and sterile inflammation is showed in atherosclerosis, where formation or uptake of cholesterol crystals in macrophages is involved [1].

7.5.1 History of cholesterol in MS

In the MS related neuroinflammation, there is harmful interaction between circulating cholesterol and the CNS possibly because of blood–brain barrier-breach (BBB-B). First, during the 1950s, scientists found in their studies that circulating lipoproteins were related in MS pathogenesis. Indeed they showed that a large proportion of plasma LDL-cholesterol can enter the parenchyma in MS plaques.

As long ago as 1970, many researchers found that enzymatic activity of lecithin–cholesterol acyltransferase was higher in the serum of MS groups than in controls. Also, the difference in the cholesterol levels between normal and demyelinated neurons in MS was noted in many research manuscripts. And many researchers reported that this raised cholesteryl ester, was in a higher amount around the demyelinated plaques compared with the normal-appearing white matter. As a result, cholesteryl ester accumulation in the brain is considered to be associated with neuronal demyelination during MS and similar demyelinating diseases. The whole mechanism for MS has yet to be clarifyed though. But today, the role of cholesterol in the pathogenesis of MS is better understood [53].

Cholesterol is an ambidextrous compound with many functions and important constituents of the lipid fraction of the human body. Also, cholesterol is a preferential, component in the nervous system. This implies that in order to cover the local requirement of the brain cholesterol, de novo synthesis is required. Almost, 25% of human total cholesterol is present in the brain. Inside the brain, cholesterol is available in two different pools. One pool of cholesterol is highly intensive, metabolically stable and present in high quantities (~70% of total residing in brain), mostly in myelin membranes of white matter, while the second pool is smaller in amount (~30% of total residing in the brain), but metabolically active.

However, because of the presence of tight junctions between brain capillary endothelial cells, only a small amount of nutritional lipids can reach to the brain from the periphery blood. Cholesterol is synthesized in the brain entirely in the isoprenoid pathway, and starts from Acetyl-CoA including a wide and energy-consuming pathway containing multiple intermediates and mediating enzymes [54, 55]. This synthesis is balanced mostly by the secretion of slightly hydrophilic 24*S*-hydroxycholesterol (which is synthesized by cholesterol 24-hydroxylase), predominantly mediated by the P450 enzyme and gene encoding CYP46A1, and it can easily pass the intact BBB. Cholesterol metabolism in the brain and cholesterol periphery differ in some important aspects; for example, in their half-life. Interestingly, the half-life of cholesterol in the neurons is between 6 months to 5 years, whereas that of periphery cholesterol is just a few days [54, 56].

The main part of cholesterol in the brain is present as free (unesterified) cholesterol, and set in myelin membranes with its primary function being in supporting myelin membrane growth and maintaining the insulator property of the myelin. However, lipids comprise over 70% of the myelin sheath. Assorted levels of cholesterol have been set in different types of MS. CNS cholesterol biosynthesis is high during development, and declines after myelination is complete. The auto-antigenic property of the cholesterol is possibly causing demyelination in MS. The unforeseen link between lipid metabolisms and demyelination provides opportunities for the development of regenerative medicines for re-myelination. As expected, it may be useful to reduce cholesterol synthesis *in vivo* in MS patients; for example, inhibition of the HMG-CoA-reductase has resulted in diminished demyelination and diminished neuroinflammation [54, 57].

7.5.2 Oxidative stress and cholesterol in MS

Experimentally, ROS and RNS, highly reactive lipid soluble mediators, play an important part in the neuroinflammatory demyelination. Undoubtedly demyelination is an important step in MS. As expected, it is reported that OS has been associated with demyelination in many reports by scientists [45]. During the process of the immune-mediated demolition of the myelin sheaths, cholesterol molecules in myelin are exposed to ROS resulting in the generation of oxidized derivatives of cholesterol, some of which are neurotoxic, possibly resulting into neuroinflammatory degeneration [58].

The feature of cholesterol to cross the BBB and finding a correlation between cholesterol and disease activity helps to form the hypothesis of the role of cholesterol and lipoproteins as a biomarker in MS. LDL in the brain is oxidatively modified in the MS plaque lesion and plays a major role in MS pathogenesis. LDL and its oxidized form (OxLDL) cause damage through OS triggering neuroinflammatory processes, as lipids, and especially the OxLDL, are the core agents of the immune response during acute neuroinflammation [54–58].

It is speculated that the MS disease processes start with increased migration of auto-reactive blood OxLDL across the damaged BBB. So, the dysfunction of the BBB in MS makes it leaky, and the danger is that OxLDL might find a way to enter the brain. However, the exact mechanism of how these dangerous lipids enter the brain is not completely understood yet. In addition, researchers found native LDL and degraded peptides of myelin basic protein to be co-localized within foamy macrophages in early and actively demyelinating MS plaques, which suggests OxLDL uptake by macrophages in MS plaques and possible demyelination. Scientists also reported that the macrophages from MS have increased production of superoxide radicals and H_2O_2 [58, 59].

In the experimental model for MS, it was seen that ROS, in particular H_2O_2, play a role in its pathogenesis. Also, dangerous lipids, including high cholesterol and high OxLDL, have a significant correlation with a higher level of clinical disability in MS. Oxysterols (hydroxylated cholesterol metabolites) such as 24*S*- and 27-hydroxycholesterol are endogenous ligands for the liver X receptor (LXR), thereby controlling the expression of genes involved in cholesterol efflux in cholesterol-loaded cells. Therefore, accumulation of these cholesterol waste product in phagocytes may pose a barrier for successful myelin regeneration [60]. For example, increased levels of 24*S*-hydroxycholesterol were seen in the active stage of RRMS, whereas the chronic stage disease was shown to have reduced levels of 24*S*-hydroxycholesterol in plasma. Although these results conclude that cholesterol and lipids could cause OS in the brain in the situation of BBB breach, and thus play an important role in MS pathogenesis, there is still potential for more investigation to be carried out to find out the exact mechanism behind MS pathogenesis. Cholesterol has been found to act in significant beneficial roles in brain improving and synaptic plasticity. A better understanding of how cholesterol exists in the CNS cells will help us to understand the harm potential of cholesterol in MS [54–59].

Th1 effector cell activation is of the accepted hypotheses of MS immune pathogenesis. For example, OxLDL is essential for main regulatory plasma T cells generation. Another useful example is given for 25-hydroxycholesterol; a cholesterol autoxidation product has been shown to amplify inflammatory signaling and regulate interleukin-1 as well as decreasing inflammatory activation in macrophages. There are other mechanisms in which OxLDL can cause neuronal damage. The action of the most abundant myelin further supports the notion of the possible auto antigenic property of OxLDL in neurons. Galactocerebroside is an immune-dominant myelin lipid, structurally similar to natural killer cells (NK) [58–61].

Another effective mechanism seems reasonable, as the oxidized lipid antigens, such as OxLDL and oxidized phosphatidylcholine, are noticed by cluster of differentiation1 (CD1) molecules, and these CD1 molecules are also found on microglia and some B cells [58, 59].

Therefore, the CNS's neurons meet their cholesterol main requirements through an ApoE-dependent mechanism. After synthesis of de novo cholesterol in the brain, glial cells secrete cholesterol, which is assimilated within ApoE for distributing to the neurons, and ultimately incorporated into the neuronal membranes. The therewithal for myelin debris clearance is also required cholesterol transporters, including ApoE. Likewise, ApoE is involved in the distribution and recycling of cholesterol during neuronal growth and death. Cholesterol cannot be broken down, it is transferred from the phagocytes back to the extracellular space via the transporters adenosine triphosphate–binding cassette (ABCA1 and ABCG1) in the plasma membrane where cholesterol binds APOE [54–62].

Recently, many studies have shown that the innate immune response in the brain is regulated by the cholesterol carrier, ApoE, by the suppression of microglial activity. It is so important, ApoE plays a principal role in the modulation of neuronal inflammation [61, 62].

Furthermore, ApoE modulates inflammatory and immune responses in an isoform-dependent manner. Therefore, the lack of ApoE induces a pro-inflammatory state overwhelmed with Th1 cells in subjects. This Th1 predominance in immune imbalance might favor MS basic pathogenesis. The protective effect of HDL cholesterol MS must also be studied more widely. Regeneration of myelin is possible, but in MS it is inadequate. Finally, in MS patients, overall down regulation of genes associated with cholesterol biosynthesis has also been seen, which further strengthens the opinion that the down regulation of cholesterol biosynthesis is related to demyelination in MS [54–58].

7.5.3 Myeline and cholesterol in MS

Neurons must have a sustained supply of cholesterol, because the myelin sheath is mainly formed of cholesterol, with the major lipid types being present in roughly equal proportions: glycerophospholipids, sphingolipids and cholesterol. Plenty of the lipids of the CNS are localized in myelin sheaths, neurons and glial cells, and therefore responsible for a number of key functions, such as synaptogenesis, neurogenesis and rapid nerve impulse conduction. In the inner leaflet of presynaptic membranes, the availability of cholesterol is almost eightfold higher than the outer side. This cholesterol concentration is, however, seen to reduce as we age. Recently studies have found that ApoE and the LDL receptor seem to influence the dispersion of cholesterol in the synaptic membrane bilayer. In fact neurons produce enough cholesterol to survive and grow, but the formation of countless mature synapses demands additional amounts that must be provided by glia cells [54, 62].

Therefore, cholesterol has been established as a rate-limiting factor for synaptogenesis in the CNS. It was also seen that cholesterol excited the neurons to form synapses. A likely explanation might be that cholesterol bound to ApoE containing lipoprotein particles is released by astrocytes and taken up by neurons, where it then encourages an increase in synapse number. These findings supply us with enough evidence to be confident that cholesterol indeed has a larger role in neurosignaling [63, 64].

The myelin formation plays a decisive role in the function of the neurons. The myelin sheath certainly cannot be synthesized without cholesterol, and cholesterol also helps in consolidating the myelin framework. Indeed, myelin is a specialized membrane enriched in cholesterol, which insulates nerve fibers so that electrical signals can be passed on quickly and efficiently. Besides, to facilitate the transport of action potentials, the distinct mission of myelin is the stabilization and organization of the axonal cytoskeleton. Disruptions in cholesterol homeostasis lead to an augmentation of inflammatory responses through increasing Toll-like receptors signaling. This abnormal cholesterol balance to cholesterol may be hazardous to the myelin. Unfortunately, in the pathologic situation, discordance in cholesterol balance may result in the dangerous accumulation of cholesterol in the myelin sheath. Moreover, cholesterol functions in the conservation of the axonal cytoskeleton in neurons. Internalized cholesterol is useful in the regional mounting of new axonal membrane, and thus participates in axon growth [54–61].

Today, cholesterol crystallization in structure of the neurons is considered to be a major factor in many neurological diseases believed to be worsening the violence of neuroinflammation and demyelinating diseases [63].

It can also withstand chronic degeneration of cholesterol, lymphocytes and macrophage-myeloid cells within the CNS, as well as microglia and astrocytes [63]. Although the suitability of lipid related immune mechanisms in MS is indisputable, it is not yet very well understood.

7.5.4 Oligodendrocyte and cholesterol

Cholesterol is not only necessary for myelin sheath formation, but also for oligodendrocyte maturation, and thus is relevant in much of the operation of CNS functioning. Oligodendrocytes are specialized glial cells that are responsible for myelination in the CNS.

Oligodendrocytes wrap several layers of their plasma membrane around axons to create myelin, providing electrical insulation to increase nerve conduction. A recently asserted hypothesis is that epigenetic changes within aging oligodendrocyte progenitor cells have been identified as possible mechanisms for cholesterol accumulation [4, 57, 64].

Oligodendrocyte and myelin development progresses along a typical chronological and topographic sequence, starting in areas related to basic homeostasis and progressing to regions controlling more complex functions in CNS [3, 64].

Scientists have found a new oligodendroglial cell type named BCAS1-positive oligodendrocytes. BCAS1-positive oligodendrocytes are found in the brain of newborns, which generate myelin at a high rate, whereas BCAS1-positive oligodendrocytes cells disappear in adults, but fortunately they can be re-formed when myelin has been damaged and needs to be regenerated. Moreover, Astrocytes are able to synthesize cholesterol tenfold higher as compared with neuronal cells, and they take over the cholesterol synthesis in adulthood. But oligodendrocytes are responsible for a strong increase in brain cholesterol content during myelination, with its peak throughout the first postnatal weeks. Because the chemical structure of cholesterol is very suitable for sterile inflammation, crystalline cholesterol in the CNS may be responsible for myelin damage in the pathogenesis of MS [52, 64].

7.6 Cholesterol needle-shaped crystals and sterile inflammation in MS

What could be the trigger of sterile inflammation that could lead to damage to neurons? Each neurodegenerative disease comes with its unique pathogenesis and etiologies, although the inflammasome response has been implicated in several neurodegenerative diseases.

Such inflammatory damage generally may be mentioned as sterile inflammation because microbial pathogens are not typically involved, but rather, the inflammasome response is directed by damage-associated inflammatory inducers [3, 4].

Many studies conducted in recent years have identified mainly two endogenous trigger agents in MS. According to the findings, these endogenous triggers may be cholesterol crystals and monosodium urate crystals [63–66].

As is well known now, neuron's myelin contains a very high amount of cholesterol. Unfortunately, if too much cholesterol accumulates in the cell, cholesterol can form needle-shaped crystals, which cause damage to the cell. Recently, scientists hypothesized that the accumulation of cholesterol may overwhelm the cholesterol transport capacity of phagocytes, thereby forming a bottleneck for successful repair in the CNS. An overdose of cholesterol crystalline derived from myelin, which is not carried away rapidly enough by phagocytes can trigger chronic neuroinflammation that in turn impedes myelin regeneration. Consequently, crystalline damage might be an incessant irritation case in the neuronal sores. Myelin damage in the nerve cell may occur if the brain cannot get rid of these pointed dangerous crystals [63, 64].

The first crystalline irritation results in immediate myelin injury and potentially neuronal death, but unfortunately also triggers a secondary cascade of events such as ROS production, which further exacerbate neuroinflammation [63, 65].

So, in MS, there is a mechanical multifocal neuronal irritation related autoimmune attack against the myelin sheath in the CNS. However, of course, these dangerous needle-shaped cholesterol crystals are cleared by microglia and macrophages also referred to as phagocytosis. These sweeper cells take up the damaged myelin, digest it and transport the non-digestible remainder, such as damaged cholesterol, out of the cell by transport molecules. But how well these sweeper cells such as microglia and macrophages do their job depends on the age of the living organism. Aged phagocytes are accumulating unnecessary amounts of myelin debris, which initiated cholesterol crystal formation and phagolysosomal membrane rupture and stimulated inflammasomes. Age-associated decline in remyelination capacity limits the restoration of nervous system functionality after irritation. Thus, cholesterol-rich myelin debris can overwhelm the efflux capacity of phagocytes, resulting in a phase transition of cholesterol into more crystals and thereby inducing a maladaptive immune response that impedes tissue regeneration. It appears that the inability of aged phagocytes to clear the enormous amounts of cholesterol that are released from myelin after myelin breakdown in demyelinating diseases results in a phase transition of free cholesterol into crystals, inducing lysosomal rupture and inflammasome stimulation [63, 67].

7.6.1 Inflammasomes and MS

Although previous studies have suggested a T cell-based immunologic pathology, additional characteristics of MS include BBB-B, demyelination and oligodendrocytes and neuronal defects. Consequently, MS may be considered to be a T cell-mediated demyelinating disease which immunologically results in the demyelination and death of neurons. Although the progression and pathology associated with all crystalline related diseases vary, these inflammasome response diseases share commonalities in that their basic pathologies are heterogeneous and initiated by innate immunology [25, 50, 59].

In MS, the demyelination is considered to begin many years before the disease becomes clinically obvious, mainly because of the strong compensatory scavenging mechanism of neurons. For this reason, some scientists put forward that in aged individuals, there is less effective needle-shaped cholesterol crystalline clearance [54, 63]. More recently, a few studies have begun to validate the demyelination role of the inflammasome in neurodegenerative diseases. Inflammasome-driven demyelination and neuronal inflammation is postulated to play a role in MS, but there is no clearly direct evidence that the nucleotide-binding domain, leucine-rich-containing family, pyrin domain-containing-3 or nod-like receptor protein 3 (NLRP3) inflammasome is involved in MS demyelination [65]. So, the inflammasome represents a potential critical mediator of neuro-inflammation and a potential therapeutic target of neurodegenerative diseases. Thus, cholesterol derived from myelin debris can activate the NLRP3 inflammasome in macrophages when toxic levels build up intracellularly in the absence of sufficient lipoprotein carriers. This could be a genuinely exciting approach because of the sterile neuro-inflammation that exists. Basically, the NLRP3 inflammasome can be activated by a broad range of stimulators, including pathogens, crystalline form of cholesterol and UA. In the last two years, a few studies have linked the NLRP3 inflammasome to neurological disorders such as MS. No doubt inflammasomes provide substantial new information about the pathogenesis of MS. Eventually, dangerous crystalline molecules activate the so-called inflammasome in phagocytes, which results in the release of inflammatory mediators, attracting even more immune cells [65, 67, 68]. Very similar problems occur in arteriosclerosis, but also in CNS, not only in blood vessels. Likewise, in atherosclerosis, irrigative needle-shaped cholesterol crystals may be able to induce inflammation by phagolysosome membrane rupture and subsequent stimulation of the caspase-1-activating NLRP3 inflammasome and secretion of IL-1 cytokines [67, 68]. Toxic overload of cholesterol drives the formation of foamy macrophages and maladaptive immune responses in atherosclerosis [1].

Hereby, NLRP3 may form a vicious cycle that causes myelin damage in CNS. Now a well known type amongst the inflammasomes, NLRP3 appears to play the strongest pathogenic role in MS. Also, other inflammasome-forming NLRs such as NLRP1 may play a role in MS but their functional role will need to be further elucidated [3, 4, 68].

Remyelination restores rapid transmission of nerve impulses and axonal function in MS. Certainly, the regeneration of intact myelin sheaths is a necessary prerequisite for patients to recover from MS relapses. Although remyelination can occur in MS, age-associated decline in myelin repair contributes to chronic progressive disease and disability.

Certainly, the regeneration of intact myelin sheaths is a necessary prerequisite for patients to recover from MS relapses. Definitely recovery of myelin is conceivable; however, in MS it is insufficient. This is presumably one of the reasons persistent irritation and chronic inflammation occur in the needle-shaped crystalline lesions. More recently, researchers have now discovered that after the irritation of myelin by needle-shaped cholesterol crystalline it can trigger persistent inflammation which prevents regeneration, similar to that in arteriosclerosis. Let us examine this issue a little more broadly [13, 14].

Nucleotide-binding leucine-rich repeat containing (NLR), also known as NOD-like, receptors are a class of cytosolic sensors or receptors. These receptors that respond to a variety of pathogen associated molecular patterns (PAMPs), which are linked to various microbes as well as damage-associated molecular patterns (DAMPs), have a very interesting role in MS. So, NLRs may be classified into various subgroups each with their own unique responses to PAMPs and DAMPS. One of the most extensively studied classes of NLRs are the inflammasome-forming NLRs. Upon sensing DAMPs and PAMPs, these NLRs mediate the release of pro-inflammatory cytokines IL-1β and IL-18. The signal specificity and functional roles of inflammasome-forming NLRs have yet to be fully elucidated. However, there are more than 20 NLR genes in humans. The constitution of NLRs consists of a tripartite domain including a variant N-terminal effector domain, a central nucleotide-binding domain, and a C-terminal domain consisting of variable leucine-rich repeats [4, 13, 68].

Usually, functional inflammasome are composed of three proteins: a sensor (NLRP3, NLRP1, NLRC4, and AIM2), an adaptor [apoptosis-associated speck like protein containing CARD (ASC)], and catalytic proteins (pro-caspase-1, pro-caspase-8). The assembly of the three proteins results in the generation of a complex that mediates the self-cleavage of pro-caspase-1 and pro-caspase-8 to their active analogs. Caspase-1 and caspase-8 will then cleave the immature forms of the pro-inflammatory cytokines IL-1β and IL-18 into the mature bioactive forms. Previous studies using MS animal models have shown that the presence of inflammasome-associated proteins such as ASC, caspase-1, IL-β, and IL-18 may play an exacerbating role in the pathogenesis of MS. Although the certain etiology of the MS remains unknown, clinical studies have suggested that elevated expression of caspase-1, IL-1 β, and IL-18 may be associated with the susceptibility, progression, and severity of MS patients. The hyper-activation of IL-1β and IL-18 by an inflammasome-forming protein complex can lead to excess production of IL-1β and IL-18 cytokine production which can impact MS pathology [25, 52, 67].

Now the products that are formed, i.e. the cytokines, may be the abundant determinant molecules for the sterile inflammatory diseases. IL-1β is known to cause the proliferation of macrophages, and neuroinflammatory cells such as microglia and astrocytes. The cytokines IL-1β and IL-18 have been implicated in the pathogenesis of MS and MS models. These cytokines are critical in the proliferation of neuroimmuno reactive cell types such as microglia and astrocytes which are cell types that respond immediately to neuronal injury and death which may occur in all three MS disease states. These cells are mostly recruited to the site of damage or sterile inflammation within the CNS. Today in MS, it has been shown that the up regulation of caspase-1, IL-1β, and IL-18 associates with the progression and severity of disease. Consequently, regulation of IL-1β and IL-18 may play a major role in attenuating and or balancing the innate immune response during neuro-inflammation.

A few scientists reported that responsive MS patients treated with interferon-beta (IFN-β) had down regulated NLRP3 and IL-1β expression. The mechanism by which IFN-β works as a therapeutic has not been fully elucidated [61, 63, 65].

It has long been known that factors like IL-1β are key inducers of interferon regulatory factor 1 (IRF-1) expression, yet the biological significance of this activity was unclear until recently. Once activated, IRF1 induces potent chemokines that recruit most immune cells to sites of sterile inflammation in neurons. These findings support that MS is a chronic inflammatory demyelinating disease characterized by activation of immune cells and phagocytes involved in the autoimmune response [63, 65].

Caspase-1 expression, in particular, is elevated in MS plaques and, together with that of cytokines, in peripheral mononuclear cells of MS patients. Recent results, nevertheless, indicate that T cell intrinsic inflammasome activity can drive IL-1β and IL-18 production via caspase-8 activation independently from caspase-1 activation. Indeed: most but not all authors have found increases of IL-1β in the CSF of MS patients and IL-1β staining was shown to be localized to resident microglia or differentiated macrophages but not to infiltrating monocytes, suggesting that IL-1β expression is induced within the CNS [48, 66, 67].

IL-1β is known to promote the differentiation of naive CD4+ T cells into Th17 T lymphocytes, whereas IL-18 is a potent activator of polarized Th1 cells for IFN-γ production and lymphocytes proliferation. Notably, whereas augmented serum and CSF IL-18 concentration was shown to be present in MS individuals, not all authors have found increases of IL-1β in the CSF of these patients. The possible involvement of these cytokines in the pathogenesis of MS was reinforced by the observations that cytokines production by immune cells of MS patients is increased and that interleukins is expressed by oligodendrocytes in brain tissues from patients with active MS. There is also an added complexity in that the pathogenesis of MS may involve more than one inflammasome-forming protein in response to a multitude of signals (such as ROS), which occur concurrently during sterile neuroinflammation [3, 4, 63].

A crucial prerequisite for the development of therapies that promote repair is a better understanding of myelin formation. Nevertheless, the body's ability to regenerate myelin decreases with age. Recently, findings of researchers have demonstrated that axons with functional impairment, including axonal transport disturbances can still be remyelinated. Fortunately, when treated with a drug that facilitates the transport of cholesterol crystalline out of the cells, neuroinflammation was reduced and myelin was regenerated by repair of myelin damage caused by sterile neuronal inflammation. Needle-shaped cholesterol crystalline might also have a causal relationship in MS, although this still remains speculative [14, 22, 24].

In recent years, in a promising study, a small molecule, MCC950, was defined as the NLRP3 antagonist of IL-1b secretion. Inflammasome-forming proteins such as AIM2, NLRP1, NLRP3, and NLRC4 play a critical role in mediating the release of the cytokines IL-1b and IL18 and thus represent potential ideal therapeutic targets. The confirmation that inflammasomes functionally contribute to the demyelination process, the identification of other inflammasome-forming NLRs that are involved in MS and the design of therapeutics targeting these molecules may be a prime target to researchers in MS [69].

7.7 Monosodium urate crystals and sterile inflammation in MS

MS has a sophisticated pathogenesis with numerous pathogenic processes (including OS) that are not monotonously dispersed in patient populations. As mentioned above, autoimmune reactions in the CNS play a critical role in the chronic neuroinflammation and demyelination that occurs in MS. From a pathogenic point of view, MS is a heterogeneous condition consisting of neuroinflammatory, autoimmune, and neurodegenerative processes that are the result of an inappropriate activation of the immune system toward myelin '*self-antigens*' [3, 4, 7]. The role of UA in the CNS remains poorly understood. UA not only activates immune effectors in the innate and adaptive immune systems but also enhances antibody immunity [27].

Naturally, UA is a spontaneous product of the purine metabolic pathway, but it is also a principal endogenous danger signal released from injured cells. Recently, researchers showed that the expression of inflammasome proteins was up regulated upon MSU crystalline stimulation in neuron cells of MS patients [66].

So, UA was demonstrated to be one of the '*danger*' signals involved in the activation of NLRP3 inflammasome; notably, the concentration of UA is increased in the serum and in the CSF of MS patients. Indeed, UA can act as a DAMP and stimulate the mounting of the inflammasome and, thus, can be one of the suspects for the activation of inflammasome-responsive sterile inflammation in MS. Upon detection of dangerous signals from UA, the inflammasome sensor molecule induces a rapid polymerization of the adaptor protein ASC into large helical filaments, which represent the hallmark of inflammasome activation [27, 66, 69]. However, the availability of hyperuricemia in MS is not confirmed by all researchers, notably, though, even if a relationship has been shown between serum levels of UA and susceptibility to the disease, hyperuricemia was not observed in every analyzed cohort of MS patients [27].

NLRP3 inflammasome is therefore suggested to play a pivotal role in development of MSU neuroinflammation in MS. So, the canonical NLRP3 inflammasome requires caspase-1 activation for IL-1β and IL-18 processing. Thus caspase-1, IL-1β, and IL-18 upregulation was shown to associate with the progression and severity of MS, and caspase-1 expression was observed to be elevated in MS plaques and in peripheral mononuclear cells (PMNC) of MS patients. NOD3 inflammasome assemblies lead to the production of pro-inflammatory cytokines; IL-18, in particular, is an inflammasome-derived cytokine whose accumulation was observed to be increased in serum and CSF of MS patients [65, 66].

IL-18 is first synthesized as an inactive precursor; the precursor can be cleaved into the biologically active form of the protein, or can be stored intracellularly. Following its cleavage by caspases, the mature and biologically active form of IL-18 is secreted from monocytes/macrophages, even if over 80% of the IL-18 precursor remains unprocessed inside the cell.

Notably, IL-18 mRNA was significantly increased in MSU stimulated cells of MS patients. Secreted IL-18 initiates multiple signaling pathways and drives inflammatory responses, which result in demyelination or death. IL-18 plays an important role in Th1 response via its ability to induce IFN-gamma production in T lymphocytes and NK cells, and numerous reports confirm that Th1 responses directed toward self-antigens are activated in MS. Based on these data it is most tempting to speculate that, in MS, MSU would be responsible for the chronic activation of NLRP3 inflammasome and, as a consequence, the persistent activation of NF-κB and an excessive generation of proinflammatory cytokines [3, 65].

This importantly suggests that in MS patients a possibly MSU related prolonged and chronic stimulation would result in the up regulation of mRNA expression of NLRP3, ASC, caspase-8, and IL-18 genes. If this scenario is correct, therapeutic strategies aimed at inhibiting MSU formation and, as a consequence, down regulating inflammasome activity might result in clinical benefit in these patients [65–68].

7.7.1 Uric acid and OS in MS

The CNS is particularly susceptible to oxidative damage. The CNS's tissue is richest in lipids and highly oxygenated. Of course, the exact reason for reduced serum UA in MS remains unclear, and researchers might suggest a pathogenic role, an association with MS, or a consequence to MS. In particular, mechanisms of increased OS in MS have not been fully understood yet, and there is no clear evidence whether OS is a primary pathogenic phenomenon inducing MS progression or a consequence of MS activity [27, 70].

As OS emerges among other culprits, antioxidative defense of the human body attracts more attention. UA, the most potent internal antioxidant, is responsible for about 60% of total plasma antioxidant capacity. In 1982 scientists hypothesized UA as a primary defense against human cancer. They focused on the capacity of the UA to scavenge FRS and ROS high serum concentration in humans. Currently, UA is a potent antioxidant therapeutic option under research, not only for cancer but for any disease under the threat of OS. Interestingly, UA is a strong natural scavenger of ROS and RNS and has been found useful to treat animal models of MS. The retrospective study revealed that MS and gout diseases were almost mutually exclusive [27, 70, 71].

It has been observed that some patients with MS exhibit lower serum UA levels. The molecule circulates at high concentrations suggesting a rearrangement of major antioxidant UA in MS patients in order to keep oxidative/antioxidative balance. Hence, the inhibition of neuroprotective effects, as a result of low UA levels, is a possible mechanism for triggering the neurodegenerative processes in patients with MS. Moreover, it is likely that the inflammatory process could be related with the consumption of UA to remove the excess of FRs produced in MS, resulting in decreased concentrations of UA [27, 72].

As mentioned above, UA is the major internal source of antioxidants. The intermediate molecule of purine metabolism in most mammals, has become an end product due to a mutation in the corresponding gene in humans. Loss of activity in uricase enzyme blocks the flow of the metabolic process after UA. It seems to be an evolutionary step that warrants humans to host high UA levels, whereas higher ROS and RNS might play a key role in disease development by contributing to myelin and oligodendroglia degeneration, which are pathological hall marks of MS. The peroxynitrite as well as other species of FRs are involved in the inflammation, demyelination, and axonal damage process that occur in MS. The FRs production may increase the inflammatory response leading to increased neuronal damage. It has been proposed that peroxynitrite plays an important role in the demyelination process during MS progression by inducing lipid peroxidation of fatty acids in the myelin sheath produced by oligodendrocytes. Some studies have also suggested that UA is a strong peroxynitrite scavenger and antioxidant, while others have shown that UA reflects xanthine oxidase activity with its subsequent production of FRs and is associated with OS and glutamate-mediated excitotoxicity in neurological patients. UA is a natural scavenger of peroxynitrite, a toxic product of the nitric oxide and superoxide that induces inflammation, demyelination, and axonal damage that occur in the pathogenesis of MS [27, 66, 70, 71].

The majority of studies show a lower level of UA in plasma of MS patients. It is not known whether low plasma UA concentrations are a cause or a consequence of MS. There is a possibility that persons with low plasma UA levels are unable to prevent FRs generation and OS, leading to the development of inflammation and the destruction of CNS cells. Moreover, it has been proposed that MSU levels may be a clinical indicator of disease activity in patients with MS; nonetheless, the role of MSU in the disease pathology is unclear [66, 71].

In this regard, results of epidemiological studies have reported decreased serum levels of UA in patients with MS, supporting the hypothesis that UA is involved in the pathogenesis of MS, in a way that the reduced concentration of UA seems to be a biomarker rather than a consequence of MSU related demyelination. Conversely, the failure to achieve such a balance or failure to keep the balance may be the break point to an active state of disease. Oxidants and antioxidants are generally permeable molecules, and disease states that cause a shift in their levels in any media will probably cause a comparable shift in their physiologic levels in serum [27, 72]. The manipulation of serum antioxidant levels has become a popular strategy in the treatment of MS and a variety of diseases. Consequently, the efficiency of measuring OS markers in follow up of therapy should be investigated.

Scientists observed the therapeutic efficiency of UA treatment in animal models. This mechanism of axonal damage by ROS and reduction of natural antioxidants in the CNS could be related with the lower levels of UA in patients with MS. Nevertheless, whether the reduction of UA levels in active MS is a cause or consequence of disease activity is a phenomenon still uncertain. Female MS patients had even lower UA values than male patients. Also, it has been reported that administration of UA may be capable of reducing inflammatory demyelization in MS. Some experimental studies have described a decrease of inflammation in the CNS and of tissue damage, by UA administration in MS. Interestingly, inosine treatment, a UA precursor, induced clinical improvement and no disease progression in patients with MS. Finally, treatment of patients with a UA precursor, inosine, and prevented progression of MS in patients tested and improved the symptoms of some patients.

Recently, studies demonstrated that administration of glatiramer acetate for six months increases serum levels of UA in MS patients, suggesting a beneficial effect of UA as a natural peroxynitrite scavenger and mitigating disease activity. Thus, UA could decrease the inflammatory process in the CNS as well as tissue damage produced by ROS resulting in a lower progression of disability in MS [26, 72].

Moreover, MS patients host an excess of iron in their brains which is a potent catalyst for ROS formation. In the last ten years, several studies evaluated serum UA levels in patients with MS, reporting conflicting results. After all, there is still no consensus if UA is a protector or a risk factor in MS. It seems that the quantity and the duration of the concentration of the MSU in the CNS is essential for this answer. However, acute elevation of UA seems to be a protective factor, whereas chronic elevation seems to be a risk factor for MSU production. The contradictory results can easily be assigned to the highly organized complexity of the antioxidant defense system of the human body [27, 66].

The debate may sound much more reasonable considering the basics of the antioxidative defense system. The degree of external antioxidants like vitamin C, vitamin E or levels of internal ones like albumin or bilirubin, is a major determinant of MSU.

7.8 Conclusion

What we do not know about MS disease is much more than we know, but we must continue to look forward to the future, because scientific researches have helped us to better understand the main pathology of MS. The response of crystal-based sterile inflammation may constitute the risk of MS in the evolutionary process. Moving away from natural life and living in a toxic environment threatens humanity with chronic diseases. Cholesterol and UA crystals probably constitute the basic pathophysiological mechanism of MS. With all this information, we hope new MS treatments will probably be implemented in the near future.

References

[1] Eren E, Ellidag H Y, Aydin O and Yilmaz N 2015 HDL functionality and crystal-based sterile inflammation in atherosclerosis *Clin. Chim. Acta* **15** 18–23

[2] Bove R M 2018 Why monkeys do not get multiple sclerosis (spontaneously): An evolutionary approach *Evol. Med. Public Health* **2018**

[3] Lang Y, Chu F, Shen D, Zhang W, Zheng C, Zhu J and Cui L 2018 Role of inflammasomes in neuroimmune and neurodegenerative diseases: a systematic review *Mediators Inflamm.* **2018** 1549549

[4] Freeman L C and Ting J P 2016 The pathogenic role of the inflammasome in neurodegenerative diseases *J. Neurochem.* **136** 29–38

[5] Jiang X, Olsson T and Alfredsson L 2018 Age at Menarche and risk of Multiple Sclerosis: current progress from epidemiological investigations *Front. Immunol.* **9** 2600

[6] Valadkeviciene D, Kavaliunas A, Kizlaitiene R, Jocys M and Jatuzis D 2018 Incidence rate and sex ratio in multiple sclerosis in Lithuania *Brain Behav.* **28** e01150

[7] Patejdl R and Zettl U K 2017 Spasticity in multiple sclerosis: Contribution of inflammation, autoimmune mediated neuronal damage and therapeutic interventions *Autoimmun. Rev.* **16** 925–36

[8] Zeinali H, Baluchnejadmojarad T, Fallah S, Sedighi M, Moradi N and Roghani M 2018 S-allyl cysteine improves clinical and neuropathological features of experimental autoimmune encephalomyelitis in C57BL/6 mice *Biomed. Pharmacother.* **97** 557–63

[9] Ibitoye R, Kemp K, Rice C, Hares K, Scolding N and Wilkins A 2016 Oxidative stress-related biomarkers in multiple sclerosis: a review *Biomark. Med.* **10** 889–902

[10] Ohl K, Tenbrock K and Kipp M 2016 Oxidative stress in multiple sclerosis: Central and peripheral mode of action *Exp. Neurol.* **277** 58–67

[11] Barbour C *et al* 2017 Molecular-based diagnosis of multiple sclerosis and its progressive stage *Ann. Neurol.* **82** 795–812

[12] Misra M K, Damotte V and Hollenbach J A 2018 The immunogenetics of neurological disease *Immunology.* **153** 399–414

[13] Voet S, Prinz M and van Loo G 2018 Microglia in central nervous system inflammation and multiple sclerosis pathology *Trends Mol. Med.* 18 pii: S1471-4914(18)30223-5
[14] Lassmann H, Brück W, Lucchinetti C and Rodriguez M 1997 Remyelination in multiple sclerosis *Mult. Scler.* **3** 133–6
[15] Wingerchuk D M, Lucchinetti C F and Noseworthy J H 2001 Multiple sclerosis: current pathophysiological concepts *Lab. Invest.* **81** 263–81
[16] Briggs F B S, Yu J C, Davis M F, Jiangyang J, Fu S, Parrotta E, Gunzler D D and Ontaneda D 2018 Multiple sclerosis risk factors contribute to onset heterogeneity *Mult. Scler. Relat. Disord.* **28** 11–6
[17] Ransohoff R M, Hafler D A and Lucchinetti C F 2015 Multiple sclerosis-a quiet revolution *Nat. Rev. Neurol.* **11** 134–42
[18] Rolak L A 2003 MS: the basic facts *Clin. Med. Res.* **1** 61–2
[19] Medaer R 1979 Does the history of multiple sclerosis go back as far as the 14th century? *Acta Neurol. Scand.* **60** 189–92
[20] Didonna A and Oksenberg J R 2017 The genetics of multiple sclerosis *Multiple Sclerosis: Perspectives in Treatment and Pathogenesis [Internet]* ed I S Zagon and P J McLaughlin (Brisbane (AU): Codon Publications) ch 5, p 27
[21] Milo R and Kahana E 2010 Multiple sclerosis: geoepidemiology, genetics and the environment *Autoimmun. Rev.* **9** A387–94
[22] Saidha S, Eckstein C and Calabresi P A 2012 New and emerging disease modifying therapies for multiple sclerosis *Ann. N. Y. Acad. Sci.* **1247** 117–37
[23] Perga S *et al* 2015 Vitamin D binding protein isoforms and apolipoprotein e in cerebrospinal fluid as prognostic biomarkers of Multiple Sclerosis *PLoS One* **10** e0129291
[24] Wendel-Haga M and Celius E G 2017 Is the hygiene hypothesis relevant for the risk of multiple sclerosis? *Acta Neurol. Scand.* **136** 26–30
[25] Miranda-Hernandez S and Baxter A G 2013 Role of toll-like receptors in multiple sclerosis *Am. J. Clin. Exp. Immunol.* **2** 75–93
[26] Adamczyk B and Adamczyk-Sowa M 2016 New insights into the role of oxidative stress mechanisms in the pathophysiology and treatment of Multiple Sclerosis *Oxid. Med. Cell Longev.* **2016** 1973834
[27] Aydin O, Kurtulus F, Eren E, Ellidag H Y, Yılmaz N and Yaman A 2015 Balanced oxidative stress index in spite of decreased uric acid levels in multiple sclerosis patients *Neurochem. J.* **9** 153–8
[28] Sies H, Berndt C and Jones D P 2017 Oxidative stress *Annu. Rev. Biochem.* **86** 715–48
[29] Jones D P and Sies H 2015 The redox code *Antioxid. Redox Signal.* **23** 734–46
[30] Bortz W M 2007 We Live too Short and Die too Long: How to Achieve and Enjoy Your Natural 100-year-plus Life Span Rev. edn. (New York: Bantam Books)
[31] Betteridge J 2000 What is oxidative stress? *Metabolism* **49** 3–8
[32] Selye H 1936 A syndrome produced by diverse nocuous agents *Nature* **138** 32
[33] Selye H 1955 Stress and disease *Science* **122** 625–31
[34] Harman D 2009 Origin and evolution of the free radical theory of aging: a brief personal history, 1954–2009 *Biogerontology* **10** 773–81
[35] Matschke V, Theiss C and Matschke J 2019 Oxidative stress: the lowest common denominator of multiple diseases *Neural Regen. Res.* **14** 238–41
[36] Sies H 2018 On the history of oxidative stress: concept and some aspects of current development *Curr. Opin. Toxicol.* **7** 122–6

[37] Mattson M P 2008 Hormesis defined *Ageing Res. Rev.* **7** 1–7

[38] McCord J M 2000 The evolution of free radicals and oxidative stress *Am. J. Med.* **108** 652–9

[39] Hybertson B M, Gao B, Bose S K and McCord J M 2011 Oxidative stress in health and disease: the therapeutic potential of Nrf2 activation *Mol. Aspects Med.* **32** 234–46

[40] Galano A and Raúl Alvarez-Idaboy J 2019 Computational strategies for predicting free radical scavengers' protection against oxidative stress: Where are we and what might follow? *Int. J. Quantum Chem.* **119** e25665

[41] Stamati K, Mudera V and Cheema U 2011 Evolution of oxygen utilization in multicellular organisms and implications for cell signaling in tissue engineering *J. Tissue Eng.* **2** 2041731411432365

[42] Oliveira M F, Geihs M A, França T F A, Moreira D C and Hermes-Lima M 2018 Is 'Preparation for Oxidative Stress' a Case of Physiological Conditioning Hormesis? *Front. Physiol.* **9** 945

[43] Go Y M and Jones D P 2017 Redox theory of aging: implications for health and disease *Clin. Sci.* **131** 1669–88

[44] Nakamura J, Mutlu E, Sharma V, Collins L, Bodnar W, Yu R, Lai Y, Moeller B, Lu K and Swenberg J 2014 The endogenous exposome *DNA Repair* **19** 3–13

[45] Tarafdar A and Pula G 2018 The role of NADPH oxidases and oxidative stress in neurodegenerative disorders *Int. J. Mol. Sci.* **19** pii: E3824

[46] Dunham J, van de Vis R, Bauer J, Wubben J, van Driel N, Laman J D, Hart B A and Kap Y S 2017 Severe oxidative stress in an acute inflammatory demyelinating model in the rhesus monkey *PLoS One* **12** e0188013

[47] Palumbo S 2017 Pathogenesis and progression of multiple sclerosis: the role of arachidonic acid-mediated neuroinflammation *Multiple Sclerosis: Perspectives in Treatment and Pathogenesis* ed I S Zagon and P J McLaughlin (Brisbane (AU): Codon Publications) ch 7, p 27

[48] Adamczyk B, Niedziela N and Adamczyk-Sowa M 2017 Novel Approaches of oxidative stress mechanisms in the multiple sclerosis pathophysiology and therapy *Multiple Sclerosis: Perspectives in Treatment and Pathogenesis* ed I S Zagon and P J McLaughlin (Brisbane (AU): Codon Publications) ch 10, p 27

[49] Vidaurre O G *et al* 2014 Cerebrospinal fluid ceramides from patients with multiple sclerosis impair neuronal bioenergetics *Brain* **137** 2271–86

[50] Levite M 2017 Glutamate, T cells and multiple sclerosis *J. Neural Transm.* **124** 775–98

[51] Rajda C, Pukoli D, Bende Z, Majláth Z and Vécsei L 2017 Excitotoxins, mitochondrial and redox disturbances in Multiple Sclerosis *Int. J. Mol. Sci.* **8** 18

[52] Chandra A and Xu Y M 2016 Cholesterol: A necessary evil from a multiple sclerosis perspective *Clin. Exp. Neuroimmunol.* **7** 145–57

[53] Newcombe J, Li H and Cuzner M L 1994 Low density lipoprotein uptake by macrophages in multiple sclerosis plaques: implications for pathogenesis *Neuropathol. Appl. Neurobiol.* **20** 152–62

[54] Zhang J and Liu Q 2015 Cholesterol metabolism and homeostasis in the brain *Protein Cell* **6** 254–64

[55] Dietschy J M and Turley S D 2004 Cholesterol metabolism in the central nervous system during early development and in the mature animal *J. Lipid Res.* **45** 1375–97

[56] Mukhopadhyay S, Fellows K, Browne R W, Khare P, Krishnan Radhakrishnan S, Hagemeier J, Weinstock-Guttman B, Zivadinov R and Ramanathan M 2017

Interdependence of oxysterols with cholesterol profiles in multiple sclerosis *Mult. Scler.* **23** 792–801
[57] Zhornitsky S, McKay K A, Metz L M, Teunissen C E and Rangachari M 2016 Cholesterol and markers of cholesterol turnover in multiple sclerosis: relationship with disease outcomes *Mult. Scler. Relat. Disord.* **5** 53–65
[58] Toshniwal P K and Zarling E J 1992 Evidence for increased lipid peroxidation in multiple sclerosis *Neurochem. Res.* **17** 205–7
[59] Wang P, Xie K, Wang C and Bi J 2014 Oxidative stress induced by lipid peroxidation is related with inflammation of demyelination and neurodegeneration in multiple sclerosis *Eur. Neurol.* **72** 249–54
[60] Mailleux J, Vanmierlo T, Bogie J F, Wouters E, Lütjohann D, Hendriks J J and van Horssen J 2018 Active liver X receptor signaling in phagocytes in multiple sclerosis lesions *Mult. Scler.* **24** 279–89
[61] Hoppmann N, Graetz C, Paterka M, Poisa-Beiro L, Larochelle C, Hasan M, Lill C M, Zipp F and Siffrin V 2015 New candidates for CD4 T cell pathogenicity in experimental neuroinflammation and multiple sclerosis *Brain* **138** 902–17
[62] Gaillard O, Gervais A, Meillet D, Plassart E, Fontaine B, Lyon-Caen O, Delattre J and Schuller E 1998 Apolipoprotein E and multiple sclerosis: a biochemical and genetic investigation *J. Neurol. Sci.* **158** 180–6
[63] Cantuti-Castelvetri L *et al* 2018 Defective cholesterol clearance limits remyelination in the aged central nervous system. *Science* **359** 684–8
[64] Fard M K *et al* 2017 BCAS1 expression defines a population of early myelinating oligodendrocytes in multiple sclerosis lesions *Sci. Transl. Med.* **9** eaam7816
[65] Lang Y, Chu F, Shen D, Zhang W, Zheng C, Zhu J and Cui L 2018 Role of inflammasomes in neuroimmune and neurodegenerative diseases: a systematic review *Mediat. Inflamm.* 2018 1549549
[66] Piancone F, Saresella M, Marventano I, La Rosa F, Santangelo M A, Caputo D, Mendozzi L, Rovaris M and Clerici M 2018 Monosodium urate crystals activate the inflammasome in primary progressive Multiple Sclerosis *Front. Immunol.* **9** 983
[67] Freeman L, Guo H, David C N, Brickey W J, Jha S and Ting J P 2017 NLR members NLRC4 and NLRP3 mediate sterile inflammasome activation in microglia and astrocytes *J. Exp. Med.* **214** 1351–70
[68] Alcocer-Gómez E, Castejón-Vega B, López-Sánchez M and Cordero M D 2018 Inflammasomes in clinical practice: a brief introduction *Exp. Suppl.* **108** 1–8
[69] Xu L, Zhang C, Jiang N, He D, Bai Y and Xin Y 2018 Rapamycin combined with MCC950 to treat multiple sclerosis in experimental autoimmune encephalomyelitis *J. Cell. Biochem.* 15
[70] Simental-Mendía E, Simental-Mendía L E and Guerrero-Romero F 2017 Serum uric acid concentrations are directly associated with the presence of benign multiple sclerosis *Neurol. Sci.* **38** 1665–9
[71] Moccia M *et al* 2015 Uric acid in relapsing-remitting multiple sclerosis: a 2-year longitudinal study *J. Neurol.* **262** 961–7
[72] Velazquez-Villoria D, Macia-Badia C, Segura-García A, Pastor Idoate S, Arcos-Algaba G, Velez-Escola L and García-Arumí J 2017 Efficacy of immunomodulatory therapy with interferon-β or glatiramer acetate on multiple sclerosis-associated uveitis *Arch. Soc. Esp. Oftalmol.* **92** 273–79

IOP Publishing

Neurological Disorders and Imaging Physics, Volume 2
Engineering and clinical perspectives of multiple sclerosis
Ayman El-Baz and Jasjit S Suri

Chapter 8

The influence of auditory neuroprosthetics on gait and postural recovery in multiple sclerosis

Shashank Ghai and Ishan Ghai

Auditory neuroprosthetics are commonly employed to facilitate motor performance in several movement disorders. Interventions like rhythmic auditory cueing and real-time auditory feedback (sonification) have shown to facilitate gait and postural performance in patients with Parkinson's disease, cerebral palsy, stroke and more. It is presumed that the 'entrainment effect' generated by these external stimulations can enhance auditory motor coupling and instigate neuralplasticity. Nevertheless, a joint consensus concerning the influence of auditory neuroprosthetics on motor performance in patients with multiple sclerosis (MS) was lacking. Recently, a review and meta-analyses study by our group presented the current state of evidence for the beneficial influence of external auditory stimulations on gait and postural performance in patients with MS. This chapter outlines the pathophyiological mechanisms associated with cognitive and motor decline in patients with MS. Further, preliminary qualitative and quantitative data is presented that supports the incorporation of external auditory stimulations in rehabilitation interventions for patients with MS.

8.1 Introduction

MS is an autoimmune, chronic and progressive neurological disorder that damages the myelin sheath of neurons in the central and peripheral nervous system. According to the Multiple Sclerosis International Federation an average of 2 million people are affected worldwide with this debiliating disorder [1]. According to recent epidemiological studies, the average total costs for treatment of a single patient across 15 countries is approximately 41 000 USD [1–3]. Furthermore, the disorder has been extensively reported to be one of the major causes of adult disability i.e. interquartile range for the age of onset of MS is between 25.3 to 31.8 years. This imposes consideable indirect costs in terms of socioeconomic factors, i.e. work loss. MS can considerably impair cognitive and motor functioning of a person, thereby

doi:10.1088/978-0-7503-1762-7ch8

making it extremely difficult for them to continue activities of daily living and work. On average, indirect costs among 15 countries have been reported to account for 13%–74% of total costs i.e. approximately 16 800 USD. In addition, intangible costs towards quality of life and early mortality have been reported to be significant yet non-quantifiable components of the economic burden of MS [1]. Genderwise, the data from World Health Organization reports that MS is more prevalent among females than males, i.e. male/female ratio is 0.5 [3].

8.1.1 Pathophysiology of multiple sclerosis

Inflammation is the primary cause of neurological damage in MS, however, specific elements that perceptuate its onset are still unknown (possibly autoimmune response against central nervous system antigens) [4]. The main pathological characteristics of MS include progressive demyelination, axonal dysfunctions, development of sclerotic plaques in parts of the central/peripheral nervous system, for instance, brain stem, cerebrum, glial scarring and reduction in the number of oligodendrocytes [5]. Due to dysfunctions in axonal connections nerve conduction is significantly altered with substantial variations in sclerosis and inflammation, thereby causing widespread neurological symptoms [6, 7]. Progressive MS is characterised by neurodegeneration of white, grey matter areas in both the central and peripheral nervous system. These atrophic changes are mainly as a result of chronic imposed hypoxia due to deficits in energy transfer because of mitochondrial dysfunction due to considerable deficits in nitric-oxide production and oxidative phosphorylation [8]. Moreover, ageing associated oxidative damage to myelin sheath and oligodendrocytes due to aggregation of iron can add stress on already impaired neurological structures.

Previously, research suggested that inflammatory changes were mainly limited to causing demyelination. However, recent pathological studies have found incidences of significant axonal pathology. For instance, on average more than 11 000 axons (transected) per mm^3 were identified in patients with early MS, whereas control brain tissue had less than one (transected) axon per mm^3 [9]. Characteristic lesions are located in the periventricular and juxtacortical regions, in addition to spinal cord and the posterior fossa involvement i.e. brainstem, cerebellum. Despite the progressive and constrictive behavior of this disorder, studies have optimistically supported the capability of oligodendrocyte progenitor cells for remyelinating damaged axonal sheaths in patients with chronic MS (also in white matter plaques) [10]. These observations suggest a strong potential for therapeutic interventions which can target recovery even during the late stages of the disease.

8.1.2 Gait and postural disorders

The episodic decline in sensory afferents, cognition, muscular strength, tone and incoordination aggregate and cause substantial dysfunctions in gait and postural performance. The disruptions in gait and postural performance have been reported to be predominantly due to dysfunctions in pyramidal track, cerebellar and spinal cord [11, 12]. Prosperini *et al* [13] for instance, reported lesions primarily in cerebellar, supratentorial associative bundles to affect the static and dynamic stability in patients with MS. Likewise, pathological involvement of leukocortical, intracortical and subpial regions have also been reported [14, 15]. Together, these sensory, motor and cognitive dysfunctions affect motor control and coordination [16], eventually promoting falls [17], and affecting the quality of life [18]. Literature suggests that a conventional gait pattern is exhibited with reduced gait velocity, stride length, cadence, and enhanced double limb support duration, step width, asymmetric gait [19, 20] (for a detailed review see [18, 21]). Moreover, corticospinal tract pathologies have been reported to further instigate general deconditioning that additionally affects energy expenditure during locomotion.

Furthermore, kinematic analysis of gait reports modifications for joint range of motions while performing gait. For instance, a greater range of motion at hip joint [22], increased knee flexion, reducing in ankle plantar flexion [23], and higher pelvic obliquity [24] have been documented for patients with MS. Further, EMG studies have reported increased musculoskeletal co-activation rates at the ankle joint [25]. Such modifications in kinematics and co-contractions have been reported to be as a result of cautionary measures adopted by patients for promoting stability during gait [26]. These modifications in gait execution are however executed with an intention to safeguard oneself from falling. On the other hand, these modifications promote a rather slow, uneconomical, unstable, and fatigue promoting gait pattern [27–30].

8.1.3 Conventional treatment strategies

Several rehabilitative interventions are utilized by healthcare practitioners to ameliorate postural and gait dysfunctions in patients with MS. Nevertheless, the aim of these interventions is to target specific neurological manifestations which aggregate and cause gait dysfunctions, for instance, weakness, incoordination, spasticity, sensory loss, cognitive deficits and more. Common treatment strategies to curb motor dysfunctions in MS include physical exercise [31, 32], training with virtual-reality [33], joint stabilizers (assistive devices), physical/occupational therapy [34], hydrotherapy [35], functional electrical stimulations [18], martial arts [36], dual-task training [37], and external sensory cueing [38, 39]. Please see table 8.1 for the symptom specific effect of interventions.

Despite the presence of several rehabilitation interventions the prognosis of patients with MS is very poor, especially in terms of gait and postural recovery. Evidence suggests that although the abovementioned rehabilitation approaches offer symptomatic relief from motor dysfunctions, this progress in terms of recovery is often very slow and imparts huge economic burden at both individual and social level.

Best practice principles in MS indicate that in order for an intervention to be effective it should possess the following properties:

(a) Individually-tailored
(b) Task-specific
(c) Meaningful
(d) Repetitive
(e) Challenging
(f) Cost-effective

Table 8.1. Illustration of dysfunction specific interventions for MS.

Dysfunction	Intervention
Spasticity	Physiotherapy, functional electrical stimulation, hydrotherapy, physical exercise, functional assisted devices, proprioceptive neuromuscular facilitation stretching
Sensory deficits	Virtual reality (enhanced optic flow), augmented reality, external sensory cueing/stimulations
Cognitive deficits	Dual-task training, music-based training, virtual reality
Paresis	Physiotherapy, functional electrical stimulation, hydrotherapy, (passive/assisted) physical exercise, assisted joint stabilizers
Muscular imbalance	Physiotherapy, functional electrical stimulation, hydrotherapy, physical exercise, assisted joint stabilizers, martial arts, proprioceptive neuromuscular facilitation stretching

A recent systematic review demonstrated that rehabilitation from music-based external sensory cueing/stimulations has the potential to meet such guidelines and principles, while yielding improvements in motor function [40].

8.1.4 Auditory cueing and stimulations

Previous studies have reported that the predominance of sensory dysfunctions in patients with MS plays a key role in disrupting motor control and coordination [41]. Disruptions in the perception of visual [42], and proprioceptive [43], systems have been well documented. Interventions utilizing additional sensory stimulations to facilitate movement execution might serve as a viable option to counteract this deficit. Only a handful of studies have analyzed the effects of external sensory stimulations (auditory, visual) on motor performance in patients with MS [38, 39, 44, 45]. The main reasons the efficiency of auditory feedback is considered to be superior are multifaceted. Firstly, rich neuroanatomical interconnectivity has been reported between auditory and motor cortex [46–48]. Here, inference can be drawn from literature evaluating auditory startle reflex on animal models [49, 50]. Studies using double-labelling experiments have revealed that cochlear root neurons in the auditory nerve can project bilaterally to sensorimotor paths, including synapsing on reticulospinal neurons [46, 49, 51]. Likewise, patterns of thalamocortical and corticocortical inputs unique to auditory cortex have also been reported (for a detailed review see [52]). In humans, neuroimaging data confirms the presence of cortico-subcortical network involving putamen, supplementary motor area, premotor cortex and the auditory cortex especially for perceiving and processing rhythmic auditory stimuli [53–56]. Secondly, the human auditory system can consistently perceive auditory cues 20–50 ms faster as compared to its visual and tactile counterparts [57–59]. Thirdly, the auditory system has a strong bias to identify temporal patterns of periodicity and structure as compared to other sensory perceptual systems [59–61].

In the literature, however, rhythmic auditory cueing [48], and real-time kinematic auditory feedback [62], also termed as sonification, are the most widely studied approaches in upper limb stroke rehabilitation. These methods impart differential effects over both neurophysiological and musculoskeletal domains. Neuroimaging data for rhythmic auditory stimuli suggests facilitated activations in premotor cortex, insula, cuneus, supplementary motor area, cerebellum and basal ganglia [54, 61, 63–65]. Moreover, training with rhythmic auditory cueing has been reported to modulate neuromagnetic β oscillations [66, 67], biological motion perception [62, 68], auditory-motor imagery [69–71], shape variability in musculoskeletal activation patterns [72], cortical reorganization, neural-plasticity [73, 74], and also movement specific re-investment [75].

Real-time kinematic auditory feedback on the other hand is a comparatively new approach. The feedback has been reported to alleviate sensory perceptions like proprioception [76], by enhancing sensorimotor representation while facilitating activations in action observation system [68], and inducing neural plasticity [77]. Moreover, the feedback has been reported by Effenberg *et al* [62] to extend the benefits of discrete rhythmic auditory cueing stimuli. Here, the authors suggest that the continuous flow of information might allow a participant to better perceive their movement amplitudes and positioning, thereby resulting in development of both feedback and feed-forward models [62]. Moreover, by allowing additional influence over the action observation system the real-time auditory stimuli might also enrich the internal stimulation of the executed movement [30, 62, 68]. This methodology involves delivering action relevant auditory feedback, where the characteristics of stimuli (e.g. frequency, amplitude) are mapped to the specific joint kinematics in real-time, for an example see [76]. Schmitz *et al* [68] in a neuroimaging study reported that observation of a convergent audio (sonification)-visual feedback led to enhanced activations in fronto-parietal networks and the action observation system, i.e. superior temporal sulcus, Broadman area 44, 6, insula, precentral gyrus, cerebellum, thalamus and basal ganglia [68]. The authors mentioned that the multimodal nature of the stimuli can enhance the activation in areas associated with biological motion perception and in subcortical structures involving striatal-thalamic frontal motor loop. This then might improve perceptual analysis of a movement, thereby resulting in efficient motor planning and execution [68].

In the systematic review, meta-analyses study by [40], the authors attempted to segregate relevant literature revealing the influence of external auditory stimulations on gait and postural performance in patients with MS. The following steps briefly outline the systematic review procedure utilized by the authors during their data accumulation and statistical analyses.

8.2 Methods

The researchers performed a systematic review and meta-analyses according to the guidelines outlined in Preferred Reporting Items for Systematic Reviews and Meta-analysis: The PRISMA statement [78]. They performed this systematic search across seven academic database. The databases included Web of Science, PEDro, EBSCO, MEDLINE, Cochrane, EMBASE and PROQUEST. Moreover, while including the specific studies of interest in the systematic review the authors also critically assessed the quality of the studies while using a PEDro (Physiotherapy Evidence Database) methodological quality scale [79]. The PEDro quality scale consists of 11 items addressing external validity, internal validity, and interpretability, and can detect potential bias with fair-to-good reliability [80], and validity [79]. The assessment and rating of the quality of the studies initially was done by the primary reviewer in a blinded manner completely independent of the second reviewer. Moreover, in situations where the ambiguous issues were encountered, discussions between the 1st (SG) and the 2nd (IG) reviewer took place and a consensus was reached. The studies were initially appraised, rated, and interpreted according to scoring of 9–10, 6–8 and 4–5 considered of 'excellent', 'good' and 'fair' quality [81], respectively. Inadequate randomization, non-blinding of assessors, no intention to treat analysis and no measurement of compliance were considered as major threats to biasing [82].

Table 8.2 provides a detailed list of the search terms utilized by the authors in their search strategy on EMBASE academic database.

While performing the systematic search across different databases, the authors followed an inclusion criteria for identifying the studies of interest. The inclusion criteria that the authors followed are mentioned as follows:

(a) Performed studies were either randomized controlled trials, cluster randomized controlled trials or controlled clinical trials.
(b) Studies reporting reliable and valid spatiotemporal gait parameters.
(c) Studies including static and/or dynamic aspects of gait stability.
(d) Studies qualified a minimal ration on PEDro methodological quality scale ($\geqslant$4 score) i.e. the studies were of at least 'good' quality.
(e) Studies were conducted on human participants.
(f) Studies were published in peer-reviewed academic journals.
(g) Studies were published either in English, German or Korean language.

However, the authors provided a narrative synthesis of the findings structured around the intervention, population characteristics, methodological quality and the type of outcome. This systematic review also included a meta-analysis approach [83], with an aim to develop a better understanding of the incorporated interventions [84].

In the included studies rhythmic auditory cueing was subjected to patients according to their comfortable cadence. The evaluated parameters while using a meta-analysis approach were spatiotemporal parameters of gait i.e. gait velocity, stride length and cadence. Likewise, dynamic postural stability was analyzed by computing the effects on a Timed 25-foot walking test. The presence and lack of

Table 8.2. Sample search strategy EMBASE (from [40]).

DATABASE	**EMBASE**
STRATEGY	**#1 AND #2 AND #3 AND #4 AND #5 AND #6**
#1	('rhythmic auditory cueing' OR 'rhythmic auditory cueing' OR 'rhythmic acoustic cueing' OR 'rhythmic auditory entrainment' OR 'metronome cueing' OR 'metronome' OR 'rhythmic metronome cueing' OR 'acoustic stimulus' OR 'acoustic cueing' OR 'acoustic cueing' OR 'external stimuli' OR 'external cueing' OR 'external cueing' OR 'music therapy' OR 'Neurological music therapy' OR 'tempo' OR 'beat' OR 'rhythm' OR 'RAC' OR 'NMT' OR 'real-time auditory cueing' OR 'sonification')/de OR (rhythmic auditory cueing OR rhythmic auditory cueing OR rhythmic acoustic cueing OR rhythmic auditory entrainment OR metronome cueing OR metronome OR rhythmic metronome cueing OR acoustic stimulus OR acoustic cueing OR acoustic cueing OR external stimuli OR external cueing OR external cueing OR music therapy OR Neurological music therapy OR tempo OR beat OR rhythm OR RAC OR NMT OR real-time auditory cueing OR sonification)ti,ab
#2	('MS' OR 'Multiple sclerosis' OR 'Acute fulminating sclerosis' OR 'disseminated sclerosis')/de OR (MS OR Multiple sclerosis OR Acute fulminating sclerosis OR disseminated sclerosis)ti,ab
#3	('walking' OR 'gait' OR 'locomotion' OR 'range of motion' OR 'ROM' OR 'ambulation' OR 'mobility' OR 'treadmill gait' OR 'balance' OR 'stability' OR 'stride' OR 'gait training' OR 'gait rehabilitation')/de OR (walking OR gait OR locomotion OR range of motion OR ROM OR ambulation OR mobility OR treadmill gait OR balance OR stability OR stride OR gait training OR gait rehabilitation);ti,ab
#4	('rehabilitation' OR 'treatment' OR 'rehab' OR 'management' OR 'therapy' OR 'physiotherapy' OR 'physical therapy' OR 'prevention' OR 'risk prevention')/de OR (rehabilitation OR treatment OR rehab OR management OR therapy OR physiotherapy OR physical therapy OR prevention OR risk prevention);ti,ab
#5	('age groups' OR 'adolescent' OR 'young' OR 'elderly' OR 'old' AND) ('gender' OR 'male' OR 'female')/de OR (age groups OR adolescent OR young OR elderly OR old AND (gender OR male OR female));ti;ab
#6	('intervention study' OR 'cohort analysis' OR 'longitudinal study' OR 'cluster analysis' OR 'crossover trial' OR 'cluster analysis' OR 'randomized trial' OR 'major clinical study')/de OR (longitudinal OR cohort OR crossover trial OR cluster analysis OR randomized trial OR clinical trial OR controlled trial);ti,ab

heterogeneity determined whether either random or fixed effect meta-analysis approach would be used [85]. The authors utilized CMA (Comprehensive meta-analysis V 2.0, USA) software to perform meta-analysis. Moreover, the authors also analyzed the extent of heterogeneity between the pooled studies while using

I^2 statistics. The authors reported effect sizes that were adjusted as Hedge's *g* [86]. The thresholds for interpretation of such 'weighted' effect size is as follows:

(a) Standard mean effect size of 0 means no change.
(b) Standard mean effect size of 0.2 is considered as a *small* effect.
(c) Standard mean effect size of 0.5 is considered as a *medium* effect.
(d) Standard mean effect size 0.8 as a *large* effect [87].

The interpretation of heterogeneity via I^2 statistics was as follows:

(a) Heterogeneity statistics at 0% were considered to be negligible.
(b) Heterogeneity statistics up to 25% were considered to be moderate.
(c) Heterogeneity statistics from 25%–75% were considered to have substantial heterogeneity.

Additionally, an analysis for publication bias was performed. The graph plots the evaluated weighted effect size i.e. Hedge's *g* values against standard error on a random effect model. For the statistical analysis a significance level of 0.05 was adopted.

8.3 Results

The systematic search across seven academic databases yielded a total of 602 studies. Thereafter, upon implementation of the inclusion criteria a total of five studies were left. Figure 8.1 illustrates the review procedure according to the PRISMA guidelines. In the five included studies, one was a randomized controlled trial, whereas four were controlled clinical trials.

In the five included studies a total of 188 participants were analyzed in the incorporated studies (144 females/ 40 males). All the studies evaluated a mixed gender sample size.

The average PEDro score for the five included studies were computed to be 5.2 out of 11, indicating fair-quality of the overall studies. One study scored 7, one scored 6, one scored 5, and two studies scored 4. Asymmetries concerning mean in the funnel plot might suggest bias (either positive or negative), in which case results are published. Figure 8.2 illustrates the results of publication bias outcome for the included studies.

Furthermore, the risk of bias across the studies for specific evaluated parameters during appraisal by PEDro scale has been illustrated in figure 8.3. likewise, table 8.3 mentions the individual PEDro score for each evaluated parameter on the scale.

8.3.1 Outcomes

The subjective outcome suggests a positive evidence for the beneficial influence of rhythmic auditory cueing on spatiotemporal gait parameters patients affected by MS. In the five included studies, they all reported significant enhancements in gait parameters with application of rhythmic auditory cueing. Table 8.4 mentions the

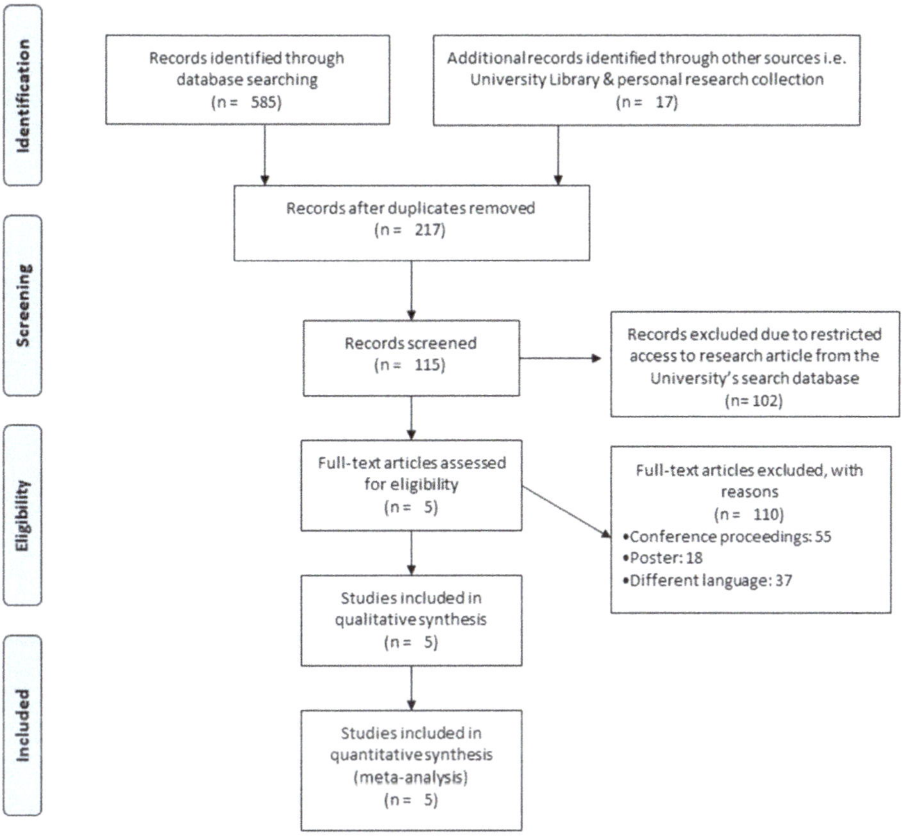

Figure 8.1. Illustrates PRISMA search strategy and the outcome. (Taken from [40]. CC. BY. 3.0.)

details for all of the included studies, their participant characteristics, PEDro methodology quality, research design, evaluated parameters, auditory signal characteristics and results.

8.3.2 Meta-analyses reports

8.3.2.1 Gait velocity (metre per second)

A meta-analysis was performed among three studies that evaluated the effects of rhythmic auditory cueing on gait velocity for patients with MS. The analysis revealed (figure 8.4) a *medium* effect size in positive direction with moderate heterogeneity (Hedge's g: 0.67, 95% CI: 0.14–1.20, I^2: 71.6%, $p = 0.02$).

8.3.2.2 Stride length (metres)

A meta-analysis was performed among three studies that evaluated the effects of rhythmic auditory cueing on gait velocity for patients with MS. The analysis revealed (figure 8.5) a *medium* effect size in positive domain with substantial heterogeneity (Hedge's g: 0.71, 95% CI: 0.17–1.26, I^2: 82.3%, $p = 0.03$).

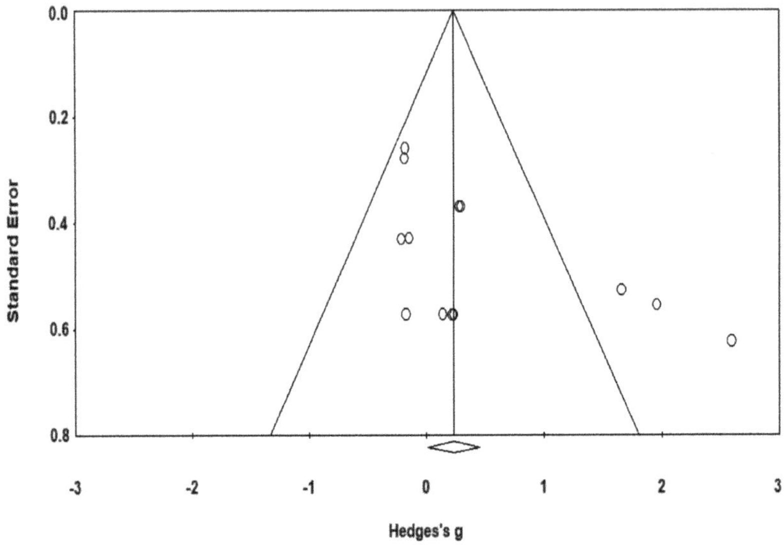

Figure 8.2. Funnel plot for Hedge's *g* and standardized effect for each effect in the meta-analysis. Each of the effects is represented in the plot as a circle. Funnel boundaries represent the area where 95% of the effects are expected to abstain if there were no publication bias. The vertical line represents mean standardized effect of zero. Absence of publication bias is represented when the effects should be equally dispersed on either side of the line. (Taken from [40]. CC. BY. 3.0.)

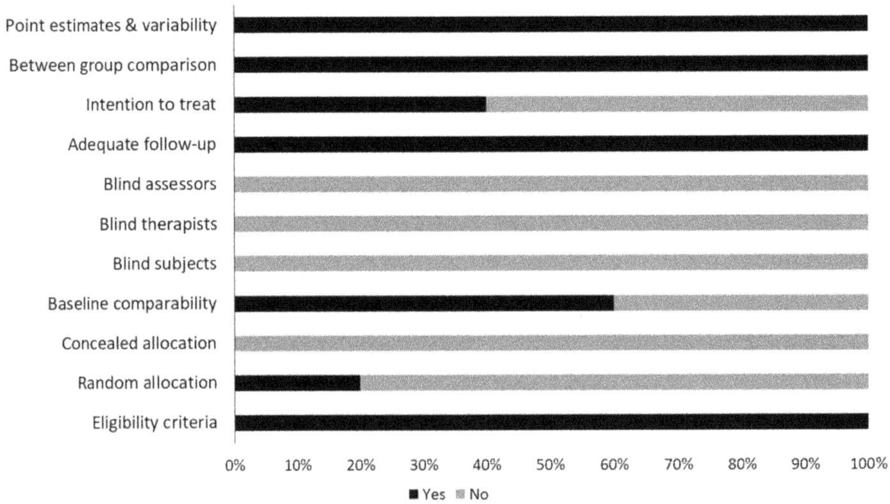

Figure 8.3. Risk of bias across studies according to PEDro quality scale appraisal. (Taken from [40]. CC. BY. 3.0.)

8.3.2.3 Cadence (number of steps per minute)

A meta-analysis was performed among two studies that evaluated the effects of rhythmic auditory cueing on gait velocity for patients with MS. The analysis revealed (figure 8.6) a *large* effect size in positive domain with substantial heterogeneity (Hedge's *g*: 1.00, 95% CI: 0.24–1.76, I^2: 70.3%, $p = 0.06$).

Table 8.3. Individual Pedro scores for studies (1: point awarded, 0: no point awarded). (Taken from [40]. CC. BY. 3.0.)

Study	Pedro score	Point estimates variability	Between group comparison	Intention to treat	Adequate follow-up	Blind assessors	Blind therapists	Blind subjects	Baseline comparability	Concealed allocation	Random allocation	Eligibility criteria
Shahraki *et al* [88]	4	1	1	0	1	0	0	0	0	0	0	1
Seebacher *et al* [89]	7	1	1	0	1	0	0	0	1	1	1	1
Seebacher *et al* [90]	6	1	1	0	1	1	0	0	0	0	1	1
Conklyn *et al* [44]	5	1	1	0	1	1	0	0	0	0	0	1
Baram and Miller [45]	4	1	1	0	1	0	0	0	0	0	0	1

Table 8.4. Studies analysing the effects of rhythmic auditory cueing on gait in patients with MS. (Taken from [40]. CC. BY. 3.0.)

Author	Research question(s)/ hypothesis	Sample description, age: (M ± S.D)	Assessment	Research design	Auditory signal characteristics	Conclusions
Shahraki *et al* [88]	Effects of auditory cueing on gait in patients affected from MS	Exp: 7F, 2M (40.3 ± 6.6) Ct: 7F, 2M (38.1 ± 12.1)	Stride length, stride time, double support time, cadence and gait velocity	Pre-test, gait training with rhythmic auditory cueing at +10% of preferred cadence for 30 min/session, 3 times/week for 3 weeks, post-test	Rhythmic metronome cueing at +10% of preferred cadence	Significant enhancement in stride length, gait speed, cadence in Exp as compared to Ct and after training with auditory cueing. Significant reduction in stride time & double support time after training with auditory cueing. Significantly reduced stride time in Exp as compared to Ct.
Seebacher *et al* [89]	Effects of rhythmic auditory cueing and motor imagery on gait in patients affected from MS	Exp I: 25F, 9M (43.8) Exp II: 29F, 5M (45.4) Ct: 31F, 2M (43.1)	Timed 25 foot walk test, 6 min walk test, multiple sclerosis walking scale 12, modified fatigue impact scale, short-form 36 health survey, multiple sclerosis impact scale 29 and Euroquol 5D 3L questionnaire	Pre-test, motor imagery training (internal gait simulation with fast gait, wider steps…) with rhythmic auditory cueing for 17 min' session, 6 times/ week for 4 weeks, post-test	Rhythmic auditory cueing at preferred cadence Exp I: Instrumental music: cueing at 2/4, 4/4 m, emphasis on 1st and 3rd beat. Exp II: metronome cueing at 2/4, 4/4 m, emphasis on 1st and 3rd beat.	Significant enhancement in 6 min walking distance in both Exp I and II after receiving auditory cueing, as compared to Ct. Significant reduction in timed 25 foot walking time, modified fatigue impact scale in

					Rhythmic verbal cues by researcher (heel off, toe off…)	both Exp I and II after receiving auditory cueing, as compared to Ct. However, Exp I had better benefits as compared to Exp II. Significant enhancement in short-form 36 health survey, MS impact scale 29 and Euroquol 5D 3L questionnaire i.e. quality of life, in both Exp I and II after receiving auditory cueing, as compared to Ct. However, Exp I had better benefits as compared to Exp II.
Seebacher *et al* [90]	Effects of rhythmic auditory cueing and motor imagery on gait in patients affected from MS	Exp I: 10F (47.3) Exp II: 7F, 3M (41.8) Ct: 5F, 5M (46.1)	Timed 25 foot walk test, 6 min walk test, modified fatigue impact scale	Pre-test, motor imagery training (internal gait simulation with fast gait, wider steps) with rhythmic auditory cueing for 17 min' session, 6 times/	Rhythmic auditory cueing at preferred cadence Exp I: Instrumental music: cueing at 2/4, 4/4 m, emphasis on 1st and 3rd beat.	Significant enhancement in 6 min walking distance in both Exp I and II after receiving auditory cueing, as compared to Ct. Significant reduction in timed 25 foot

(*Continued*)

Table 8.4. (*Continued*)

Author	Research question(s)/ hypothesis	Sample description, age: (M ± S.D)	Assessment	Research design	Auditory signal characteristics	Conclusions
				week for 4 weeks, post-test	Exp II: metronome cueing at 2/4, 4/4 m, emphasis on 1st and 3rd beat. Rhythmic verbal cues by researcher (heel off, toe off…)	walking time, modified fatigue impact scale in both Exp I and II after receiving auditory cueing, as compared to Ct
Conklyn *et al* [44]	Effect of rhythmic auditory cueing on gait in patients affected from MS	Exp: 3F, 2M (47 ± 10.5) Ct: 4F, 1M (50.2 ± 5.4)	Functional ambulation performance, double support percentage (right/ left), cadence, stride length (right/left), gait velocity, step length (right and left), norm velocity and timed 25-foot walking test	Exp: Pre-test, gait performance for 20 min per day for 4 weeks with rhythmic auditory cueing increased by 10% of attained cadence on every evaluation of test, post-tests at week 1, week 2, week 3, week 6 Ct: same procedure but rhythmic auditory cueing only for 2 latter weeks	Rhythmic auditory cueing in music at +10% of preferred cadence on each evaluation post-test	Significant enhancement in cadence, stride length (right/left), gait velocity, step length (right and left), norm velocity after training with rhythmic auditory cueing for 1 week. Significant reduction in double support percentage (right/ left) in Exp as compared to Ct.

Baram and Miller [45]	Effect of auditory on gait in patients affected from MS	Exp: 10F, 4M (48.5 ± 8) Ct: 6F, 5M (25.4 ± 1.9)	Gait velocity, stride length, 10 m walking test	Pre-test, followed by rhythmic auditory cueing and 10 min follow-up short term residual performance test	Rhythmic auditory cueing modified in real-time with steps	Significant enhancement in gait speed and stride length with rhythmic auditory cueing. Significant enhancement in short-term residual performance with auditory cueing.

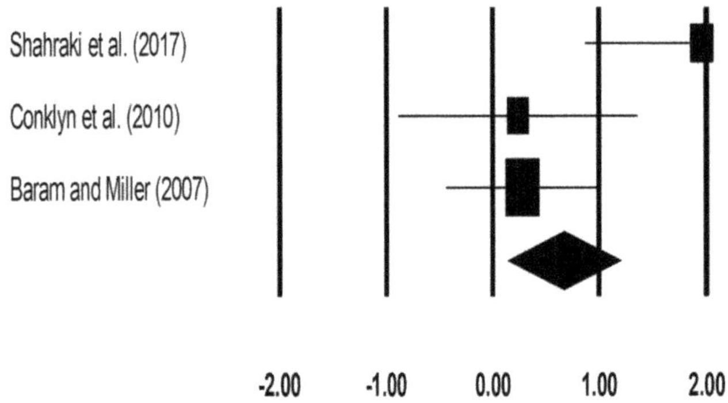

Figure 8.4. Illustrates forest plots for the studies reporting the effects of rhythmic auditory cueing, on gait velocity (metre per second) for patients with MS. Weighted effect sizes; Hedge's *g* (boxes) and 95% CI (whiskers) are presented, demonstrating performance for individual studies. The black diamond represents the combined pooled effect size and 95% confidence interval. (Taken from [40]. CC. BY. 3.0.)

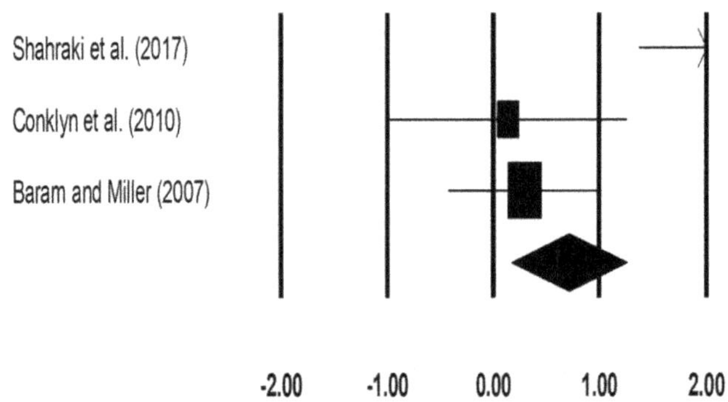

Figure 8.5. Illustrates forest plots for the studies reporting the effects of rhythmic auditory cueing, on stride length (metres) for patients with MS. Weighted effect sizes; Hedge's *g* (boxes) and 95% CI (whiskers) are presented, demonstrating performance for individual studies. The black diamond represents the combined pooled effect size and 95% confidence interval. (Taken from [40]. CC. BY. 3.0.)

8.3.2.4 Timed 25-foot walking test (seconds)

A meta-analysis was performed among three studies that evaluated the effects of rhythmic auditory cueing on gait velocity for patients with MS. Additional data was extracted from two studies. The analysis revealed (figure 8.7) a *small* effect size in negative domain with substantial heterogeneity (Hedge's g: −0.17, 95% CI: −0.48 to 0.12, I^2: 0%, $p > 0.05$).

8.4 Discussion

This systematic review and meta-analysis study by [40] presents the current state of knowledge for the influence of rhythmic auditory cueing on gait performance and dynamic postural stability in patients with MS. The review reports that all the included studies observed significant enhancements in performance of spatiotemporal gait parameters and dynamic postural stability post training with auditory

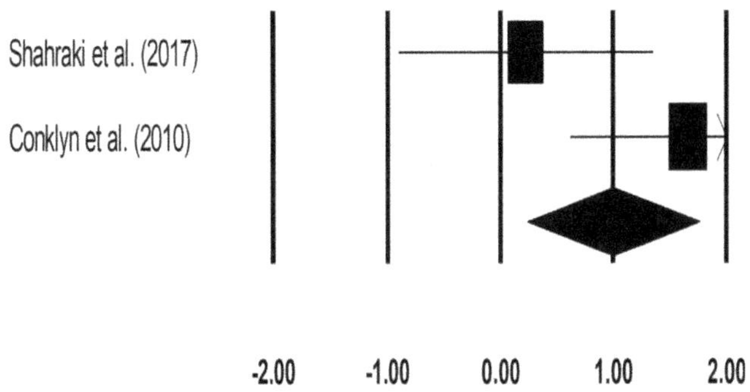

Figure 8.6. Illustrates forest plots for the studies reporting the effects of rhythmic auditory cueing, on cadence (number of steps per minute) for patients with MS. Weighted effect sizes; Hedge's *g* (boxes) and 95% CI (whiskers) are presented, demonstrating performance for individual studies. The black diamond represents the combined pooled effect size and 95% confidence interval. (Taken from [40]. CC. BY. 3.0.)

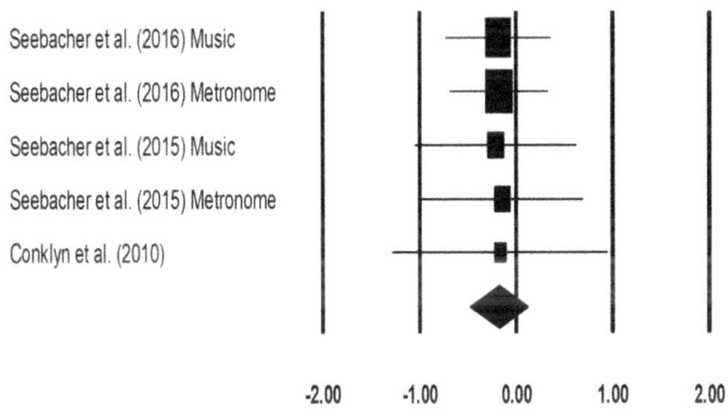

Figure 8.7. Illustrates forest plots for the studies reporting the effects of rhythmic auditory cueing, on Timed 25-foot walking (seconds) test for patients with MS. Weighted effect sizes; Hedge's *g* (boxes) and 95% CI (whiskers) are presented, demonstrating performance for individual studies. The black diamond represents the combined pooled effect size and 95% confidence interval. (Taken from [40]. CC. BY. 3.0.)

cueing. Moreover, the meta-analysis revealed significant *small*-to-*large* standardized effects suggesting the beneficial effects of rhythmic auditory cueing on spatiotemporal gait parameters.

Conventionally, MS has an adverse impact on spatiotemporal gait parameters [18] and dynamic postural stability. Muratori *et al* [91], for instance, have reported that reductions in gait velocity, cadence and stride length are strong predictors for reduced quality of life, and increased fall related morbidity or mortality. In addition, a strong correlation was reported by the researchers between gait velocity and the severity of MS (quality of life outcome). Similarly, step length and cadence had a strong correlation with the Community Balance and Mobility scale [91]. The current systematic review and meta-analysis reveals that training with rhythmic auditory cueing enhances gait velocity (Hedge's *g*: 0.67), stride length (0.70), and cadence (1.0). The evaluation of dynamic postural stability was done while using a Timed 25-foot walk test. This test has been characterized as an important predictor to determine quality of life by focusing on the functional independence of a patient and its impact on occupation and social life [92]. In the meta-analysis, a decrease in the Timed 25-foot walking test (−0.17) was observed, i.e. the patient needed less time to perform the test. Therefore, suggesting potential benefits of rhythmic auditory cueing for directly enhancing the quality of life and reducing morbidity/mortality ratios in patients with MS.

8.4.1 Neurophysiological impact

The underlying mechanisms due to which auditory cueing seems to facilitate gait and dynamic postural performance in patients with MS are not well understood [18, 39, 45]. Typically, MS is characterized with onset of movement disorders due to dysfunctions in white matter regions [18, 39, 93]. In this instance, inferences can be drawn for the beneficial effects of auditory cueing from studies analyzing the influence of auditory-motor training while playing musical instruments on white matter plasticity [94, 95]. Bengtsson *et al* [94], for instance reported that auditory-sensorimotor training can increase myelination due to increased neural activity in the fiber tracts during training. The authors reported significantly enhanced fractional anisotropic changes (usually reduced in MS [96, 97]) in corpus callosum, cortico-spinal, cortico-cortical tracts and the posterior limb of the internal capsule. Literature suggests that these neural structures are of critical importance when performing tasks incorporating fine motor performance, bimanual coordination, auditory processing and motor learning [98, 99]. Therefore, we hypothesize that training with auditory cueing could have enhanced the gait performance by facilitating the deficit white matter regions.

Moreover, previous studies for instance by Grimaud *et al* [93], have reported that involvement of deep gray matter regions such as basal ganglia is unusual in patients with MS [100]. Accordingly, literature reports that diffused neurodegenerative lesions in gray matter structures like, basal ganglia, thalamus are important precursors for contributing in development of neurological disabilities [7, 100–105], cognitive dysfunctions [104, 106], and the onset of fatigue [107, 108]. Accordingly, research has also revealed a strong correlation between the quantitative susceptibility mapping of putamen and caudate nucleus with the severity of disease [104], thereby suggesting larger involvement of gray matter structures with disease progression. Here, inferring from the literature pertaining to the beneficial influence of rhythmic auditory cueing on patients with Parkinson's disease (similar deficits in basal ganglia circuitry) offers an additional explanation to enhance gait performance, reduce the level of depression, anxiety and fatigue in patients with MS [57]. In this instance, the application of external auditory stimulations could assist in movement execution by providing an external cue to time movements. The external cueing can effectively bypass the deficit internal cueing pathway (cerebellum–putamen–thalamus–pre-supplementary motor area–supplementary motor area–primary motor area) through an alternative preserved pathway between (cerebellum–thalamus–parietal cortex–premotor area–primary motor area) and facilitate motor activity [57]. Figure 8.8 illustrates the neurophysiological change that could provide such enhancements.

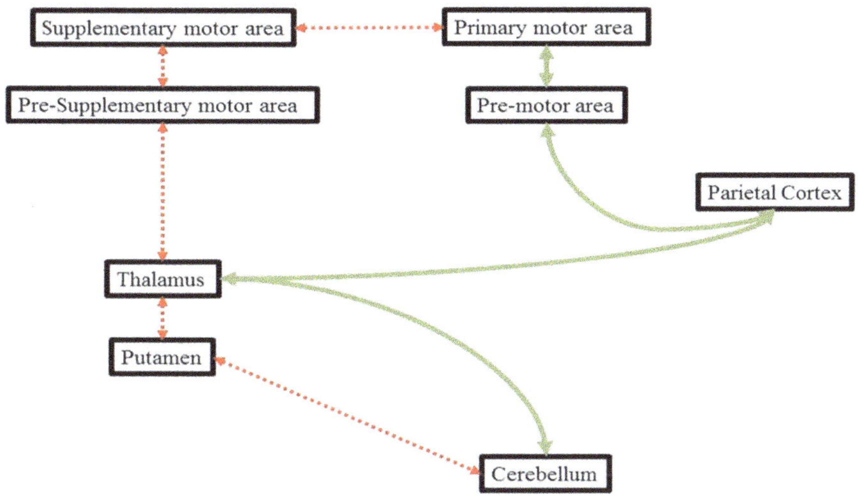

Figure 8.8. Illustrating the deficit basal ganglia circuitry (dotted red line) and how external cueing might bypass this deficit pathway via an alternative route (green line). Adapted from Nombela *et al* [57] and Ghai *et al* [29].

Furthermore, deficits in cerebellum (both grey and white matter regions [109]) have also been extensively documented in patients with MS [110, 111]. Music-based training interventions have been reported to impart beneficial influence in patients with cerebellar dysfunctions. Molinari *et al* [112] suggested that cerebellar dysfunctions such as in MS might impair the capability to consciously detect rhythmic variations for stabilizing motor response. However, the authors presume that unconscious effects to entrain movements with external auditory cues might still be preserved in such patients. Therefore, the motor entrainment to auditory cueing under such circumstances might be induced unconsciously, independent of cerebellar processing at either the spinal or the cortical level. Moreover, the external cueing might allow peripheral computation of the temporal information to execute movements. Thereafter, this information can then be transferred directly into adjacent motor structures, which entrain with the neural motor codes and allow enhanced synchronization between the auditory stimuli and motor response [112].

In addition, recent research findings suggest that application of auditory cueing can facilitate cortical reorganization in patients with MS [48]. To date, only one research has analysed the influence of rhythmic auditory cueing on cortical activation in patients with MS [113]. The researchers reported enhanced activation in the left superior frontal gyrus, left anterior cingulate, and left superior temporal gyrus after gait training with the application of rhythmic auditory cueing [39, 113]. This increased neuronal activation was further correlated with enhancements in executive functioning, auditory-motor entrainment, attention and motivation [48, 114]. Similarly, enhanced activations in inferior colliculi [115], brainstem [116, 117], sensorimotor cortex [118, 119], premotor areas [120] have been reported post application of rhythmic auditory cueing in other movement disorders such as stroke and Parkinson's disease. Enhanced activation in these neuronal structures could have also facilitated recovery in patients with MS.

Furthermore, modulation of neuromagnetic β oscillations (functional parameter for coordination between auditory-motor systems) with application of auditory cueing has been reported in auditory cortex, inferior frontal gyrus, somatosensory area, sensorimotor cortex and cerebellum [66]. This ability of auditory cueing has been recently demonstrated by Ross *et al* [67] to facilitate immediate neural plasticity by facilitating feedforward mechanisms. Studies also suggest that training with rhythmic auditory cueing might offer reorganization of cortical and cerebellar circuits [73]. Schaefer [121] for instance, suggested that auditory cueing infused with regularity and repetition of movement can result in an accelerated learning and neuroplasticity. Patients with MS have been reported to possess similar rapid-onset motor plasticity levels to that of healthy controls [122]. Together, the current state of evidence suggests robust potential of auditory cueing interventions to facilitate both gait and postural recovery in patients with MS. However, lack of conclusive evidence limits our interpretations, therefore future studies are strongly recommended to analyse these components in neuroimaging studies.

8.4.2 Physiological effects

Shahraki *et al* [88] hypothesized that external auditory cueing could also facilitate postural stability by stimulating the vestibular system (through medial geniculate nuclei—organ of Corti) [123]. The researchers reported substantial increments in spatiotemporal gait parameters with the application of external auditory in patients with MS. Likewise, Baram and Miller [45] too reported the beneficial aspects of external auditory cueing as compared to visual cueing. The researchers reported increased gait velocity with the application of external auditory stimulations (real-time) as compared to visual cueing. The researchers suggested that reduced reaction time (lower threshold for temporal perception by auditory system) facilitated increments with auditory stimulations during voluntary movements. Moreover, significant enhancements in stride length (8.3% versus 0.3%) were also reported with the application of real-time rhythmic auditory cueing. Moreover, the authors reported enhanced learning during residual performance (without auditory cueing) for both gait velocity (18.7% versus 2.4%), and stride length (9.9% versus 4.0%).

Likewise, based on the existing literature we strongly believe that the external auditory cueing could have also guided the gait of patients by explicitly synchronizing their ground contact and lift-off times [124]. The cueing could have allowed the patients to effectively plan their movements before executing them [125]. This could have also enhanced kinematic efficiency and reduced variability in musculoskeletal activation patterns post-training with rhythmic auditory cueing [28]. Similarly, modifications in tempi of the external auditory stimulation could have played a substantial role for facilitating gait performance and adaptations. In the current review, only one study [88] trained their participants with a faster tempo (+10%) of rhythmic auditory cueing as compared to tempo paired according to their preferred cadence. This 'change in tempo' characteristic, although not evaluated in the meta-analysis due to lack of data, can serve as a crucial factor in rehabilitation of gait. For example, change in tempo has been related with various neurophysiological changes, i.e. increased neuronal activation in frontal–occipital cortical networks [126], and increased excitability of spinal motor neurons (via reticulospinal pathways). Moreover, it has been reported that prolonged training with a constant pattern of rhythm can decrease fractal scaling of stride times from healthy $1/f$ structure [127–129]. Here, we strongly recommend the future studies to analyze the influence of modified tempo for auditory cueing on motor performance in patients with MS. We presume that changing the tempo regularly during training can promote the development of a stable, and adaptable gait pattern. From a rehabilitative perspective, teaching this adaptation pattern is very crucial as it might teach fall-prone patients to regulate gait speeds when passing through fall prone environments, e.g. traffic signals, escalators etc.

Another crucial aspect analysed in the current review is the effects of auditory cueing induced mental imagery in patients with MS [89, 90]. Labriffe *et al* [130] reported higher activations in primary sensorimotor cortex and secondary somato-sensory cortex bilaterally during the imagination of gait. The authors correlated the enhancements with facilitated activations in bilateral somatosensory area and right pre-somatosensory area during mental imagery of gait. This training regime seems plausible in patients with MS where physical fatigue is a major concern for medical practitioners [131]. Seebacher *et al* [89] in their randomized controlled trial, asked the patients to kinaesthetically imagine gait from the first-person perspective with music and metronome induced rhythmic auditory cueing [90]. Researchers reported that the ability to imagine movements is adversely affected in patients with MS, but this diminished ability can be counteracted with the application of external auditory stimulations. Further, their study revealed significant enhancements spatiotemporal gait parameters such as Timed 25- foot walking test, and 6 min walking test with the application of metronome/music-cued motor imagery groups. Here, comparable enhancements during the 6 min walking test in music-cued (512.6 m), and metronome-cued (533.9 m) groups as compared to control group (471.2 m) clearly demonstrate beneficial effects of training with auditory cueing for enhancing physiological performance, i.e. reduced fatigue. Similarly, improvements in MS related quality of life, pain, physical and mental health related quality of life were larger both in music- or metronome-based cueing groups as compared to a control group. We would like to propose that the beneficial effects of mental imagery here can also be effectively incorporated in home-based interventions. For example, fatigue can force patients with MS to train specific skill sets less and further adversely impact the prognostic outcome of the disorder. However, in such cases the patients can be taught to imagine themselves performing gait, while also imagining auditory cues. Previous studies suggest that the retention of enhancements in rehabilitation is dependent on how much the patient follows the treatment protocol at home [29, 30, 132].

One of the included studies incorporated a home-based training intervention with external auditory cueing [44]. Conklyn *et al* [44] utilized a simple mp3 player to deliver rhythmic auditory cueing for practising gait as a home-based intervention. Researchers reported significant increments in the performance of spatiotemporal gait parameters and also suggested enhanced patient adherence towards the intervention. This type of home-based intervention could possibly be beneficial for people lacking proper exposure to medical interventions in developing countries [133]. For instance, patients lacking effective medical resources can utilize smartphone devices with metronome applications for example Walkmate [128], Listenmee [134], or imagine gait with external stimulations or even imagine gait with auditory stimulations (joint audio-motor imagery).

Finally, a quantitative assessment for analysing specific training dosage could not be performed in this study because of the limited amount of data and substantial heterogeneity in between the studies. Nevertheless, four of the included studies used a training regime that lasted for more than 17 min per session and was performed for at least three times a week for more than three weeks [44, 88–90]. Likewise, based on the current evidence of training dosage for other movement disorders this dosage seems viable. Ghai *et al* [29] for instance, suggested a dosage of 25–40 min/session, for 3–5 sessions per week for patients with Parkinson's disease. Moreover, according to the findings of Bangert and Altenmüller [74] this training dosage seems plausible. The authors investigated cortical activation patterns during an audio-motor task and reported auditory-sensorimotor EEG co-activity after at least 20 min of training. Bangert and Altenmüller [74] speculate that this time frame is crucial for sensitive auditory monitoring, forming associations with the auditory target image in the working memory, during motor execution. Therefore, we suggest future studies to design training regimes with external auditory stimulations with at least 20 min training sessions.

The review by [40], presents preliminary evidence for beneficial effects of training with rhythmic auditory cueing on gait and postural performance in patients with MS. Our results are consistent with the findings of review studies suggesting the beneficial effects of rhythmic auditory cueing in the healthy population [30], and population groups with movement disorders such as parkinsonism [57], stroke [135], and cerebral palsy [136]. In conclusion, the findings from the review and meta-analysis by [40] recommend the incorporation of rhythmic auditory cueing for enhancing gait performance in patients with MS.

8.4.3 limitations

Two major limitations were identified in the present review.

(a) The meta-analysis in this study was performed on a limited number of studies. Although, the main aim for conducting a meta-analysis was to allow a better understanding of the effects of auditory cueing over different spatiotemporal gait parameters for medical practitioners, patients and future researchers.

(b) This present systematic review and meta-analysis was not pre-registered in a prospective register for systematic reviews, such as PROSPERO.

8.4.4 Future directions: applications of real-time auditory feedback (sonification)

Based on the current state of evidence which suggests beneficial influence of ecologically valid, action relevant auditory stimulations as compared to conventional isosynchronous metronomes, we recommend future studies to analyse the effects of such modified auditory stimulations on gait and postural performance in patients with MS. As mentioned before, MS is characterized by substantial deficits in sensory perception and therefore action relevant auditory stimulus delivered at higher than the usual threshold could impart beneficial effects for patients. Therefore, using ecologically valid action related sounds (walking on gravel, snow) conveying spatio-temporal information can possibly enhance saliency of sensory information for patients with MS [137–140]. Similarly, analysing the effects of methods providing real-time auditory information could possess considerable benefits for enhancing gait performance as well. This type of feedback allows converting the movement parameters in real-time to sound (mapping with pitch, amplitude). Here, the aim is to enhance motor perception and performance by targeting areas associated with biological motion perception [68, 141, 142].

Moreover, Effenberg *et al* [62] have shown that the synchronization of cyclic movement patterns with real-time auditory feedback can reduce variability and increase consistency of movements when compared with isosynchronous rhythmic stimulations [143]. According to Ghai *et al* [29] this feedback can enable the patients to identify their own movement amplitudes and compare their produced sound patterns with the sound of an auditory movement model, thereby creating a new auditory reference framework. This then can possibly allow a better comparison between instructed and intended movement while simultaneously amplifying the internal representation of movements [144]. We also propose future studies to compare different auditory signal characteristics, i.e. ecologically valid feedback, real-time kinematic feedback. This might provide important insights as to which type of auditory stimulations could allow multifaceted benefits for patients with MS from both psychological and physiological aspects.

Furthermore, combining the effects of auditory stimulations with music therapy could also yield additional benefits in both cognitive and motor recovery for patients with MS. For instance, Thaut *et al* [145] demonstrated that musical mnemonics can facilitate a stronger oscillatory network synchronization in prefrontal regions during a word learning task in patients with MS. The researchers proposed that the musical stimuli used in the study could have facilitated ‘deep-encoding’ while learning a skill set and could have also sharpened the timings of neural dynamics in neural networks which are usually affected due to the demyelination process in MS. Interestingly, research also suggests that this enhancement in cognitive performance is proportional as the disease progresses [145, 146]. Likewise, recently enhanced cortical reorganization and regeneration in areas associated with cognition have been reported post music therapy [147, 148].

Furthermore, beneficial effects of music therapy in patients with MS have also been reported on respiratory musculature [149, 150]. Developing efficient interventions that focus on both motor recovery while also facilitating respiratory efficiency could be crucial for enhancing the prognosis of patients with MS. Last but not least, it is important to consider the important psychological support that music therapy can offer to the patients with MS by reducing anxiety, depression, improving mood, self-acceptance and motivation [151–153]. The studies can also focus on analysing these psychological aspects during the training regimes as this might allow development of a multifaceted rehabilitation approach focussing on psychophysiological recovery of patients with MS.

Acknowledgements

This chapter includes excerpts from [40] published under CC-BY, version 4.0 in *Frontiers in Neurology* journal. Figures, tables and work included from the published article have been included after due permission from the original authors and the permission of *Frontiers*.

References

[1] Trisolini M, Honeycutt A, Wiener J and Lesesne S 2010 *RTI International. Global Economic Impact of Multiple Sclerosis* (London: Multiple Sclerosis International Federation)

[2] Chen H, Kwong J C, Copes R, Tu K, Villeneuve P J and Van Donkelaar A *et al* 2017 Living near major roads and the incidence of dementia, Parkinson's disease, and multiple sclerosis: a population-based cohort study *Lancet* **389** 718–26

[3] Koch-Henriksen N and Sørensen P S 2010 The changing demographic pattern of multiple sclerosis epidemiology *Lancet Neurol.* **9** 520–32

[4] Wingerchuk D M, Lucchinetti C F and Noseworthy J H 2001 Multiple sclerosis: current pathophysiological concepts *Lab. Invest.* **81** 263

[5] Lassmann H 2011 Review: the architecture of inflammatory demyelinating lesions: implications for studies on pathogenesis *Neuropathol. Appl. Neurobiol.* **37** 698–710

[6] Tallantyre E C, Bo L, Al-Rawashdeh O, Owens T, Polman C H and Lowe J S *et al* 2010 Clinico-pathological evidence that axonal loss underlies disability in progressive multiple sclerosis *Mult. Scler. J.* **16** 406–11

[7] Prins M, Schul E, Geurts J, van der Valk P, Drukarch B and van Dam A M 2015 Pathological differences between white and grey matter multiple sclerosis lesions *Ann. N. Y. Acad. Sci.* **1351** 99–113

[8] DeLuca J, Chelune G J, Tulsky D S, Lengenfelder J and Chiaravalloti N D 2004 Is speed of processing or working memory the primary information processing deficit in multiple sclerosis? *J. Clin. Exp. Neuropsychol.* **26** 550–62

[9] Cook S D 2001 *Handbook of Multiple Sclerosis* (Boca Raton, FL: CRC Press)

[10] Chang A, Tourtellotte W W, Rudick R and Trapp B D 2002 Premyelinating oligodendrocytes in chronic lesions of multiple sclerosis *N. Engl. J. Med.* **346** 165–73

[11] Calabrese M, Poretto V, Favaretto A, Alessio S, Bernardi V and Romualdi C *et al* 2012 Cortical lesion load associates with progression of disability in multiple sclerosis *Brain* **135** 2952–61

[12] Motl R W, Goldman M D and Benedict R H 2010 Walking impairment in patients with multiple sclerosis: exercise training as a treatment option *Neuropsychiatr. Dis. Treat.* **6** 767
[13] Prosperini L, Sbardella E, Raz E, Cercignani M, Tona F and Bozzali M *et al* 2013 Multiple sclerosis: white and gray matter damage associated with balance deficit detected at static posturography *Radiology* **268** 181–9
[14] Ontaneda D, Thompson A J, Fox R J and Cohen J A 2017 Progressive multiple sclerosis: prospects for disease therapy, repair, and restoration of function *Lancet* **389** 1357–66
[15] Peterson J W, Bö L, Mörk S, Chang A and Trapp B D 2001 Transected neurites, apoptotic neurons, and reduced inflammation in cortical multiple sclerosis lesions *Ann. Neurol.* **50** 389–400
[16] Thoumie P, Lamotte D, Cantalloube S, Faucher M and Amarenco G 2005 Motor determinants of gait in 100 ambulatory patients with multiple sclerosis *Mult. Scler. J.* **11** 485–91
[17] Matsuda P N, Shumway-Cook A, Bamer A M, Johnson S L, Amtmann D and Kraft G H 2011 Falls in multiple sclerosis *Phys. Med. Rehabil.* **3** 624–32 quiz 632
[18] Bethoux F 2013 Gait disorders in multiple sclerosis *Continuum* **19** 1007–22
[19] Preiningerova J L, Novotna K, Rusz J, Sucha L, Ruzicka E and Havrdova E 2015 Spatial and temporal characteristics of gait as outcome measures in multiple sclerosis (EDSS 0 to 6.5) *J. Neuroeng. Rehabil.* **12** 14
[20] McLoughlin J V, Barr C J, Patritti B, Crotty M, Lord S R and Sturnieks D L 2016 Fatigue induced changes to kinematic and kinetic gait parameters following six minutes of walking in people with multiple sclerosis *Disabil. Rehabil.* **38** 535–43
[21] Comber L, Galvin R and Coote S 2017 Gait deficits in people with multiple sclerosis: A systematic review and meta-analysis *Gait Posture* **51** 25–35
[22] Benedetti M, Piperno R, Simoncini L, Bonato P, Tonini A and Giannini S 1999 Gait abnormalities in minimally impaired multiple sclerosis patients *Mult. Scler. J.* **5** 363–8
[23] Nogueira L A C, Teixeira L, Sabino P, Filho H A, Alvarenga R M P and Thuler L C 2013 Gait characteristics of multiple sclerosis patients in the absence of clinical disability *Disabil. Rehabil.* **35** 1472–8
[24] van der Linden M L, Scott S M, Hooper J E, Cowan P and Mercer T H 2014 Gait kinematics of people with multiple sclerosis and the acute application of functional electrical stimulation *Gait Posture* **39** 1092–6
[25] Kelleher K J, Spence W, Solomonidis S and Apatsidis D 2010 The characterisation of gait patterns of people with multiple sclerosis *Disabil. Rehabil.* **32** 1242–50
[26] Wurdeman S R, Huisinga J M, Filipi M and Stergiou N 2013 Multiple sclerosis alters the mechanical work performed on the body's center of mass during gait *J. Appl. Biomech.* **29** 435–42
[27] Cofré Lizama L E, Khan F, Lee P V and Galea M P 2016 The use of laboratory gait analysis for understanding gait deterioration in people with multiple sclerosis *Mult. Scler. J.* **22** 1768–76
[28] Ghai S, Ghai I and Effenberg A O 2018 Effect of rhythmic auditory cueing on gait in cerebral palsy: a systematic review and meta-analysis *Neuropsychiatr. Dis. Treat.* **14** 43–59
[29] Ghai S, Ghai I, Schmitz G and Effenberg A O 2018 Effect of rhythmic auditory cueing on parkinsonian gait: A systematic review and meta-analysis *Sci. Rep.* **8** 506
[30] Ghai S, Ghai I and Effenberg A O 2017 Effect of rhythmic auditory cueing on aging gait: a systematic review and meta-analysis *Aging Dis.* 131–200

[31] Motl R W and Pilutti L A 2016 Is physical exercise a multiple sclerosis disease modifying treatment? *Expert Rev. Neurother.* **16** 951–60

[32] Rachel E S, Klaren E, Chiu C-Y, Kinnett-Hopkins D, McAuley E and Motl R W 2016 Levels and rates of physical activity in older adults with Multiple Sclerosis *Aging Dis.* **7** 278–84

[33] Massetti T, Trevizan I L, Arab C, Favero F M, Ribeiro-Papa D C and de Mello Monteiro C B 2016 Virtual reality in multiple sclerosis - A systematic review *Mult. Scler. Relat. Disord.* **8** 107–12

[34] Amatya B, Khan F, Ng L and Galea M 2017 Rehabilitation for people with multiple sclerosis: an overview of Cochrane systematic reviews *Cochrane Database Syst. Rev.* **2017** CD012732

[35] Castro-Sánchez A M, Matarán-Peñarrocha G A, Lara-Palomo I, Saavedra-Hernández M, Arroyo-Morales M and Moreno-Lorenzo C 2012 Hydrotherapy for the treatment of pain in people with multiple sclerosis: a randomized controlled trial *Evid. Based Complement. Alternat. Med.* **2012** 473963

[36] Burschka J M, Keune P M, Oy U H, Oschmann P and Kuhn P 2014 Mindfulness-based interventions in multiple sclerosis: beneficial effects of Tai Chi on balance, coordination, fatigue and depression *BMC Neurol.* **14** 165

[37] Ghai S, Ghai I and Effenberg A O 2017 Effects of dual tasks and dual-task training on postural stability: a systematic review and meta-analysis *Clin. Interv. Aging* **12** 557–77

[38] Baram Y and Miller A 2010 Glide-symmetric locomotion reinforcement in patients with multiple sclerosis by visual feedback *Disabil. Rehabil.: Assist. Technol.* **5** 323–6

[39] Bethoux F 2017 Functionality, music and Multiple Sclerosis *Altern. Complement. Ther.* **23** 125–8

[40] Ghai S and Ghai I 2018 Effects of rhythmic auditory cueing in gait rehabilitation for multiple sclerosis: a mini systematic review and meta-analysis *Front. Neurol.* **9** 386

[41] Rolak L A 2003 Multiple Sclerosis: It's not the disease you thought it was *Clin. Med. Res.* **1** 57–60

[42] Sakai R E, Feller D J, Galetta K M, Galetta S L and Balcer L J 2011 Vision in Multiple Sclerosis (MS): the story, structure-function correlations, and models for neuroprotection *J. Neuro-ophthalmol.* **31** 362–73

[43] Rougier P, Faucher M, Cantalloube S, Lamotte D, Vinti M and Thoumie P 2007 How proprioceptive impairments affect quiet standing in patients with multiple sclerosis *Somatosens. Motor Res.* **24** 41–51

[44] Conklyn D, Stough D, Novak E, Paczak S, Chemali K and Bethoux F 2010 A home-based walking program using rhythmic auditory stimulation improves gait performance in patients with multiple sclerosis: a pilot study *Neurorehabil. Neural Repair* **24** 835–42

[45] Baram Y and Miller A 2007 Auditory feedback control for improvement of gait in patients with Multiple Sclerosis *J. Neurol. Sci.* **254** 90–4

[46] Ermolaeva V Y and Borgest A 1980 Intercortical connections of the auditory areas with the motor area *Neurosci. Behav. Physiol.* **10** 210–5

[47] Felix R A, Fridberger A, Leijon S, Berrebi A S and Magnusson A K 2011 Sound rhythms are encoded by postinhibitory rebound spiking in the superior paraolivary nucleus *J. Neurosci.* **31** 12566–78

[48] Thaut M H, McIntosh G C and Hoemberg V 2014 Neurobiological foundations of neurologic music therapy: rhythmic entrainment and the motor system *Front. Psychol.* **5** 1185

[49] Nodal F R and López D E 2003 Direct input from cochlear root neurons to pontine reticulospinal neurons in albino rat *J. Comp. Neurol.* **460** 80–93
[50] Mirjany M, Preuss T and Faber D S 2011 Role of the lateral line mechanosensory system in directionality of goldfish auditory evoked escape response *J. Exp. Biol.* **214** 3358–67
[51] de la Mothe L A, Blumell S, Kajikawa Y and Hackett T A 2006 Cortical connections of the auditory cortex in marmoset monkeys: core and medial belt regions *J. Comp. Neurol.* **496** 27–71
[52] Read H L, Winer J A and Schreiner C E 2002 Functional architecture of auditory cortex *Curr. Opin. Neurobiol.* **12** 433–40
[53] Chen J L, Zatorre R J and Penhune V B 2006 Interactions between auditory and dorsal premotor cortex during synchronization to musical rhythms *Neuroimage* **32** 1771–81
[54] Grahn J A and Rowe J B 2009 Feeling the beat: premotor and striatal interactions in musicians and nonmusicians during beat perception *J. Neurosci.* **29** 7540–8
[55] Tecchio F, Salustri C, Thaut M H, Pasqualetti P and Rossini P M 2000 Conscious and preconscious adaptation to rhythmic auditory stimuli: a magnetoencephalographic study of human brain responses *Exp. Brain Res.* **135** 222–30
[56] Giovannelli F, Innocenti I, Rossi S, Borgheresi A, Ragazzoni A and Zaccara G *et al* 2012 Role of the dorsal premotor cortex in rhythmic auditory–motor entrainment: a perturbational approach by rTMS *Cereb. Cortex* **24** 1009–16
[57] Nombela C, Hughes L E, Owen A M and Grahn J A 2013 Into the groove: can rhythm influence Parkinson's disease? *Neurosci. Biobehav. Rev.* **37** 2564–70
[58] Spidalieri G, Busby L and Lamarre Y 1983 Fast ballistic arm movements triggered by visual, auditory, and somesthetic stimuli in the monkey. II. Effects of unilateral dentate lesion on discharge of precentral cortical neurons and reaction time *J. Neurophysiol.* **50** 1359–79
[59] Thaut M, Kenyon G, Schauer M and McIntosh G 1999 The connection between rhythmicity and brain function *IEEE Eng. Med. Biol. Mag.* **18** 101–8
[60] Repp B H and Su Y-H 2013 Sensorimotor synchronization: a review of recent research (2006–2012) *Psychon. Bull. Rev.* **20** 403–52
[61] Grahn J A 2012 See what I hear? Beat perception in auditory and visual rhythms *Exp. Brain Res.* **220** 51–61
[62] Effenberg A O, Fehse U, Schmitz G, Krueger B and Mechling H 2016 Movement sonification: Effects on motor learning beyond rhythmic adjustments *Front. Neurosci.* **10** 219
[63] Grahn J A, Henry M J and McAuley J D 2011 FMRI investigation of cross-modal interactions in beat perception: audition primes vision, but not vice versa *Neuroimage* **54** 1231–43
[64] Grahn J A 2012 Neural mechanisms of rhythm perception: current findings and future perspectives *Top. Cogn. Sci.* **4** 585–606
[65] Hove M J, Fairhurst M T, Kotz S A and Keller P E 2013 Synchronizing with auditory and visual rhythms: an fMRI assessment of modality differences and modality appropriateness *Neuroimage* **67** 313–21
[66] Fujioka T, Trainor L J, Large E W and Ross B 2012 Internalized timing of isochronous sounds is represented in neuromagnetic beta oscillations *J. Neurosci.* **32** 1791–802
[67] Ross B, Barat M and Fujioka T 2017 Sound-making actions lead to immediate plastic changes of neuromagnetic evoked responses and induced beta-band oscillations during perception *J. Neurosci.* **37** 5948–59

[68] Schmitz G, Mohammadi B, Hammer A, Heldmann M, Samii A and Münte T F *et al* 2013 Observation of sonified movements engages a basal ganglia frontocortical network *BMC Neurosci.* **14** 1

[69] Heremans E, Nieuwboer A, Spildooren J, De Bondt S, D'hooge A-M and Helsen I W *et al* 2012 Cued motor imagery in patients with multiple sclerosis *Neuroscience* **206** 115–21

[70] Heremans E, Nieuwboer A, Feys P, Vercruysse S, Vandenberghe W and Sharma N *et al* 2012 External cueing improves motor imagery quality in patients with Parkinson disease *Neurorehabil. Neural Repair* **26** 27–35

[71] Lima C F, Lavan N, Evans S, Agnew Z, Halpern A R and Shanmugalingam P *et al* 2015 Feel the noise: relating individual differences in auditory imagery to the structure and function of sensorimotor systems *Cereb. Cortex* **25** 4638–50

[72] Miller R A, Thaut M H, McIntosh G C and Rice R R 1996 Components of EMG symmetry and variability in parkinsonian and healthy elderly gait *Electroencephalogr. Clin. Neurophysiol./Electromyogr. Motor Control* **101** 1–7

[73] Luft A R, McCombe-Waller S, Whitall J, Forrester L W, Macko R and Sorkin J D *et al* 2004 Repetitive bilateral arm training and motor cortex activation in chronic stroke: a randomized controlled trial *J. Am. Med. Assoc.* **292** 1853–61

[74] Bangert M and Altenmüller E O 2003 Mapping perception to action in piano practice: a longitudinal DC-EEG study *BMC Neurosci.* **4** 26

[75] Rochester L, Baker K, Nieuwboer A and Burn D 2011 Targeting dopa-sensitive and dopa-resistant gait dysfunction in Parkinson's disease: Selective responses to internal and external cues *Mov. Disord.* **26** 430–5

[76] Ghai S, Schmitz G, Hwang T-H and Effenberg A O 2018 Auditory proprioceptive integration: effects of real-time kinematic auditory feedback on knee proprioception *Front. Neurosci.* **12** 142

[77] Dyer J, Stapleton P and Rodger M 2017 Transposing musical skill: sonification of movement as concurrent augmented feedback enhances learning in a bimanual task *Psychol. Res.* **81** 850–62

[78] Liberati A, Altman D G, Tetzlaff J, Mulrow C, Gøtzsche P C and Ioannidis J P *et al* 2009 The PRISMA statement for reporting systematic reviews and meta-analyses of studies that evaluate health care interventions: explanation and elaboration *Ann. Intern. Med.* **151** W65–94

[79] de Morton N A 2009 The PEDro scale is a valid measure of the methodological quality of clinical trials: a demographic study *Aust. J. Physiother.* **55** 129–33

[80] Maher C G, Sherrington C, Herbert R D, Moseley A M and Elkins M 2003 Reliability of the PEDro scale for rating quality of randomized controlled trials *Phys. Ther.* **83** 713–21

[81] Teasell R, Foley N, Salter K, Bhogal S, Jutai J and Speechley M 2009 Evidence-based review of stroke rehabilitation: executive summary *Topics in stroke rehabilitation* **16** 463–88

[82] Ramsey L, Winder R J and McVeigh J G 2014 The effectiveness of working wrist splints in adults with rheumatoid arthritis: A mixed methods systematic review *J. Rehabil. Med.* **46** 481–92

[83] Longford N T 2010 Estimation of the effect size in meta-analysis with few studies *Stat. Med.* **29** 421–30

[84] Borenstein M, Hedges L V, Higgins J and Rothstein H R 2010 A basic introduction to fixed-effect and random-effects models for meta-analysis *Res. Synth. Methods* **1** 97–111

[85] Higgins J P and Green S 2011 *Cochrane Handbook for Systematic Reviews of Interventions* vol 4 (New York: Wiley)

[86] Cumming G 2013 *Understanding the New Statistics: Effect Sizes, Confidence Intervals, and Meta-analysis* (New York: Routledge)
[87] Cohen J 1988 *Statistical Power Analysis for the Behavioral Sciences* 2nd edn (Hillsdale, NJ: L. Erlbaum Associates)
[88] Shahraki M, Sohrabi M, Torbati H T, Nikkhah K and NaeimiKia M 2017 Effect of rhythmic auditory stimulation on gait kinematic parameters of patients with multiple sclerosis *J. Med. Life* **10** 33
[89] Seebacher B, Kuisma R, Glynn A and Berger T 2016 The effect of rhythmic-cued motor imagery on walking, fatigue and quality of life in people with multiple sclerosis: A randomised controlled trial *Mult. Scler. J.* **23** 286–96
[90] Seebacher B, Kuisma R, Glynn A and Berger T 2015 Rhythmic cued motor imagery and walking in people with multiple sclerosis: a randomised controlled feasibility study *Pilot Feasibility Stud.* **1** 25
[91] Muratori L, Martin E, Fafard L, Bumstead B, Zarif M and Gudesblatt M 2016 Multiple Sclerosis, EDSS and gait: putting legs that work on a walking scale (P2.126) *Neurology* **86**
[92] Goldman M D, Motl R W, Scagnelli J, Pula J H, Sosnoff J J and Cadavid D 2013 Clinically meaningful performance benchmarks in MS: Timed 25-Foot Walk and the real world *Neurology* **81** 1856–63
[93] Grimaud J, Millar J, Thorpe J W, Moseley I F, McDonald W I and Miller D H 1995 'Signal intensity on MRI of basal ganglia in multiple sclerosis *J. Neurol. Neurosurg. Psychiatry* **59** 306–8
[94] Bengtsson S L, Nagy Z, Skare S, Forsman L, Forssberg H and Ullén F 2005 Extensive piano practicing has regionally specific effects on white matter development *Nature Neurosci.* **8** 1148
[95] Imfeld A, Oechslin M S, Meyer M, Loenneker T and Jancke L 2009 White matter plasticity in the corticospinal tract of musicians: a diffusion tensor imaging study *Neuroimage* **46** 600–7
[96] Elshafey R, Hassanien O and Khalil M 2014 Diffusion tensor imaging for characterizing white matter changes in multiple sclerosis *Egypt. J. Radiol. Nucl. Med.* **45** 881–8
[97] Inglese M and Bester M 2010 Diffusion imaging in multiple sclerosis: research and clinical implications *NMR Biomed.* **23** 865–72
[98] Swinnen S P and Wenderoth N 2004 Two hands, one brain: cognitive neuroscience of bimanual skill *Trends Cogn. Sci.* **8** 18–25
[99] Tanji J 2001 Sequential organization of multiple movements: involvement of cortical motor areas *Annu. Rev. Neurosci.* **24** 631–51
[100] Haider L, Simeonidou C, Steinberger G, Hametner S, Grigoriadis N and Deretzi G *et al* 2014 Multiple sclerosis deep grey matter: the relation between demyelination, neurodegeneration, inflammation and iron *J. Neurol. Neurosurg. Psychiatry* **85** 1386–95
[101] Minagar A, Barnett M H, Benedict R H B, Pelletier D, Pirko I and Sahraian M A *et al* 2013 The thalamus and multiple sclerosis: Modern views on pathologic, imaging, and clinical aspects *Neurology* **80** 210–9
[102] Pirko I, Lucchinetti C F, Sriram S and Bakshi R 2007 Gray matter involvement in multiple sclerosis *Neurology* **68** 634–42
[103] Krutenkova E, Aitmagambetova G, Khodanovich M, Bowen J, Gangadharan B and Henson L *et al* 2016 Demyelination of subcortical nuclei in multiple sclerosis *J. Phys. Conf. Ser.* **677** 012006

[104] Schmalbrock P, Prakash R S, Schirda B, Janssen A, Yang G K and Russell M *et al* 2016 Basal ganglia iron in patients with multiple sclerosis measured with 7T quantitative susceptibility mapping correlates with inhibitory control *Am. J. Neuroradiol.* **37** 439–46

[105] Hasan K M, Walimuni I S, Abid H, Frye R E, Ewing-Cobbs L and Wolinsky J S *et al* 2011 Multimodal quantitative magnetic resonance imaging of thalamic development and aging across the human lifespan: implications to neurodegeneration in multiple sclerosis *J. Neurosci.* **31** 16826–32

[106] Cui F, Zhou L, Wang Z, Lang C, Park J and Tan Z *et al* 2017 Altered functional connectivity of striatal subregions in patients with Multiple Sclerosis *Front. Neurol.* **8** 129

[107] Finke C, Schlichting J, Papazoglou S, Scheel M, Freing A and Soemmer C *et al* 2015 Altered basal ganglia functional connectivity in multiple sclerosis patients with fatigue *Mult. Scler. J.* **21** 925–34

[108] DeLuca J, Genova H M, Capili E J and Wylie G R 2009 Functional neuroimaging of fatigue *Phys. Med. Rehabil. Clin. North Am.* **20** 325–37

[109] Koppelmans V, Hirsiger S, Merillat S, Jancke L and Seidler R D 2015 Cerebellar gray and white matter volume and their relation with age and manual motor performance in healthy older adults *Hum. Brain Mapp.* **36** 2352–63

[110] Wilkins A 2017 Cerebellar dysfunction in multiple sclerosis *Front. Neurol.* **8** 312

[111] Weier K, Banwell B, Cerasa A, Collins D L, Dogonowski A M and Lassmann H *et al* 2015 The role of the cerebellum in multiple sclerosis *Cerebellum* **14** 364–74

[112] Molinari M, Leggio M G, De Martin M, Cerasa A and Thaut M 2003 Neurobiology of rhythmic motor entrainment *Ann. N. Y. Acad. Sci.* **999** 313–21

[113] Bethoux F, Lowe M and Koenig K 2014 Effects of rhythmic auditory stimulation on gait and on cortical activation with mental imagery of walking in patients with multiple sclerosis *Int. J. Mult. Scler. Care* **16** 76

[114] Thaut M H 2005 *Rhythm, Music, and the Brain: Scientific Foundations and Clinical Applications* vol 7 (New York: Routledge)

[115] Tierney A and Kraus N 2013 The ability to move to a beat is linked to the consistency of neural responses to sound *J. Neurosci.* **33** 14981–8

[116] Debaere F, Wenderoth N, Sunaert S, Van Hecke P and Swinnen S P 2003 Internal vs external generation of movements: differential neural pathways involved in bimanual coordination performed in the presence or absence of augmented visual feedback *Neuroimage* **19** 764–76

[117] Hausdorff J M, Lowenthal J, Herman T, Gruendlinger L, Peretz C and Giladi N 2007 Rhythmic auditory stimulation modulates gait variability in Parkinson's disease *Eur. J. Neurosci.* **26** 2369–75

[118] Asanuma H and Keller A 1991 'Neuronal mechanisms of motor learning in mammals,' *Neuroreport* **2** 217–24

[119] Suh J H, Han S J, Jeon S Y, Kim H J, Lee J E and Yoon T S *et al* 2014 Effect of rhythmic auditory stimulation on gait and balance in hemiplegic stroke patients *NeuroRehabilitation* **34** 193–9

[120] Grahn J A and Brett M 2007 Rhythm and beat perception in motor areas of the brain *J. Cogn. Neurosci.* **19** 893–906

[121] Schaefer R S 2014 Auditory rhythmic cueing in movement rehabilitation: findings and possible mechanisms *Philos. Trans. R. Soc. B: Biol. Sci.* **369** 20130402

[122] Zeller D, aufm Kampe K, Biller A, Stefan K, Gentner R and Schutz A *et al* 2010 Rapid-onset central motor plasticity in multiple sclerosis *Neurology* **74** 728–35
[123] Horak F B 1987 Clinical measurement of postural control in adults *Phys. Ther.* **67** 1881–5
[124] Ford M P, Malone L A, Nyikos I, Yelisetty R and Bickel C S 2010 Gait training with progressive external auditory cueing in persons with Parkinson's disease *Arch. Phys. Med. Rehabil.* **91** 1255–61
[125] Thaut M H, Leins A K, Rice R R, Argstatter H, Kenyon G P and McIntosh G C *et al* 2007 Rhythmic auditory stimulation improves gait more than NDT/Bobath training in near-ambulatory patients early poststroke: a single-blind, randomized trial *Neurorehabil. Neural Repair* **21** 455–9
[126] Thaut M H, Gardiner J C, Holmberg D, Horwitz J, Kent L and Andrews G *et al* 2009 Neurologic music therapy improves executive function and emotional adjustment in traumatic brain injury rehabilitation *Ann. N. Y. Acad. Sci.* **1169** 406–16
[127] Delignières D and Torre K 2009 Fractal dynamics of human gait: a reassessment of the 1996 data of Hausdorff *et al J. Appl. Physiol.* **106** 1272–9
[128] Hove M J, Suzuki K, Uchitomi H, Orimo S and Miyake Y 2012 Interactive rhythmic auditory stimulation reinstates natural 1/f timing in gait of Parkinson's patients *PLoS One* **7** e32600
[129] Hausdorff J M, Purdon P L, Peng C, Ladin Z, Wei J Y and Goldberger A L 1996 Fractal dynamics of human gait: stability of long-range correlations in stride interval fluctuations *J. Appl. Physiol.* **80** 1448–57
[130] Labriffe M, Annweiler C, Amirova L E, Gauquelin-Koch G, Ter Minassian A and Leiber L-M *et al* 2017 Brain activity during mental imagery of gait versus gait-like plantar stimulation: a novel combined functional MRI paradigm to better understand cerebral gait control *Front. Hum. Neurosci.* **11** 106
[131] Demougeot L and Papaxanthis C 2011 Muscle fatigue affects mental simulation of action *J. Neurosci.* **31** 10712–20
[132] Ghai S, Ghai I and Effenberg A O 2017 Effects of dual tasks and dual-task training on postural stability: a systematic review and meta-analysis *Clin. Interv. Aging* **12** 557–77
[133] Browne P, Chandraratna D, Angood C, Tremlett H, Baker C and Taylor B V *et al* 2014 Atlas of Multiple Sclerosis 2013: A growing global problem with widespread inequity *Neurology* **83** 1022–4
[134] Lopez W O, Higuera C A, Fonoff E T, Cde O S, Albicker U and Martinez J A 2014 Listenmee and Listenmee smartphone application: synchronizing walking to rhythmic auditory cues to improve gait in Parkinson's disease *Hum. Mov. Sci.* **37** 147–56
[135] Yoo G E and Kim S J 2016 Rhythmic auditory cueing in motor rehabilitation for stroke patients: systematic review and meta-analysis *J. Music Ther.* **53** 149–77
[136] Kim S J, Kwak E E, Park E S, Lee D S, Kim K J and Song J E *et al* 2011 Changes in gait patterns with rhythmic auditory stimulation in adults with cerebral palsy *NeuroRehabilitation* **29** 233–41
[137] Gaver W W 1993 How do we hear in the world? Explorations in ecological acoustics *Ecol. Psychol.* **5** 285–313
[138] Young W R, Rodger M W and Craig C M 2014 Auditory observation of stepping actions can cue both spatial and temporal components of gait in Parkinson' s disease patients *Neuropsychologia* **57** 140–53

[139] Young W, Rodger M and Craig C M 2013 Perceiving and reenacting spatiotemporal characteristics of walking sounds *J. Exp. Psychol.: Hum. Percept. Perform* **39** 464
[140] Dotov D, Bayard S, de Cock V C, Geny C, Driss V and Garrigue G *et al* 2017 Biologically-variable rhythmic auditory cues are superior to isochronous cues in fostering natural gait variability in Parkinson's disease *Gait Posture* **51** 64–9
[141] Effenberg A O 2014 Sensory systems: auditory, tactile, proprioceptive *Encyclopedia of Sport and Exercise Psychology* vol 2 ed R C Eklund and G Tenenbaum (Los Angeles, USA: SAGE Publications) pp 663–7
[142] Effenberg A O, Fehse U, Schmitz G, Krueger B and Mechling H 2016 Movement sonification: effects on motor learning beyond rhythmic adjustments *Front. Neurosci.* **10** 219
[143] Ghai S, Schmitz G, Hwang T-H and Effenberg A O 2018 Auditory proprioceptive integration: Effects of real-time kinematic auditory feedback on knee proprioception *Front. Neurosci.* **12** 142
[144] Tagliabue M and McIntyre J 2014 A modular theory of multisensory integration for motor control *Front. Comput. Neurosci.* **8**
[145] Thaut M H, Peterson D A, McIntosh G C and Hoemberg V 2014 Music mnemonics aid verbal memory and induce learning—related brain plasticity in Multiple Sclerosis *Front. Hum. Neurosci.* **8** 395
[146] Hallam S, Cross I and Thaut M 2011 *Oxford Handbook of Music Psychology* (Oxford: Oxford University Press)
[147] Särkämö T, Altenmüller E, Rodríguez-Fornells A and Peretz I 2016 Editorial: music, brain, and rehabilitation: emerging therapeutic applications and potential neural mechanisms *Front. Hum. Neurosci.* **10** 103
[148] Särkämö T, Ripollés P, Vepsäläinen H, Autti T, Silvennoinen H M and Salli E *et al* 2014 Structural changes induced by daily music listening in the recovering brain after middle cerebral artery stroke: a voxel-based morphometry study *Front. Hum. Neurosci.* **8** 245
[149] Wiens M E, Reimer M A and Guyn H L 1999 Music therapy as a treatment method for improving respiratory muscle strength in patients with advanced multiple sclerosis: a pilot study *Rehabil. Nurs.* **24** 74–80
[150] Weller C M and Baker F A 2011 The role of music therapy in physical rehabilitation: a systematic literature review *Nord. J. Music Ther.* **20** 43–61
[151] Aldridge D, Schmid W, Kaeder M, Schmidt C and Ostermann T 2005 Functionality or aesthetics? A pilot study of music therapy in the treatment of multiple sclerosis patients *Complement. Ther. Med.* **13** 25–33
[152] Raglio A, Attardo L, Gontero G, Rollino S, Groppo E and Granieri E 2015 Effects of music and music therapy on mood in neurological patients *World J. Psychiatry* **5** 68–78
[153] Lengdobler H and Kiessling W 1989 Group music therapy in multiple sclerosis: initial report of experience *Psychother. Psychosom. Med. Psychol.* **39** 369–73

IOP Publishing

Neurological Disorders and Imaging Physics, Volume 2
Engineering and clinical perspectives of multiple sclerosis
Ayman El-Baz and Jasjit S Suri

Chapter 9

Neuropsychological assessment in multiple sclerosis

Ornella Argento and Ugo Nocentini

Cognitive deficits are one of the three clinical features characterizing multiple sclerosis (MS), together with physical and affective symptoms: they are experienced by 40%–70% of people with MS [1]. MS-related cognitive impairment has a significant impact on several aspects of patients' and their relatives' lives. In this chapter, we illustrate the importance of a reliable neuropsychological assessment for all patients, particularly for those at early stages of the pathology, and the need for repeated assessments of cognitive status across the disease course.

Furthermore, we shall present the most reliable and worldwide used test batteries from the more comprehensive to the so-called 'screening tools', and their use in both clinical and research settings.

Special attention will be directed towards the ongoing debate on some methodological aspects of the neuropsychological assessment: within them the importance of having norms for parallel forms of tests to be used for repeated assessments; the statistical choice between discrete norming and regression-based norms; and the more recent ecological approach to neuropsychological assessment.

However, when considering the assessment of cognitive functioning of some clinical populations, such as MS patients, it is also important to consider two aspects that we believed it was important to treat in this chapter: the variables influencing cognition and the importance of differentiating an ongoing cognitive decline from a more widespread and disabling cognitive impairment.

We have concluded this overview in the field of the neuropsychological assessment for MS patients, with a look at future perspectives.

9.1 Cognition in multiple sclerosis

Cognitive impairment (CI) is one of the most relevant and disabling consequences of MS since it affects 40%–70% of patients [1]. As MS is a chronic, demyelinating and

doi:10.1088/978-0-7503-1762-7ch9

neurodegenerative disease with a more frequent onset in young adults, MS-related CI may affect patients and, consequently, their caregivers in the prime of their life. In fact, MS is often diagnosed between the ages of 20 and 40 years [2]. Despite the fact that upper- and lower-limb impairments are most apparent to patients, especially in early stages of the pathology, cognitive functioning involvement is often underestimated by patients, even if it is significantly disabling for everyday independence. Cognitive abilities are crucial in all the activities that young adults have to face and this make them experience independence and life satisfaction. Therefore, feeling limited in some of those activities, due to MS-related CI, may have a detrimental effect on patients and their family, as well as a negative impact on their ability to cope with this new condition. Recent studies explored the impact of MS-related CI on different personal, social, familiar, vocational and financial aspects of patients' lives.

Due to the pathology, at least 30% of MS patients require daily home care that is often provided by their spouses or partners [3]. This may be particularly challenging in a time when a couple should be managing family, relationship, children and career demands.

Consequently, cognitive changes were found to have the most burdensome impact on a caregiver's psychological wellbeing [4, 5].

Furthermore, recent studies also confirmed that in MS patients cognitive decline is among the several factors associated with fall risk and home accidents [6–8]. Of note, these studies suggested that even mild decline in a specific cognitive domain may make everyday activities, such as housekeeping or moving in a familiar environment, harder and this may call for changes in the habits of patients and their relatives. The results of a recently performed research on cognitive-motor interference confirms previously cited studies by focusing the attention on a specific aspect: the real disabling impact of MS may not be reliably ascertained without considering the interaction between cognitive and motor aspects [9]. In fact, little changes in cognitive status may not be detected with only cognitive assessment but may have a significant impact when patients are asked to perform a cognitive task when moving or walking, since the attention, in this case, has to be divided between two concurrent tasks.

CI also seems to influence driving behaviors, since it can result in an increased risk of being involved in motor vehicle accidents [10] and information processing speed, memory and executive functioning are the most relevant predictors of driving safety [11].

The vocational status of MS patients is another aspect that is influenced by cognitive deficits. In particular, several studies have evidenced that information processing speed and memory deficits are two of the variables contributing to job withdrawal [12] and work-related changes and that patients with lower performance on cognitive tests are more likely to have negative work-related events [13].

Therefore, the social functioning of these patients is strongly affected by the occurrence of a cognitive decline and its consequences, requiring patients to adapt to a decline in their standards of living. Coping with this new condition often forces a reduction in the level of activity and participation in daily activity and a withdrawal from social and leisure activities [14]. Furthermore, the MS-related CI causes a reduction in the interaction with healthcare providers and decreases the compliance with therapies and rehabilitation programs [15].

All this evidence together gives the idea of how the MS-related cognitive decline negatively affects patients' and caregivers' quality of life in a wide range of aspects of activity, independence and life satisfaction. Therefore, to face all the consequences of cognitive decline is essential.

An adequate and objective neuropsychological assessment, even in the early stages of the pathology, is essential in order to identify and follow-up cognitive abilities of MS patients.

9.2 Neuropsychological batteries for MS

Although in the early descriptions of the disease by Charcot in 1877 [16] the presence of a memory enfeeblement was already noticed, the first attempt to perform a specific assessment of cognitive deficits in MS was not made until 1991 by Rao and colleagues [17]. Since then, a strong effort has been devoted to both define the incidence and the characteristics of cognitive deficits in MS patients, and propose test batteries specifically built for MS patients' assessment.

As a consequence of the heterogeneous neuropathology of MS, CI can involve multiple domains with various combinations of deficits, and cause different impairment patterns depending on pathology courses [18]. The most frequently affected domains are information processing speed and episodic memory followed by executive functioning, verbal fluency and visual processing [17, 19].

Probably due to that prevalent profile of cognitive impairment, it has been demonstrated that the most used screening tests for the identification of senile dementia (such as the Mini Mental State Examination) [20] are not sensitive in detecting MS-related cognitive deficits [21]. Therefore, due to the high prevalence and the relevant impact of CI in MS, it is important to have different neuropsychological tests for a reliable and valid assessment and for the quantification of CI in MS patients. The evaluation approach has to account for confounding factors such as depression, anxiety and fatigue; it should also be cost effective for use in routine clinical settings [22].

The first attempt to build a neuropsychological assessment battery specifically dedicated to identify MS-related CI was proposed by Rao and colleagues with both the *Neuropsychological Screening Battery* and the *Brief Repeatable Battery for Multiple Sclerosis* (BRB-N) [23, 24]. The first proposed version of the battery was composed of 5 tests selected within a pool of 23 tests following the guidelines for Neuropsychological Research in MS. The assessed cognitive domains and the chosen tests were: information processing speed (Symbol Digit Modalities Test; SDMT) [25], working memory (Paced Auditory Serial Addition Test; PASAT) [26], verbal memory (Selective Reminding Test; SRT) [27], visuo-spatial memory (7/24 Spatial Recall Test; 7/24 SPART) [28], and executive functions (Controlled Oral Word Association Test; COWAT) [29]. In a revised version of the Rao's battery (BRB-N) the Word List Generation test (WLG) [30] replaced the COWAT test and the 10/36 SPART replaced the 7/24 SPART. The BRB-N has good psychometric properties (sensitivity range: 67%–71%; specificity range: 85%–94%) and the total time required for the assessment by the BRB-N is about 30 min [31]. This battery has been translated and validated in several languages for use in different countries and has two parallel forms available. Then, numerous studies have ascertained the correlation between the BRB-N and damage measured by brain magnetic resonance imaging [32, 33]. The BRB-N is still considered one of the most valid neuropsychological test batteries for the assessment of CI in an MS patient though uncertainties were raised on two aspects: the first is that the BRB-N battery did not cover all the cognitive domains that may be involved in MS-related impairment; the second is related to the insufficiency in psychometric properties information for test–retest assessments and parallel forms [34].

To give an overview of these limits, a consensus conference was proposed by the Consortium of MS Centers with a panel of 16 neuropsychologists and clinical psychologists with ascertained experience in clinical evaluation and/or research in MS in order to recommend a minimal set of neuropsychological tests to be included in a routine assessment [35]. The aims of these experts were both to include currently available tests with good psychometric properties covering all the cognitive domains involved in MS and to identify strategies for improving neuropsychological assessment of MS patients in the future [35]. As a result of their work, this panel proposed the *Minimal Assessment of Cognitive Function in MS* (MACFIMS) which was composed of seven tests: the PASAT (3 and 2 s versions); the SDMT (only the oral version of the test); the California Verbal Learning test-II (a verbal learning and memory test; CVLT-II) [36]; the Brief Visuo Spatial Memory test-Revised version (a visuo-spatial memory test; BVMT-R) [37]; the Benton Judgment of Line Orientation test (measuring the accuracy of spatial orientation judgments; BJLO) [38]; the COWAT and the Delis–Kaplan Executive Function System Sorting Test (measuring concept-formation skills, modality-specific problem-solving skills in both verbal/ nonverbal aspects, and the ability to explain sorting concepts abstractly) [39].

Following the consensus conference, the MACFIMS battery was conceived as an assessment tool for both detecting CI in MS and monitoring the changes in cognitive status over time. The time required for the whole administration of the battery was about 90 min and its appropriate application and interpretation needs adequate training in neuropsychological testing [35]. Several studies have been carried out in order to assess test–retest reliability and validity of the MACFIMS battery. In the first case, a study by Benedict and colleagues [40] showed a test–retest reliability ranging from good to excellent and recommended the use of the alternative forms at follow-up evaluations. Concerning the validity of the battery, another study by Benedict and colleagues [19] confirmed the good construct validity and its good ability in predicting a patient's vocational condition. Furthermore, the MACFIMS battery has been cross-culturally validated for patients with MS in several populations [41–44].

Since the development of the MACFIMS, others consensus standards on cognitive testing in MS and other neuropsychological assessments have been suggested, such as the *Brief International Cognitive Assessment for MS* (BICAMS)

[45, 46]; the *National Institute of Neurological Disorders and Stroke-Common Data Elements* (NINDS-CDE) [47]; the *Multiple Sclerosis Cognition Assessment Battery* (MS-COG) [48]. Interestingly all of them are included in the MACFIMS battery combined in different ways.

9.2.1 From comprehensive to brief neuropsychological batteries

Although the MACFIMS battery has an ascertained relevance as neuropsychological assessment battery for MS-related CI, the long time needed for the administration and interpretation, the associated high costs and the need of a specific expertise, make its use difficult outside of specialized centers. Therefore, in 2010 an expert committee of seven neurologists and five neuropsychologists developed recommendations for a tool for clinicians working with MS patients: the BICAMS [45]. Their recommendations were justified by the need for short, well-validated and widely accepted tools that can be used in everyday practice and that can be administered by a neurologist as well as by other healthcare workers [49]. As the BICAMS battery was conceived to be incorporated in routine clinical practice and to be used for baseline evaluations and regular follow-up assessments the experts recommended that the battery should be completed within 15 min, should not require any special equipment and could be appropriately translated for international use [50].

After an accurate selection on the tests available, their psychometric properties and their feasibility the panel of experts choose to include in the battery the SDMT, the first five trials of the CVLT-II and the first three trials of the BVMT-R and then published an international validated protocol. This protocol was then validated in several languages [51–53] but a considerable effort is still ongoing in order to further extend this validation process to other cultures and languages (http://www.bicams.net/).

On the other side, Erlanger and colleagues have built up the MS-COG, an *a priori* composite endpoint to be used to determine efficacy of disease modifying drugs in the improvement of cognitive functioning in MS patients. This battery was composed by the SDMT, the PASAT (3′ and 2′), the SRT (learning and delayed recall trials) and the BVMT-R (total learning and delayed recall trials). The results confirmed that the MS-COG is a reliable (test–retest reliability of 0.91), repeatable measure of MS cognitive functioning; it is also sensitive to CI in MS patients with both secondary-progressive and relapsing–remitting courses and could be useful for multicenter clinical trials [48].

9.2.2 Screening tools

In clinical settings, it is necessary to screen for CI without resort to a comprehensive neuropsychological assessment. Therefore, a large number of short screening tools have been suggested across the years. Within these, in 2001 Benedict and colleagues developed a questionnaire that could be completed by both patients and their informant or caregivers in a few minutes: the Multiple Sclerosis Neuropsychological Questionnaire (MSNQ) [54]. The MSNQ has been developed in two versions, self-report and informant ones, in order to obtain information on the presence and the impact of cognitive symptoms. It has been shown that the MSNQ has a sensitivity of 83%–87% and a specificity of 68%–84% [54]. However, other studies have found that the self-report version of the questionnaire is strongly related to depressive symptoms [55]. Even anxiety, fatigue and self-efficacy as they are related to cognition, strongly influence MSNQ self-report questionnaire because they shape attitude, beliefs and expectations of patients on their CI [56]. In contrast, the informant version of the questionnaire is mostly related to objective cognitive testing and is more reliable, with a minor number of false-positive results [57].

Unfortunately, it is not always possible to rely on an informant in routine clinical visits [56]. More recently, a first attempt to validate a web based version of the questionnaire has been proposed by Akban and colleagues [58]. As a consequence of the modest sensitivity and specificity values of this version, the authors suggest further researches before it can be confidently used.

Within screening tools for CI detection in MS, an important role was played for a long time by the PASAT as part of the Multiple Sclerosis Functional Composite (MSFC) [59]. It has been considered a gold standard screening test for cognition in MS as it involves information processing speed, working memory and complex attention, although the administration of the test raises some difficulties. First of all, it requires a trained examiner and the use of audio equipment; furthermore, the administration of the PASAT is not easily accepted by patients since it causes anxiety; finally, it is strongly affected by practice effects, mathematical skills, and dysarthria [15].

Due to all these difficulties, an alternative test has been considered as a reliable minimal screening tool: the SDMT, oral version. In fact, this test that assesses information processing speed, working memory, complex attention and visual scanning, has good psychometric properties (82% sensitivity, 60% specificity and good test–retest reliability); and it is subject to limited practice effects due to the presence of alternative forms available for repeated assessments. Furthermore, a recent study confirmed that the SDMT is more valid and reliable compared to PASAT 3′ as a single assessment tool, it is easier to perform in everyday practice and more pleasant from the patient's perspective [60].

Interestingly, in the recent study of Pardini and colleagues the authors included a reduction of 4 points in the SDMT within the criteria to define the 'Isolated Cognitive Relapse' [61].

To conclude, at present several studies support the use of SDMT as the most reliable screening measure for MS-related CI, even if further effort should be made in order to identify the best screening tool to use.

9.3 Cognitive assessment: the relevance in clinical and research fields

MS-related CI occurs in all the phenotypes of the disease, including Cognitive Isolated Syndrome (CIS) [62] and Radiologically Isolated Syndrome (RIS) [63]. However, research and clinical practice confirm that the higher prevalence and severity of CI is registered in patients with secondary-progressive (SP) or primary-progressive (PP) courses [18]. The most commonly affected cognitive domains are information processing speed and memory [1] even though there is evidence of a frequent involvement of complex attention, executive functions, verbal fluency, visuo-spatial perception; more recently the impairment of social cognition competences has been also identified [64]. Therefore, the availability of reliable and repeatable cognitive assessment tools, for a complete exam, for screening or monitoring purposes is relevant in both clinical and research settings.

As recommended in the recent study of Kalb and colleagues [65], the screening of cognitive functioning in a clinical setting should be performed even in newly diagnosed patients. As cognitive dysfunctions can be found also in the early stages of the disease, a cognitive screening should be included early in patients' workup. This is what the London (Ontario, Canada) MS Clinic has performed since 2012. In particular, they provide all newly diagnosed MS patients with a baseline cognitive testing in order to compare it with future assessments. This fixed procedure can also give important and reliable information on the prevalence of cognitive impairment in a newly diagnosed population. Therefore, a recent study of DiGiuseppe and colleagues [66] in which those data were used, found that CI, especially of processing speed, is frequent in persons with newly diagnosed MS.

The presence of CI may also have an impact on the adherence to pharmacological treatments making harder clinician work. A recent study has shown that the percentage of MS patients adhering to treatment recommendations is between 49%–93% [67]. Part of the reason for patients' non-adherence is their difficulty in remembering to follow clinicians' recommendations [68] that relies on memory functioning as well as on attention and executive functions. Furthermore, Gerstenecker and colleagues [69] found that MS patients in the progressive courses and with deficits in verbal learning, memory, and verbal fluency, perform worst on appreciation, reasoning, and understanding consent standards and, therefore, may have some trouble in making decisions on their treatments. Again, a multicenter observational study on the adherence to disease-modifying therapies in patients with relapsing–remitting MS has also found that adherent patients reported better quality of life and fewer neuropsychological issues compared to non-adherent patients [70].

A relevant effort is actually focused on the interventions specifically directed to counteract cognitive decline by the use of both pharmacological and other approaches. In particular, several studies have tried to explore the impact of Disease Modifying Therapies (DMT) and Symptomatic Drugs (SD) on CI in patients with MS and showed weak and variable positive effects of DMT. These results may be due to two factors: the time point of treatment in the disease course, as early treatment by both DMT and SD may have better effects in preserving cognitive functioning or slow down the development of CI compared to the late treatments; the cognitive assessment varies significantly across the studies in terms of domains assessed and repeatability of assessments [71, 72].

Despite the evidence supporting the efficacy of cognitive rehabilitation interventions, the absence of objective, systematic and uniform neuropsychological assessment across research studies also affects these programs in terms of extent and reproducibility of results [73]. An account of this variety of outcome measures across cognitive-focused rehabilitation studies can be found in the recent review of Gromisch and colleagues in 2018. In this meta-analysis study the authors, exploring 33 studies on cognitive rehabilitation in MS patients, grouped 10 objective outcome categories with around thirty assessment tests used across them [74].

To conclude, it is well known how MS patients frequently show a pattern of co-occurring CI but whether deficits in one cognitive domain may contribute to the dysfunction in other possibly correlated domains is still to be explored [75]. Therefore, the use of a comprehensive neuropsychological assessment before and after undergoing a cognitive rehabilitation program may help clinician and researcher in choosing between single- or multiple-domain rehabilitation programs and in understanding the effectiveness and extent of benefits.

9.4 Methodological issues

Despite the high prevalence of CI in MS patients and the efforts made to propose a reliable and uniform neuropsychological assessment, several issues of debates and difficulties still remain challenging. In this part of the chapter, we aimed to present some of these issues and to show the related discussion on them.

9.4.1 Discrete norms versus regression-based norms

After having administered a test to a patient, their performance has to be interpreted, mainly by placing the performance at a pathological level or not. This interpretation should be made taking into account the contribution given by all the variables that may influence that performance. Among them, the most relevant are the demographic ones: age, sex and level of education. For example, the impact of sex on cognitive functioning in healthy people has widely been reported in literature with evidence showing that women outperform men on verbal memory tasks [76], and men outperform women in visuo-spatial abilities [77, 78]. Furthermore, it is well known how age is generally linearly and inversely related to cognitive performance [79] and how the level of education contributes to the formation of cognitive reserve, which contributes to the brain's resilience in the presence of injury influencing the performance on some cognitive tests [80].

Typically, two types of norms have been employed to interpret cognitive performance in the light of demographic influences: the discrete norms and the continuous norms. The level of appropriateness of these two procedures still remains an issue of debate.

Discrete norms include sets of descriptive statistics for specific age groups [81]. However, these groups are often based on arbitrary age ranges. The same procedure can be applied for all demographic variables that may influence the performance, obtaining a wide range of age/sex/education groups with a minimum number of participants each as performed, for example, in several studies [79, 82]. The use of discrete norms was considered valid when the mean and standard deviation of the normative sample group are approximately near to those of the target population and when the raw scores are normally distributed [81].

However, some problems have been raised on this procedure. For example, patient performance upon becoming 35 years old may be submitted to a different correction depending on the passage from the 25–34 to the 35–44 range: this may not correspond to a real change in their cognitive profile.

For this reason, several studies suggested an alternative approach: the continuous norms using multiple regression equations. In this approach, it is suggested to add the age-squared to the common predictive demographic variables in order to evaluate the influence of non-linear age effects on normal cognitive performance [83].

Following the procedure of previous studies, raw scores obtained by healthy controls should be converted first into scaled scores using the cumulative frequency distribution of each measure in order to normalize all test scores distributions. Then, the obtained scaled scores have to be entered as dependent variables en bloc into the multiple regression analyses with demographics. Predicted scaled scores deriving from this analysis should be subtracted from each participant's raw score and the difference should be divided by standard deviation of participants' raw residual for each measure. To conclude, the resulting values have to be converted into T scores (for a more complete statistical procedure explanation, see [84–86]).

The regression-based norms permit one to account for demographic influences on test performance as well as to use the entire normative sample influence rather than divide it into smaller subgroups accounting for sex-, age- or education-combinations.

Parmenter and colleagues [84] constructed regression-based norms for the MACFIMS battery and tried to compare their regression-based *T*-scores with those based on discrete published norms for each single test. Then, authors evaluated the rates of impairment detected by each type of norm. It was found that regression-based norms yield significantly different *T*-scores from those obtained by the discrete norms published for each test, with published norms detecting significantly lower rates of impairment than regression-based ones.

Although the use of regression-based norms may be unfamiliar to clinicians, the use of computer spreadsheets may overcome this limitation, as suggested in several works [84, 85].

The regression-based approach has shown its reliability in considering the influence of demographic variables on test performances, but an issue still to be solved is whether this approach may be applied to other variables too: some authors suggest including not only demographic variables, but also neurological ones when considering the cognitive performance of specific clinical samples. This might be particularly important in an MS patient for which we need to take into account several variables such as: clinical phenotype, disease duration, ongoing depression etc. Therefore, currently the challenge has moved from a discrete versus regression-based approach, to determining which variables are reasonable predictors, and have to be included within those influencing patients' performance.

9.4.2 An ecological approach: the cognitive-motor interference and the actual reality

The need for a more ecological approach to neuropsychological testing stems from the observation that the performance assessed by the various neuropsychological tests does not correspond to what is routinely required in everyday life. For example, in their everyday life, people often perform a cognitive task while walking (e.g. talking or remembering lists) in a so-called Dual-Task (DT) condition. Therefore, the real disabling impact of the MS-related CI may be hard to detect without considering the mutual interaction between cognitive and motor aspects: the cognitive-motor interference. This is particularly true for patients, such as those with MS, that are affected by decrease in both motor and cognitive efficiency. In the clinical routine assessment, cognitive and motor aspects are explored separately and, in particular, the neuropsychological assessment is often performed asking patients to stay sit in a quiet room without any disturbance.

Furthermore, the study of Allalì and colleagues [87] evidenced that subtle changes due to the administration of a certain therapy could not be detected when the assessment of motor/cognitive aspects is performed separately. This could justify the discrepancy between self-perceived cognitive deficit and an objective measured one. The self-perceived impairment is linked to the loss of efficiency observed by patients in their everyday life activities (which often requires the use of both motor and cognitive functions); conversely, the objective measurement is performed by the assessment of the two aspects separately requiring the whole attention completely dedicated to one function per time. In fact, the recent study of Beste and colleagues [88] underline that executive functions, often affected in MS patients, are relevant in the concurrent performance of two or more tasks. So, the authors suggest that the use of a dual-tasking paradigm in the routine neuropsychological assessment may help in detecting early and subtle cognitive dysfunction in MS.

In line with the need for a more ecological evaluation of cognitive efficiency in MS patients, it has been proposed to use the so-called 'actual reality', which is a performance-based approach to assess real, everyday life activities by the use of the internet [89]: for example, to purchase an airline ticket paying with a credit card. The performance in 'actual reality' tests correlated with that on BICAMS [90] showing a relationship between cognitive skills and everyday life performance. In particular, BICAMS seems to have a certain clinical utility as a short cognitive screening tool able to predict functional performance in patients with MS.

Ecological tools seem to detect executive function deficits that are underestimated by the common neuropsychological assessments [91], and have raised the interest of patients since they can easily understand the meaning of the test [22].

The preservation or deterioration of cognitive functioning in MS patients is also dependent on the intellectual enrichment, the level of education and the intellectual lifestyle of patients: the so-called 'cognitive reserve'. In fact, several studies have demonstrated that higher levels of education and continuous cognitive exercise may slow the MS-related cognitive decline even when significant brain volume loss is already present [92]. These results suggest the need to consider a questionnaire assessing cognitive reserve within a complete neuropsychological assessment.

9.4.3 Repeated assessments

During the course of the pathology, patients are often exposed to relapses that may have an impact on cognition, in isolation or together with other symptoms: in the first case, the term 'isolated cognitive relapse' has been coined; otherwise, patients can have changes in cognitive efficiency due to increasing brain damage not evidenced by a relapse.

Furthermore, cognitive efficiency may go through positive changes due to the use of disease-modifying therapies or rehabilitation programs.

Therefore, repeated assessments are needed in order to detect these changes.

Even in normal aging or other pathologies affecting cognition, it is important to detect cognitive function changes that may occur, for example, after the introduction of treatments, or for the spontaneous evolution of the pathology. Therefore, in clinical practice, it is quite common to use repeated neuropsychological assessments: the first problem to face regarding these repetitions is the practice effect, particularly for memory tests. In fact, as already pointed out by Benedict and Zgaljiardic in 1998, when a memory test is repeatedly proposed to a patient there are two potential sources of practice-related measurement biases: the test-taking strategies that may be developed by a patient during the course of repeated assessments; and the item-specific practice effect which depends on the possibility to memorize the information presented more than one time and remember it in the next test administration [93].

The item-specific practice effect may be controlled by the use of alternative forms of the same test.

Several studies have been made to assess the impact of practice effects on the most used cognitive tests for MS and to develop alternative forms. This is the case of Benedict and colleagues [40] who assessed the practice effect of the CVLT-II in patients with MS and found that patients receiving an alternative form at a one week follow-up showed a smaller practice effect compared with those who received the same form at the same time interval [40]. Subsequently, the study performed in 2006 by Woods and colleagues in a sample of 195 healthy adults showed comparable results: in this study the practice effects of the CVLT-II were investigated by attributing the participants to one of the two conditions: standard/standard and standard/alternative forms, before and after a delayed time of at least one week [94]. These results suggest the need for alternative lists of the CVLT-II to reduce practice effects across repeated clinical assessments.

Concerning the BVMT-R, the possibility to have six alternative forms with a good intra-form reliability have increased the usefulness of this test for repeated assessments [95].

The practice effect has also been observed on SDMT performance when the same form is administered repeatedly, although this test requires rapid processing and adjusting visual gaze, making it difficult for participants to memorize specific symbol/number pairings [96]. For this reason, a recent study has tried to assess the reliability and equivalence of five alternative forms of the SDMT: it has been obtained that at least three of them are statistically equivalent, with the same degree of difficulty in healthy adults. Furthermore, the authors confirmed the reliability of these forms and suggested their implementation in clinical trials in order to ameliorate the evaluation of cognitive outcomes [97].

As stated previously, repeated assessments are frequent and needed in MS patients. It is important to underline that the panel of experts, who suggested the use of the MACFIMS battery, have included in the selection criteria the need to have alternative forms of equivalent difficulty for each test (even if this standard is not equally applicable to all cognitive domains) [19]. At the time of the selection of the tests to include in the MACFIMS, those who did not have published alternative forms were the PASAT and the SDMT-oral version. However, the introduction of SDMT alternative forms guarantees the improvement of the MACFIMS battery.

Another often underestimated aspect regarding the repeated assessment is the minimal distance between assessments needed to avoid, or at least reduce, the test-taking strategies. However, to our knowledge, no studies have ever assessed this aspect.

On the other hand, as patients with MS may experience a decrease in cognitive functioning for various occurrences (e.g. isolated cognitive relapse, relapses involving both cognition and other functions, disease progression without relapses), it is hard to decide when a neuropsychological re-assessment should be performed.

Both the UK National Institute for Health and Care Excellence and the American Academy of Neurology suggest that at least an annual routine assessment should be performed even in clinically stable patients, although the debate on this topic remains still unsolved [98, 99].

However, considering the difficulties, already treated elsewhere, in performing annual routine complete assessment of all MS patients, a fast screening could be an acceptable alternative [100]. Interestingly, an Italian study has assessed the test-retest reliability after three weeks from the baseline assessment and confirmed the suitability of the BICAMS battery for longitudinal assessments [51].

9.5 Variables influencing cognition

When considering the performance in a neuropsychological assessment it is important to collect information on the other variables that may influence that performance.

Within these variables, mood and, particularly, depressive episodes are relevant as they are frequently associated with MS. This can be justified by the relevance of being diagnosed as affected by MS, by the severity of the pathology, by its disabling impact, and by the consequences on everyday lives of patients.

The estimate frequency of depressive symptoms in the MS population is around 26% of patients following a community based study [101]. These data are confirmed by the study of Strober and Arnett [102] by the use of self-report measures of depression. In the light of the high prevalence of both depression and cognitive impairments in MS patients, different studies have tried to ascertain the correlation between the two aspects with divergent findings. On the one hand, a study has not found any correlation between the two aspects [103]. However, some authors supposed that this absence of correlations may be due to overlap between the neuro-vegetative symptoms of depression and the MS symptoms. Considering this overlap, a wide range of tools specifically developed for the assessment of non-somatic symptoms of depression in MS have been developed.

On the other hand, other studies have found this relationship as in the case of Arnett and colleagues studies [104–107]. In these studies, Arnett and colleagues found that depression worsened memory, processing speed, and executive functions in patients with MS [104–107]. More recently, other studies [108, 109] confirmed the link between depression and MS patients' performance on memory tests and that MS patients' performance on information processing speed and attention tests correlated with a higher level of anxiety and depression.

Several other studies have confirmed the link between depression and cognitive status of patients with MS by the use of both objective and subjective measures [110, 111].

Moreover, the relationship between depression and cognition seems relevant in a rehabilitative perspective: it can be expected that therapies focused on cognition may reduce depression levels or, otherwise, depression-focused intervention may have an impact on some cognitive performance.

Another aspect that may influence cognitive performance is the MS-related self-perceived fatigue.

Fatigue is frequently reported by MS patients. It has been generally differentiated into: 'physical fatigue' versus 'cognitive fatigue'. One of the aspects characterizing MS-related fatigue is that it is usually self-reported by patients and its relationship between objective measures is hard to explore. Some studies have tried to find an association between cognitive fatigue and the objective measurement of cognitive domains impairment in MS. However, just a few studies have found this relationship. This is the case for the study performed by Krupp and Elkins [112], which found an effect of fatigue on the decline in cognitive performance during a task or across a testing session. Another study supporting the link between fatigue and cognition is that of Diamond and colleagues, in which slower processing speed was found to be correlated with higher levels of depressed mood and fatigue [110]. However, other studies do not confirm this correlation, undermining the idea that 'fatigue' results in a decrease of cognitive performance except for a weak relationship with alert/vigilance aspects as shown in the recent review of Hanken and colleagues [113]. In general, both depression and subjective/cognitive fatigue seem to be confounding factors in assessing patients' cognitive performance: therefore, they should both be taken into account during a cognitive assessment for understanding the severity of cognitive symptoms [114].

However, in their recent work, Kalb and colleagues [65] confirm the existence of a complex interrelation between mood, fatigue, sleep disturbances and cognition.

Furthermore, sleep disturbances in MS patients with depression, fatigue or pain contribute to the perception of cognitive problems above and beyond the impact of depression [115]. Concerning the role of sleep and its impact on cognitive functioning, two recent studies found that both sleep disturbances and obstructive sleep apnea are associated with performances on visual and verbal memory, executive function, attention, processing speed and working memory tests in patients with MS

[116, 117]. Thus, as suggested, taking care of the adequate management of sleep in MS patients may improve the accuracy of objective measurement of cognitive impairment.

Another aspect affecting cognition in patients with MS is apathy. Apathy is one of the major neuropsychiatric symptoms in patients with MS. Few studies have explored the relationship between cognitive impairment and apathy: the study of Figved and colleagues [118] found that apathy was significantly associated with intrusions in memory tests. Furthermore, a recent study by Niino and colleagues [109] confirmed that, in patients with MS, most test scores of the BRB-N are correlated with the scores on the apathy scale.

Finally, recent studies have also found an impact of some personality traits, such as neuroticism, extraversion and conscientiousness, on the path of cognitive decline in MS [119, 120].

9.6 Cognitive impairment and cognitive decline

In clinical assessment it is important to define the performance of a patient on neuropsychological tests in terms of 'preserved' or 'impaired'. What is often underestimated is that the performance of a patient with a progressive neurodegenerative disease can be located in a continuum from 'preserved' to heavily 'impaired'. Furthermore, as described elsewhere in this chapter, each single patient with MS may have a specific pattern of cognitive involvement derived by both the ongoing neurodegeneration and the influence of several other variables influencing cognition. It is possible to have situations in which a slight decline in more than one score or cognitive function may not be considered as relevant in terms of global impairment; otherwise, a more prominent global impairment may be completely due to the involvement of one cognitive function but the preservation of the others.

It is important, to clarify both the difference between the cognitive impairment and the cognitive decline and underline the difference between single domain-impairment and global cognitive impairment.

Usually, the 'impairment' is attributed when the obtained score is located below a defined SD from the performance of matched healthy controls. However, the choice of which SD to use has always been arbitrary so that, for example, the estimated rates of prevalence of CI are often strongly variable across studies [75]. For example, in the validity study on the MACFIMS performed by Benedict and colleagues [16], the authors have arbitrarily established the threshold of below 1.5 SD for each score [16]. However, it is important to focus attention on the changes in cognitive efficiency from the previous functioning level, that patients may experience and that do not exceed the established threshold of 'cognitive impairment' [75]. These changes show that a certain level of ongoing 'decline' is present and this may be underestimated or untreated before reaching a given threshold. Therefore, it is clear how this under-evaluation may have a detrimental impact on patients' lives as they may often not have access to specific treatments in the moment when they could most benefit from them.

As suggested by Sumowski and colleagues [75], it is important to consider and include the accurate assessment of decline from previous functioning level into neuropsychological assessments in order to monitor the possible progression of deficits as well as to evaluate the efficiency of treatments.

A recent study by our group, addressing the validation of an Italian version of the MACFIMS battery, has tried to overcome both these limitations by (1) defining graduation level of impairment depending on different SDs; (2) proposing a global Cognitive Impairment Index graduated into three levels of impairments in order to also detect a patient not-preserved but not yet severely impaired, which are those patients that may negatively evolve as well as benefit the most from cognitive rehabilitation and/or pharmacological treatments; (3) identifying the specific cognitive profile of patients; (4) increasing the knowledge on the rates of co-occurring deficits [41]. One of the first attempts to propose a Cognitive Impairment Index was made by Camp and colleagues in 1999 with greater impairment corresponding to higher scores [121].

Another aspect that is currently interesting both clinician and researcher is the 'clinically meaningful change', which concerns the ability to detect a minimal clinically meaningful change by using a neuropsychological assessment. Across the studies, different standards have been suggested, but the primary question that should be posed is how to translate this minimum change into an advantage or disadvantage for everyday efficiency of patients. So, first of all, one should identify those assessment tools that may have a strong relationship with the everyday efficiency outcome. Currently, three of these assessment tools have been identified as a potential target: the SDMT, the Multiple Sclerosis Functional Composite (MSFC) [122], and the BICAMS. The SDMT has shown great reliability and good correlation with magnetic resonance imaging as well as good association with daily working activities so that recently a change of 3 or 4 points on the SDMT raw score was found to be able to discriminate patients' work status [123, 124]. The performance on the 25-foot walk test of the MSFC was found to be associated with occupational disability and trouble with instrumental activity [125]. Finally, a more recent study found that a benchmark composed by both MSFC and BICAMS is associated with impairment in work activities [126].

Finally, we know that the MS-related cognitive decline that does not reach the threshold of 'impairment' is still something that affects patients' everyday efficiency in several ways. Routine repeated assessment may help in detecting these little changes before they significantly increase. On the other side, we need to consider the performance more in terms of degrees than as preserved/impaired, in order to catch more accurately these changes.

9.7 Future perspectives

The adequate management of cognitive dysfunction in MS patients is still missing some important points. Among them are education for people with MS and their caregivers about common cognitive changes related to the disease and their impact in terms of activity limitations and participation restrictions [127]. People with MS should be made aware of the cognitive symptoms they may incur and of the importance of a routine baseline assessment as well as of longitudinal repeated assessments.

Then the appropriate approach to cognitive impairment in MS should be to make patients aware of the importance of early screening and ongoing monitoring throughout the disease course, as well as of the remediation by rehabilitation programs, compensatory strategies and drugs impacting on cognitive functioning.

Of note is the approach suggested by some recent studies with an algorithm for the management of cognitive function in MS [100]. This algorithm starts from an unavoidable brief annual assessment of cognitive functioning and assesses mood, fatigue, disease activity and comorbidities when a cognitive decline is suspected. Therefore, if the suspect of cognitive decline is confirmed one can decide to perform a more extended neuropsychological examination before directing patients to the correct intervention. This assessment should be performed by the most widely applied, validated and reliable tools, which have been described in this chapter.

We believe that following this approach may help the clinician in the management of the cognitive consequences of MS while maintaining the cost-effectiveness relationship in everyday clinical practice.

References

[1] Chiaravalloti N D and DeLuca J 2008 Cognitive impairment in multiple sclerosis *Lancet Neurol.* **7** 1139–51

[2] Rodriguez M, Siva A, Ward J, Stolp-Smith K, O'brien P and Kurland L 1994 Impairment, disability, and handicap in multiple sclerosis A population-based study in Olmsted County, Minnesota *Neurology* **44** 28

[3] Minden S L, Frankel D, Hadden L S, Srinath K P and Perloff J N 2004 Disability in elderly people with multiple sclerosis: An analysis of baseline data from the Sonya Slifka Longitudinal Multiple Sclerosis Study *NeuroRehabilitation* **19** 55–67

[4] Figved N, Myhr K M, Larsen J P and Aarsland D 2007 Caregiver burden in multiple sclerosis: the impact of neuropsychiatric symptoms *J. Neurol. Neurosurg. Psychiatry* **78** 1097–102

[5] Appleton D, Robertson N, Mitchell L and Lesley R 2018 Our disease: a qualitative meta-synthesis of the experiences of spousal/partner caregivers of people with multiple sclerosis *Scand. J. Caring Sci.* **32** 1262–78

[6] D'Orio V L, Foley F W, Armentano F, Picone M A, Kim S and Holtzer R 2012 Cognitive and motor functioning in patients with multiple sclerosis: neuropsychological predictors of walking speed and falls *J. Neurol. Sci.* **316** 42–6

[7] Sosnoff J J, Balantrapu S, Pilutti L A, Sandroff B M, Morrison S and Motl R W 2013 Cognitive processing speed is related to fall frequency in older adults with multiple sclerosis *Arch. Phys. Med. Rehabil.* **94** 1567–72

[8] Argento O, Incerti C C, Pisani V, Magistrale G, Di Battista G, Romano S, Ferraro E, Caltagirone C and Nocentini U 2014 Domestic accidents and multiple sclerosis: an exploratory study of occurrence and possible causes *Disabil. Rehabil.* **36** 2205–9

[9] Wajda D A, Motl R W and Sosnoff J J 2013 Dual task cost of walking is related to fall risk in persons with multiple sclerosis *J. Neurol. Sci.* **335** 160–3

[10] Schultheis M T, Garay E, Millis S R and DeLuca J 2002 Motor vehicle crashes and violations among drivers with multiple sclerosis *Arch. Phys. Med. Rehabil.* **83** 1175–8
[11] Lincoln N B and Radford K A 2008 Cognitive abilities as predictors of safety to drive in people with multiple sclerosis *Mult. Scler. J.* **14** 123–8
[12] Strober L, Chiaravalloti N, Moore N and DeLuca J 2014 Unemployment in multiple sclerosis (MS): utility of the MS functional composite and cognitive testing *Mult. Scler. J.* **20** 112–5
[13] Clemens L and Langdon D 2018 How does cognition relate to employment in multiple Sclerosis? A systematic Review *Mult. Scler. Relat. Disord.* **26** 183–91
[14] Hakim E, Bakheit A M O, Bryant T N, Roberts M W H, McIntosh-Michaelis S A, Spackman A J, Martin J P and McLellan D L 2000 The social impact of multiple sclerosis-a study of 305 patients and their relatives *Disabil. Rehabil.* **22** 288–93
[15] Amato M P, Morra V B, Falautano M, Ghezzi A, Goretti B, Patti F, Riccardi A and Mattioli F 2018 Cognitive assessment in multiple sclerosis—an Italian consensus *Neurol. Sci.* **39** 1317–24
[16] Charcot J M 1877 *Leçons sur les maladies du système nerveux: faites à la Salpêtrière* vol 2 (Paris: Adrien Delahaye)
[17] Rao S M, Leo G J, Bernardin L and Unverzagt F 1991 Cognitive dysfunction in multiple sclerosis.: I. Frequency, patterns, and prediction *Neurology* **41** 685–91
[18] Johnen A, Landmeyer N C, Buerkner P C, Wiendl H, Meuth S G and Holling H 2017 Distinct cognitive impairments in different disease courses of multiple sclerosis—a systematic review and meta-analysis *Neurosci. Biobehav. Rev.* **83** 568–78
[19] Benedict R H, Cookfair D, Gavett R, Gunther M, Munschauer F, Garg N and Weinstock-Guttman B 2006 Validity of the minimal assessment of cognitive function in multiple sclerosis (MACFIMS) *J. Int. Neuropsychol. Soc.* **12** 549–58
[20] Folstein M F, Folstein S E and McHugh P R 1975 Mini-mental state: a practical method for grading the cognitive state of patients for the clinician *J. Psychiatr. Res.* **12** 189–98
[21] Beatty W W and Goodkin D E 1990 Screening for cognitive impairment in multiple sclerosis: an evaluation of the Mini-Mental State Examination *Arch. Neurol.* **47** 297–301
[22] Ruet A and Brochet B 2018 Cognitive assessment in patients with multiple sclerosis: From neuropsychological batteries to ecological tools *Ann. Phys. Rehabil. Med.*
[23] Rao S M 1991 A manual for the brief *Repeatable Battery of Neuropsychological Tests in Multiple Sclerosis*
[24] Rao S M 1991 Neuropsychological screening battery for multiple sclerosis *Unpublished manuscript section of Neuropsychology, Department of Neurology, Medical College of Wisconsin. Cognitive Impairment in Multiple Sclerosis*
[25] Smith A 1982 *Symbol Digit Modality Test (SDMT): Manual (revised)* (Los Angeles, CA: Psychological Services)
[26] Gronwall D M A 1977 Paced auditory serial-addition task: a measure of recovery from concussion *Percept. Mot. Skills* **44** 367–73
[27] Buschke H 1984 Cued recall in amnesia *J. Clin. Exp. Neuropsychol.* **6** 433–40
[28] Rao S M, Hammeke T A, McQuillen M P, Khatri B O and Lloyd D 1984 Memory disturbance in chronic progressive multiple sclerosis *Arch. Neurol.* **41** 625–31
[29] Spreen O and Strauss E 1991 *Controlled oral word association (word fluency) A Compendium of Neuropsychological Tests* ed O Spreen and E Strauss (Oxford: Oxford University Press) pp 219–27

[30] Wepman J M 1972 The assessment of aphasia and related disorders *Psyccritiques* **17** 614
[31] Rao S M 1990 The cognitive function study group of the national multiple sclerosis society *A Manual for the Brief Repeatable Battery of Neuropsychological Tests in Multiple Sclerosis*
[32] Christodoulou C *et al* 2003 Cognitive performance and MR markers of cerebral injury in cognitively impaired MS patients *Neurology* **60** 1793–8
[33] Amato M P, Zipoli V and Portaccio E 2006 Multiple sclerosis-related cognitive changes: a review of cross-sectional and longitudinal studies *J. Neurol. Sci.* **245** 41–6
[34] Roy S and Benedict R H B 2018 Assessment of cognitive impairment in multiple sclerosis *Cognition and Behaviour in Multiple Sclerosis* ed J DeLuca and B M Sandroff (Washington, DC: American Psychological Association) pp 7–31
[35] Benedict R H *et al* 2002 Minimal neuropsychological assessment of MS patients: a consensus approach *Clin. Neuropsychol.* **16** 381–97
[36] Delis D C 2000 *CVLT-II: California Verbal Learning Test: Adult Version* (San Antonio, TX: Psychological Corporation)
[37] Benedict R H, Schretlen D, Groninger L, Dobraski M and Shpritz B 1996 Revision of the Brief Visuospatial Memory Test: studies of normal performance, reliability, and validity *Psychol. Assess.* **8** 145
[38] Benton A L, Sivan A B, deS Hamsher K and Spreen O 1994 *Contributions to Neuropsychological Assessment: A Clinical Manual* (New York: Oxford University Press)
[39] Delis D C 2001 *Manual for the Delis-Kaplan Executive Function System (D-KEFS)* (San Antonio, TX: The Psychological Corporation)
[40] Benedict R H 2005 Effects of using same-versus alternate-form memory tests during short-interval repeated assessments in multiple sclerosis *J. Int. Neuropsychol. Soc.* **11** 727–36
[41] Argento O, Incerti C C, Quartuccio M E, Magistrale G, Francia A, Caltagirone C, Pisani V and Nocentini U 2018 The Italian validation of the minimal assessment of cognitive function in multiple sclerosis (MACFIMS) and the application of the Cognitive Impairment Index scoring procedure in MS patients *Neurol. Sci.* **39** 1237–44
[42] Walker L A, Marino D, Berard J A, Feinstein A, Morrow S A and Cousineau D 2017 Canadian normative data for minimal assessment of cognitive function in multiple sclerosis *Can. J. Neurol. Sci.* **44** 547–55
[43] Eshaghi A *et al* 2012 Validity and reliability of a Persian translation of the Minimal Assessment of Cognitive Function in Multiple Sclerosis (MACFIMS) *Clin. Neuropsychol.* **26** 975–84
[44] Dusankova J B, Kalincik T, Havrdova E and Benedict R H 2012 Cross cultural validation of the minimal assessment of cognitive function in multiple sclerosis (MACFIMS) and the brief international cognitive assessment for multiple sclerosis (BICAMS) *Clin. Neuropsychol.* **26** 1186–200
[45] Langdon D W *et al* 2012 Recommendations for a brief international cognitive assessment for multiple sclerosis (BICAMS) *Mult. Scler. J.* **18** 891–8
[46] Benedict R H *et al* 2012 Brief International Cognitive Assessment for MS (BICAMS): international standards for validation *BMC Neurol.* **12** 55
[47] Benedict R H B, Krupp L and Francis G 2012 *NINDS common data elements, multiple sclerosis, neuropsychology/cognition recommendations* (Washington, DC: National Institute for Neurological Diseases and Stroke)

[48] Erlanger D M, Kaushik T, Caruso L S, Benedict R H, Foley F W, Wilken J, Cadavid D and DeLuca J 2014 Reliability of a cognitive endpoint for use in a multiple sclerosis pharmaceutical trial *J. Neurol. Sci.* **340** 123–9
[49] Langdon D *et al* 2011 The Brief International Cognitive Assessment for Multiple Sclerosis (BICAMS): first consensus steps towards a brief universal cognitive assessment for MS *Neurology* **76** A479
[50] Corfield F and Langdon D 2018 A systematic review and meta-analysis of the Brief Cognitive Assessment for Multiple Sclerosis (BICAMS) *Neurol. Ther.* **7** 287–306
[51] Goretti B *et al* 2014 The brief international cognitive assessment for multiple sclerosis (BICAMS): normative values with gender, age and education corrections in the Italian population *BMC Neurol.* **14** 171
[52] O'Connell K, Langdon D, Tubridy N, Hutchinson M and McGuigan C 2015 A preliminary validation of the brief international cognitive assessment for multiple sclerosis (BICAMS) tool in an Irish population with multiple sclerosis (MS) *Mult. Scler. Relat. Disord.* **4** 521–5
[53] Polychroniadou E *et al* 2016 Validation of the Brief International Cognitive Assessment for Multiple Sclerosis (BICAMS) in Greek population with multiple sclerosis *Mult. Scler. Relat. Disord.* **9** 68–72
[54] Benedict R H, Munschauer F, Linn R, Miller C, Murphy E, Foley F and Jacobs L 2003 Screening for multiple sclerosis cognitive impairment using a self-administered 15-item questionnaire *Mult. Scler. J.* **9** 95–101
[55] O'Brien A, Gaudino-Goering E, Shawaryn M, Komaroff E, Moore N B and DeLuca J 2007 Relationship of the Multiple Sclerosis Neuropsychological Questionnaire (MSNQ) to functional, emotional, and neuropsychological outcomes *Arch. Clin. Neuropsychol.* **22** 933–48
[56] Kim S, Zemon V, Rath J F, Picone M, Gromisch E S, Glubo H, Smith-Wexler L and Foley F W 2017 Screening instruments for the early detection of cognitive impairment in patients with multiple sclerosis *Int. J. MS Care* **19** 1–10
[57] Benedict R H, Cox D, Thompson L L, Foley F, Weinstock-Guttman B and Munschauer F 2004 Reliable screening for neuropsychological impairment in multiple sclerosis *Mult. Scler. J.* **10** 675–8
[58] Akbar N, Honarmand K, Kou N, Levine B, Rector N and Feinstein A 2010 Validity of an internet version of the Multiple Sclerosis Neuropsychological Questionnaire *Mult. Scler. J.* **16** 1500–6
[59] Fisher J S, Rudick R, Cutter G and Reingold S C 1999 The Multiple Sclerosis Functional Composite measure (MSFC): an integrated approach to MS clinical outcome assessment *Mult. Scler.* **5** 244–50
[60] Sonder J M, Burggraaff J, Knol D L, Polman C H and Uitdehaag B M 2014 Comparing long-term results of PASAT and SDMT scores in relation to neuropsychological testing in multiple sclerosis *Mult. Scler. J.* **20** 481–8
[61] Pardini M, Uccelli A, Grafman J, Yaldizli Ö, Mancardi G and Roccatagliata L 2014 Isolated cognitive relapses in multiple sclerosis *J. Neurol. Neurosurg. Psychiatry* **85** 1035–7
[62] Diker S, Has A C, Kurne A, Göçmen R, Oğuz K K and Karabudak R 2016 The association of cognitive impairment with gray matter atrophy and cortical lesion load in clinically isolated syndrome *Mult. Scler. Relat. Disord.* **10** 14–21
[63] Labiano-Fontcuberta A *et al* 2016 A comparison study of cognitive deficits in radiologically and clinically isolated syndromes *Mult. Scler. J.* **22** 250–3

[64] Langdon D W 2011 Cognition in multiple sclerosis *Curr. Opin. Neurol.* **24** 244–9
[65] Kalb R *et al* 2018 Recommendations for cognitive screening and management in multiple sclerosis care *Mult. Scler. J.* **24** 1665–80
[66] DiGiuseppe G, Blair M and Morrow S A 2018 Prevalence of cognitive impairment in newly diagnosed relapsing-remitting multiple sclerosis *Int. J. MS Care* **20** 153–7
[67] Di Battista G, Bertolotto A, Gasperini C, Ghezzi A, Maimone D and Solaro C 2014 Multiple Sclerosis State of the Art (SMART): a qualitative and quantitative analysis of therapy's adherence, hospital reliability's perception, and services provided quality *Mult. Scler. Int.* **2014** 752318
[68] Kołtuniuk A and Rosińczuk J 2018 Adherence to disease-modifying therapies in patients with multiple sclerosis *Patient prefer. Adherence* **12** 1557
[69] Gerstenecker A, Lowry K, Myers T, Bashir K, Triebel K L, Martin R C and Marson D C 2017 Medical decision-making capacity and its cognitive predictors in progressive MS: Preliminary evidence *J. Neurol. Sci.* **380** 38–43
[70] Devonshire V *et al* 2011 The Global Adherence Project (GAP): A multicenter observational study on adherence to disease-modifying therapies in patients with relapsing-remitting multiple sclerosis *Eur. J. Neurol.* **18** 69–77
[71] Foley F W, Benedict R H, Gromisch E S and DeLuca J 2012 The need for screening, assessment, and treatment for cognitive dysfunction in multiple sclerosis: results of a multidisciplinary CMSC consensus conference, September 24, 2010 *Int. J. MS Care* **14** 58–64
[72] Amato M P, Langdon D, Montalban X, Benedict R H, DeLuca J, Krupp L B, Thompson A J and Comi G 2013 Treatment of cognitive impairment in multiple sclerosis: position paper *J. Neurol.* **260** 1452–68
[73] Messinis L *et al* 2017 Efficacy of a computer-assisted cognitive rehabilitation intervention in relapsing-remitting multiple sclerosis patients: a multicenter randomized controlled trial *Behav. Neurol.* **2017** 5919841
[74] Gromisch E S, Fiszdon J M and Kurtz M M 2018 The effects of cognitive-focused interventions on cognition and psychological well-being in persons with multiple sclerosis: A meta-analysis *Neuropsychol. Rehabil.* 1–20
[75] Sumowski J F *et al* 2018 Cognition in multiple sclerosis: State of the field and priorities for the future *Neurology* **90** 278–88
[76] Kimura D and Clarke P G 2002 Women's advantage on verbal memory is not restricted to concrete words *Psychol. Rep.* **91** 1137–42
[77] Piber D, Nowacki J, Mueller S C, Wingenfeld K and Otte C 2018 Sex effects on spatial learning but not on spatial memory retrieval in healthy young adults *Behav. Brain Res.* **336** 44–50
[78] Gale S D, Baxter L, Connor D J, Herring A and Comer J 2007 Sex differences on the Rey Auditory Verbal Learning Test and the Brief Visuospatial Memory Test–Revised in the elderly: Normative data in 172 participants *J. Clin. Exp. Neuropsychol.* **29** 561–7
[79] Argento O, Pisani V, Incerti C C, Magistrale G, Caltagirone C and Nocentini U 2015 The California Verbal Learning Test-II: normative data for two Italian alternative forms *Clin. Neuropsychol.* **28** 42–54
[80] Rahn K, Slusher B and Kaplin A 2012 Cognitive impairment in multiple sclerosis: a forgotten disability remembered *Cerebrum: the Dana Forum on Brain Science* vol 2012 (New York: Dana Foundation)

[81] Zachary R A and Gorsuch R L 1985 Continuous norming: Implications for the WAIS-R *J. Clin. Psychol.* **41** 86–94
[82] Caffarra P, Vezzadini G, Dieci F, Zonato F and Venneri A 2002 Rey-Osterrieth complex figure: normative values in an Italian population sample *Neurol. Sci.* **22** 443–7
[83] Van der Elst W, Van Boxtel M P, Van Breukelen G J and Jolles J 2006 The Stroop color-word test: influence of age, sex, and education; and normative data for a large sample across the adult age range *Assessment* **13** 62–79
[84] Parmenter B A, Testa S M, Schretlen D J, Weinstock-Guttman B and Benedict R H 2010 The utility of regression-based norms in interpreting the minimal assessment of cognitive function in multiple sclerosis (MACFIMS) *J. Int. Neuropsychol. Soc.* **16** 6–16
[85] Argento O, Smerbeck A, Pisani V, Magistrale G, Incerti C C, Caltagirone C, Benedict R H and Nocentini U 2016 Regression-based norms for the Brief Visuospatial Memory Test-Revised in Italian population and application in MS patients *Clin. Neuropsychol.* **30** 1469–78
[86] Testa S M, Winicki J M, Pearlson G D, Gordon B and Schretlen D J 2009 Accounting for estimated IQ in neuropsychological test performance with regression-based techniques *J. Int. Neuropsychol. Soc.* **15** 1012–22
[87] Allali G, Laidet M, Assal F, Chofflon M, Armand S and Lalive P H 2014 Dual-task assessment in natalizumab-treated multiple sclerosis patients *Eur. Neurol.* **71** 247–51
[88] Beste C, Mückschel M, Paucke M and Ziemssen T 2018 Dual-tasking in multiple sclerosis–implications for a cognitive screening instrument *Front. Hum. Neurosci.* **12** 24
[89] Goverover Y, O'Brien A R, Moore N B and DeLuca J 2010 Actual reality: a new approach to functional assessment in persons with multiple sclerosis *Arch. Phys. Med. Rehabil.* **91** 252–60
[90] Goverover Y, Chiaravalloti N and DeLuca J 2016 Brief International Cognitive Assessment for Multiple Sclerosis (BICAMS) and performance of everyday life tasks: Actual reality *Mult. Scler. J.* **22** 544–50
[91] Rouaud O, Graule-Petot A, Couvreur G, Contegal F, Osseby G V, Benatru I, Giroud M and Moreau T 2006 Contribution of ecological evaluation of executive disorders in multiple sclerosis *Rev. Neurol.* **162** 964–9
[92] Sumowski J F, Chiaravalloti N, Wylie G and DeLuca J 2009 Cognitive reserve moderates the negative effect of brain atrophy on cognitive efficiency in multiple sclerosis *J. Int. Neuropsychol. Soc.* **15** 606–12
[93] Benedict R H and Zgaljardic D J 1998 Practice effects during repeated administrations of memory tests with and without alternate forms *J. Clin. Exp. Neuropsychol.* **20** 339–52
[94] Woods S P, Delis D C, Scott J C, Kramer J H and Holdnack J A 2006 The California Verbal Learning Test–second edition: test-retest reliability, practice effects, and reliable change indices for the standard and alternate forms *Arch. Clin. Neuropsychol.* **21** 413–20
[95] Benedict R H and Groninger L 1995 Preliminary standardization of a new visuospatial memory test with six alternate forms *Clin. Neuropsychol.* **9** 11–6
[96] Morrow S A *et al* 2010 Evaluation of the symbol digit modalities test (SDMT) and MS neuropsychological screening questionnaire (MSNQ) in natalizumab-treated MS patients over 48 weeks *Mult. Scler. J.* **16** 1385–92
[97] Benedict R H, Smerbeck A, Parikh R, Rodgers J, Cadavid D and Erlanger D 2012 Reliability and equivalence of alternate forms for the Symbol Digit Modalities Test: implications for multiple sclerosis clinical trials *Mult. Scler. J.* **18** 1320–5

[98] National Institute for Health and Care Excellence 2014 *Multiple sclerosis in adults: management Clinical Guidelines (CG 186)* (London: NICE)

[99] Rae-Grant A, Bennett A, Sanders A E, Phipps M, Cheng E and Bever C 2015 Quality improvement in neurology: Multiple sclerosis quality measures executive summary *Neurology* **85** 1904–8

[100] Bakirtzis C, Ioannidis P, Messinis L, Nasios G, Konstantinopoulou E, Papathanasopoulos P and Grigoriadis N 2018 The rationale for monitoring cognitive function in multiple sclerosis: practical issues for clinicians *Open Neurol. J.* **12** 31

[101] Viner R, Fiest K M, Bulloch A G, Williams J V, Lavorato D H, Berzins S, Jette N, Metz L M and Patten S B 2014 Point prevalence and correlates of depression in a national community sample with multiple sclerosis *Gen. Hosp. Psychiatry* **36** 352–4

[102] Strober L B and Arnett P A 2015 Depression in multiple sclerosis: The utility of common self-report instruments and development of a disease-specific measure *J. Clin. Exp. Neuropsychol.* **37** 722–32

[103] Fischer J S, Foley F W, Aikens J E, Ericson G D, Rao S M and Shindell S 1994 What do we really know about cognitive dysfunction, affective disorders, and stress in multiple sclerosis? A practitioner's guide *J. Neurol. Rehabil.* **8** 151–64

[104] Arnett P A, Higginson C I, Voss W D, Bender W I, Wurst J M and Tippin J M 1999 Depression in multiple sclerosis: relationship to working memory capacity *Neuropsychology* **13** 546

[105] Arnett P A, Higginson C I, Voss W D, Wright B, Bender W I, Wurst J M and Tippin J M 1999 Depressed mood in multiple sclerosis: relationship to capacity-demanding memory and attentional functioning *Neuropsychology* **13** 434

[106] Arnett P A, Higginson C I and Randolph J J 2001 Depression in multiple sclerosis: relationship to planning ability *J. Int. Neuropsychol. Soc.* **7** 665–74

[107] Arnett P A, Barwick F H and Beeney J E 2008 Depression in multiple sclerosis: review and theoretical proposal *J. Int. Neuropsychol. Soc.* **14** 691–724

[108] Heesen C, Schulz K H, Fiehler J, Von der Mark U, Otte C, Jung R, Poettgen J, Kriger T and Gold S M 2010 Correlates of cognitive dysfunction in multiple sclerosis *Brain Behav. Immun.* **24** 1148–55

[109] Niino M *et al* 2014 Apathy/depression, but not subjective fatigue, is related with cognitive dysfunction in patients with multiple sclerosis *BMC Neurol.* **14** 3

[110] Diamond B J, Johnson S K, Kaufman M and Graves L 2008 Relationships between information processing, depression, fatigue and cognition in multiple sclerosis *Arch. Clin. Neuropsychol.* **23** 189–99

[111] Demaree H, Gaudino E and DeLuca J 2003 The relationship between depressive symptoms and cognitive dysfunction in multiple sclerosis *Cogn. Neuropsychiatry* **8** 161–71

[112] Krupp L B and Elkins L E 2000 Fatigue and declines in cognitive functioning in multiple sclerosis *Neurology* **55** 934–9

[113] Hanken K, Manousi A, Klein J, Kastrup A, Eling P A T M and Hildebrandt H 2016 On the relation between self-reported cognitive fatigue and the posterior hypothalamic – brainstem network *Eur. J. Neurol.* **23** 101–9

[114] Golan D, Doniger G M, Wissemann K, Zarif M, Bumstead B, Buhse M, Fafard L, Lavi I, Wilken J and Gudesblatt M 2018 The impact of subjective cognitive fatigue and depression on cognitive function in patients with multiple sclerosis *Mult. Scler. J.* **24** 196–204

[115] Hughes A J, Parmenter B A, Haselkorn J K, Lovera J F, Bourdette D, Boudreau E, Cameron M H and Turner A P 2017 Sleep and its associations with perceived and objective cognitive impairment in individuals with multiple sclerosis *J. Sleep Res.* **26** 428–35
[116] Braley T J, Kratz A L, Kaplish N and Chervin R D 2016 Sleep and cognitive function in multiple sclerosis *Sleep* **39** 1525–33
[117] Patel V P, Walker L A and Feinstein A 2017 Processing speed and distractibility in multiple sclerosis: the role of sleep *Mult. Scler. Relat. Disord.* **11** 40–2
[118] Figved N, Benedict R, Klevan G, Myhr K M, Nyland H I, Landrø N I, Larsen J P and Aarsland D 2008 Relationship of cognitive impairment to psychiatric symptoms in multiple sclerosis *Mult. Scler. J.* **14** 1084–90
[119] Roy S, Schwartz C E, Duberstein P, Dwyer M G, Zivadinov R, Bergsland N, Powell V and Benedict R H 2016 Synergistic effects of reserve and adaptive personality in multiple sclerosis *J. Int. Neuropsychol. Soc.* **22** 920–7
[120] Sandroff B M, Schwartz C E and DeLuca J 2016 Measurement and maintenance of reserve in multiple sclerosis *J. Neurol.* **263** 2158–69
[121] Camp S J *et al* 1999 Cognitive function in primary progressive and transitional progressive multiple sclerosis *Brain* **122** 1341–8
[122] Jill S F, Jak A J and Kniker M A J E 2001 Multiple Sclerosis Functional Composite (MSFC) *Administration and Scoring Manual*
[123] Morrow S A, Drake A, Zivadinov R, Munschauer F, Weinstock-Guttman B and Benedict R H 2010 Predicting loss of employment over three years in multiple sclerosis: clinically meaningful cognitive decline *Clin. Neuropsychol.* **24** 1131–45
[124] Benedict R H, DeLuca J, Phillips G, LaRocca N, Hudson L D, Rudick R and Multiple Sclerosis Outcome Assessments Consortium 2017 Validity of the Symbol Digit Modalities Test as a cognition performance outcome measure for multiple sclerosis *Mult. Scler. J.* **23** 721–33
[125] Goldman M D, Ward M D, Motl R W, Jones D E, Pula J H and Cadavid D 2017 Identification and validation of clinically meaningful benchmarks in the 12-item Multiple Sclerosis Walking Scale *Mult. Scler. J.* **23** 1405–14
[126] Benedict R H, Drake A S, Irwin L N, Frndak S E, Kunker K A, Khan A L, Kordovski V M, Motl R W and Weinstock-Guttman B 2016 Benchmarks of meaningful impairment on the MSFC and BICAMS *Mult. Scler. J.* **22** 1874–82
[127] Bickenbach J, Cieza A, Rauch A and Stucki G (ed) 2012 *ICF Core Sets: Manual for Clinical Practice for the ICF Research Branch, in Cooperation with the WHO Collaborating Centre for the Family of International Classifications in Germany (DIMDI)* (Boston, MA: Hogrefe)

IOP Publishing

Neurological Disorders and Imaging Physics, Volume 2
Engineering and clinical perspectives of multiple sclerosis
Ayman El-Baz and Jasjit S Suri

Chapter 10

Imaging disconnection in multiple sclerosis

Riccardo Manca, Basil Sharrack and Annalena Venneri

Multiple sclerosis (MS) is an immune-mediated disease characterised by demyelination across the central nervous system (CNS). Lesions characteristic of MS are mainly detected in white matter by means of magnetic resonance imaging (MRI). The consequent disruption observed in structural brain connections favoured the conceptualization of MS as a disconnection syndrome. However, only recently researchers have started to explore with more advanced neuroimaging techniques the effects that MS-induced disconnection exerts on brain organization as well as on clinical manifestations.

Diffusion and functional MRI represent the main two techniques that offer a window into the investigation of such alterations. In particular, while structural connectivity appears to decrease throughout the disease course, functional connectivity increases associated with preserved cognitive and motor functions have been reported to occur transiently in the early phases of MS. Interesting confirmatory findings have also emerged from recently developed approaches, such as, for example, computational modelling and machine learning.

10.1 The complexity of multiple sclerosis

MS is an immune-mediated disease characterized by an abnormal inflammatory response targeting the CNS [1]. The worldwide prevalence of MS is estimated to be of about 2.3–2.5 million people affected [2, 3]. The onset of MS often occurs early in life, with a peak commonly reported around 30 years of age, and for this reason this disease is considered as one of the major causes of disability in young adulthood [4]. Although MS represents a considerable source of burden for patients and careers, its etiology is still unclear and multiple interacting factors, genetic and environmental, are considered essential in the etiology of MS and in its progression by influencing both severity of symptoms and neural damage [5, 6].

The clinical features that characterize MS are the outcome of neural damage resulting from two types of disease process: neural inflammation and

doi:10.1088/978-0-7503-1762-7ch10

neurodegeneration [7]. Inflammation has been extensively documented by the detection of different populations of autoreactive T cells in the neural tissue. In particular, these cells attack and damage the myelin sheath that surrounds axons [8, 9] and subsequently cause axonal transection and oligodendrocytes death [10]. The resulting demyelinating lesions can be visualized by means of conventional structural MRI and represent the hallmark of MS. However, with increasing and spreading myelin damage, other pathological processes are triggered and lead to neurodegeneration both in white (WM) and gray matter (GM) [11]. Indeed, the MS-related inflammatory response is associated with several different pathological mechanisms, such as astrocytes activation, microglia activation, mitochondria dysfunction, and iron accumulation [12]. As the disease progresses, these processes worsen and loss of brain volume becomes the predominant feature [13].

The course of this disease can be highly variable, but different phenotypes have been classified mainly based on the dynamic patterns of signs and symptoms [14]. At onset, about 85% of patients are diagnosed with relapsing–remitting MS (RRMS) [15], the course of which is characterized by relapses, featuring sudden increases in levels of disability, followed by partial or full recovery and general functional improvement [14]. After an average period of about 10 years from onset of RRMS, patients may transition to secondary progressive MS (SPMS) [16]. The so-called primary progressive MS (PPMS), instead, presents with a steady increase of disability from onset without definite relapses [17, 18]. Similarly to SPMS, neurodegenerative processes rather than inflammatory activity are thought to underlie this phenotype [19].

The clinical presentation of MS is characterized by multiple levels of complexity that reflect not only variable disease courses, but also heterogeneity of signs and symptoms experienced by patients, including fatigue, reported by 40%–80% of the people with MS [20–22], motor dysfunction [3], visual [23] and somatosensory dysfunctions [24], cognitive impairment [25] and mental health problems [26].

10.2 The importance of MRI in MS

The use of MRI plays a pivotal role in the process of diagnosis definition in MS. Indeed, according to the McDonald criteria, two distinct clinical attacks along with dissemination in time and space of CNS lesions must be evidenced [27]. In particular, to diagnose RRMS at least two different relapses must be reported by patients or objectively observed in the absence of fever and inflammation, over at least 24 h, and presenting either as new symptoms or worsening of existing ones.

A diagnosis of MS can be potentially made on the basis of clinical history of symptoms compatible with demyelinating pathology alone, yet at least one relapse needs to be corroborated by MRI findings. Additionally, the analysis of cerebrospinal fluid can support a diagnosis of MS if oligoclonal bands are detected, since they signal the presence of intrathecal inflammation. Imaging brain and spinal cord lesions is an essential step and different structural MRI sequences, i.e. T1-weighted, T2-weighted and fluid attenuated inversion recovery (FLAIR) images, are commonly used in clinical practice for this purpose. In particular, T1-weighted scans combined with injection of contrast agents containing gadolinium are used to enhance newly formed WM lesions. Indeed, in normal conditions gadolinium molecules cannot cross the blood–brain barrier (BBB) because of their dimensions. However, when the BBB is damaged by inflammatory processes like in MS, gadolinium can spread in the neural tissue and highlight areas of recent disease activity that may be distinguished from older non-active lesions [28, 29]. Diagnosis of PPMS, instead, depends on documented evidence of not less than 1 year progression of disease with continuous worsening of symptoms corroborated by objective MRI findings [27, 30].

Cerebral WM lesions can arise in any location throughout the neural tissue, but peaks of distribution have been consistently reported in periventricular areas and the centrum semiovale [31, 32]. Moreover, regions with high venous and low arterial density are particularly prone to lesion accumulation, probably as a result of higher susceptibility to the pathological processes of MS, such as, for example, oxidative stress [33]. Lesions can be classified into three groups on the basis of the presence of inflammation and demyelination: active lesions, characterized by ongoing demyelination and by the presence of activated macrophages and microglia; inactive lesions, without ongoing demyelination and a negligible amount of macrophages and microglia; mixed lesions, characterized by inflammatory activity in their peripheral layers only [34]. Pathological studies have shown that demyelination is a dynamic process and that during remissions oligodendrocyte precursor cells can regenerate the myelin sheath [35]. However, the remyelination process does not lead to full replacement of the axonal cover, occurs only for a proportion of patients [36] and the new oligodendrocytes are highly susceptible to further damage [37].

MS lesions also affect the spinal cord, although less attention has been given to this structure due to its mobility and smaller size that make it more difficult to investigate with MRI [38]. Similarly, demyelination can extend beyond WM to the deepest GM layers forming juxtacortical lesions [39] or even develop just within cortical or deep GM [40]. GM lesions have been traditionally difficult to detect with conventional structural MRI (T1-weighted, T2-weighted and FLAIR) because they are characterized by low inflammatory activity and have no association with significant BBB disruption. Moreover, problematic partial volume effects are present due to the proximity of cortical GM and the cerebrospinal fluid [41]. Significant improvements have been reached with the use of new MRI sequences, such as double inversion recovery [42], magnetization-prepared rapid acquisition with gradient echo [43] and phase-sensitive recovery imaging [44]. However, despite these promising results, visualization of GM pathology in MS is not considered optimal yet [30].

Along with imaging lesions that are indicative of inflammatory disease activity, the monitoring of brain macrostructural alterations occurring over time due to neurodegeneration has also been investigated in MS. In particular, GM atrophy has been extensively documented and is thought to result directly from GM lesions, but also from retrograde degeneration secondary to WM lesions causing axonal transection [45]. The annual rate of brain volume loss in people affected by MS has been observed to be about 0.7%, significantly higher than the 0.1%–0.3% found in age-matched healthy controls [46]. GM areas that are mainly affected include subcortical nuclei, thalamus and basal ganglia [47], as well as primary somatosensory and motor cortices [48]. After the transition from RRMS to SPMS, neurodegenerative changes worsen and atrophy spreads to other areas, especially the hippocampus and the cerebellum [49].

The above mentioned lesional and atrophy measures have been applied to the investigation of the impact of MS on the brain as well as to the assessment of response to various disease modifying and symptomatic treatments [50]. However, the complex symptomatology that characterizes MS and any potential treatment effects can be explained only marginally by such imaging outcome measures. Advanced neuroimaging techniques (e.g. diffusion tensor and functional MRI as well as neurophysiology measures) have also been used recently in MS research, although they present higher demands in both acquisition and analysis that currently limit their application in clinical settings. Nevertheless, these advanced techniques provide more details than lesion and atrophy quantification about the dynamic and multifaceted changes triggered by MS pathology at different neural levels and, in particular, offer a valuable opportunity to clarify how this disease alters brain architecture.

10.3 Brain organization in MS: the impact of disease on connectivity

Lesions characteristics of MS pathology may arise in both WM and GM in any part of the CNS, although some specific lesion sites have been associated with both severity [51] and evolution of clinical symptoms [52]. Radiological and clinical observations, especially of cognition [53, 54], have led to the proposal of a theoretical framework that conceives MS as a disconnection syndrome or even as a multiple disconnection syndrome to account for the high degree of variability in symptoms [55]. In MS, disconnection is predominantly observed at the structural level, since demyelination and axonal transection occurring in MS lesions deeply affect WM fiber integrity. As a consequence, communication between connected brain areas becomes, at first, inefficient and, in later stages, largely deficient [56]. Moreover, alterations in functional cerebral organization, both at rest and during active task performance, have been also documented in MS [57]. The interruption of one or more structural links supporting functional brain networks is likely to be the major cause of such changes. However, an in-depth characterization of which specific WM tracts may be preferentially interested by MS-related pathology and of the possible wider impact on brain functioning is still fragmentary. For this reason and in consideration of the central role that the concept of disconnection has assumed in this field of research, neuroimaging evidence of both structural and functional disconnection in this disease will be reviewed in this chapter.

10.3.1 Structural connectivity

Structural connections have been mainly investigated by means of MRI sequences designed to capture diffusion properties of the brain tissues. Indeed, the study of how water molecules diffuse in the brain allows the indirect *in vivo* (non-invasive) assessment of the structural alterations that may occur in the CNS and especially in WM tracts.

In the past decades, different approaches have been adopted to develop mathematical models of diffusion that could be biologically plausible. The first concepts of diffusion MRI have been introduced by Le Bihan *et al* [58] and paved the way to diffusion tensor imaging (DTI) [59, 60], which represents the most commonly used technique in the field. The diffusion tensor is a tri-dimensional model based on the assumption that water molecules in the brain diffuse following a Gaussian pattern along each direction. This behaviour is geometrically described by an ellipsoid, the main three axes of which are named eigenvectors (ε_1, ε_2, ε_3) (figure 10.1). The scalars that quantify the length of the main axes are named eigenvalues (λ_1, λ_2, λ_3) and are used to derive several DTI indices to characterize the status of the neural tissue.

In particular, three measures provide information about the amount of diffusion in different directions: mean diffusivity (MD) is calculated as the average of the three eigenvalues; axial diffusivity (AD) is equivalent to λ_1, i.e. the level of diffusion along the principal axis; radial diffusivity (RD), corresponds to the average of λ_2 and λ_3 and describes the possibility of diffusion along directions perpendicular to the principal axis.

Fractional anisotropy (FA), instead, is a scalar with a value that spans between 0 and 1 and is calculated with the following formula:

$$FA = \sqrt[2]{\frac{1}{2}} \frac{\sqrt[2]{(\lambda_1 - \lambda_2)^2 + (\lambda_2 - \lambda_3)^2 + (\lambda_3 - \lambda_1)^2}}{\sqrt[2]{\lambda_1^2 + \lambda_2^2 + \lambda_3^2}}$$

FA describes the directionality of diffusion, i.e. the higher *FA* values, the more direction-dependent is diffusion of water molecules. Therefore, when water diffuses preferentially along one main axis, *FA* approaches 1 and the ellipsoid becomes more

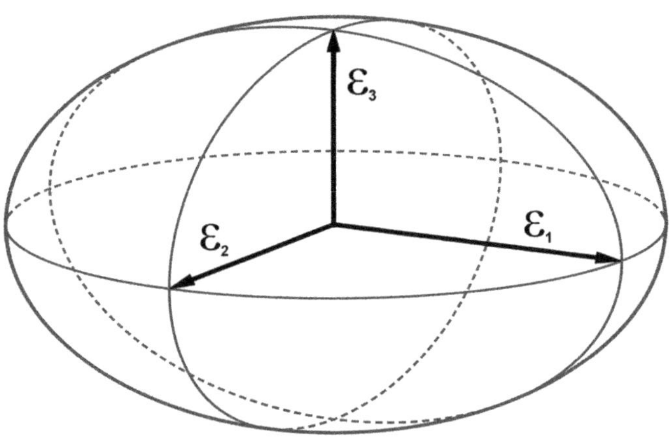

Figure 10.1. Ellipsoid that geometrically represents the diffusion tensor.

elongated due to the large difference between λ_1 and λ_2/λ_3values. In contrast, *FA* value decreases towards 0 when water is free to diffuse in any direction.

Although it provides useful information about microstructural integrity of normal appearing WM, DTI remains a simplistic model of diffusion and its application to the characterization of voxels containing multidirectional fibres shows limitations [61]. In order to overcome this issue, high angular resolution diffusion imaging (HARDI) [62, 63] has been developed by acquiring signals along a number of diffusion directions higher than standard DTI. As a result, its application has improved reconstruction of crossing fibres in brain areas characterized by the presence of intersecting WM tracts [64].

An alternative 'model-free' approach is *q*-space imaging, based on the acquisition of diffusion data at multiple *b* values. The central concept of this technique is the derivation of diffusion parameters by the Fourier transformation of signal decay [65]. The application of this technique may provide more detailed measures of neural tissue integrity and function than DTI [66]. However, to date very limited applications of these techniques to MS can be traced in the literature, probably due to their high demands in terms of technology and time needed for image acquisition [67].

More recently, new models of diffusion MRI have been elaborated to incorporate multiple compartments of brain tissue that appear to improve our ability to image WM microstructure [68, 69]. In fact, efforts have been made to develop sequences that may detect specific biological orientation properties, such as neurite dispersion and density imaging (NODDI) [70], a new diffusion technique based on HARDI optimized for clinical settings and suitable for the assessment of properties of three compartments: intra-cellular, extra-cellular and cerebrospinal fluid. Although the clinical relevance of these results has not been fully ascertained, the authors suggested the two markers identified by means of NODDI are more specific than FA and, for this reason, their possible applications to MS appear promising. Indeed, the interest for the development of new sequences that can be integrated in clinical neuroradiological protocols is continuously growing, not only to identify MS-related microstructural changes [67], but also to develop diffusion MRI outcome measures for clinical trials [71, 72].

Currently available analyses for diffusion MRI data focus on two complementary levels of investigation: indices derived from DTI and similar models are used to infer the status of microstructural integrity of brain tissue, while tractography represents a tool to characterize macrostructural changes in volume and fibre count within specific reconstructed WM tracts. Therefore, both of these two lines of research will be further discussed.

10.3.1.1 White matter diffusivity

Global measures of atrophy and lesional neural tissue are able to explain symptomatic manifestations of MS only marginally and the severity of patients' functional status does not always appear to be justified by the macrostructural alterations [73]. The lack of a straightforward association between MRI measures conventionally available in the clinic and signs observed in patients may be due to limitations in the way we image MS-related pathological changes. In fact, it is an intuitive thought that the detection of new gadolinium-enhancing lesions must be necessarily preceded by a series of pathological processes (e.g. demyelination, axonal injury etc) not reflected in the type of information acquired by means of T1-weighted, T2-weighted and FLAIR images. It follows that lesions typical of brains affected by MS may be considered as the macrostructural hallmark of a cascade of events occurring at a microstructural scale and, therefore, captured to a greater extent by diffusion MRI.

A few longitudinal DTI studies have been carried out to clarify the relationship between the emergence of new lesions and possible alterations in WM microstructure. A study found that all common indices of diffusivity, but in particular RD, increase significantly up to 10 months prior to detection of lesion enhancement in sites of normal appearing WM where lesions would later form [74]. Similarly, *FA* values would also decrease in the same areas but only 3 months prior to detection of lesion enhancement. These results are consistent with longitudinal observations of changes in magnetization transfer ratio (MTR) preceding enhancement detection [75]. MTR quantifies the interaction between protons in constrained environments, such as the macromolecules found in cell membranes and in the myelin sheath, and those whose motion is less restricted, e.g. water molecules. This phenomenon is indicative of both microstructural and macrostructural degenerative processes that may occur in the CNS, such as demyelination.

Detection of microstructural changes characteristic of MS detected by DTI appears to follow the appearance of new lesions. Increased diffusivity indices and decreased *FA* were observed in the inferior cerebellar peduncles and in the arcuate fasciculus [76]; Chiang *et al* [77], instead, found drops in *FA* values in the corticospinal tract and the forceps major, but not in the forceps minor. Therefore, the presence of enhancing lesions, sign of active inflammatory mechanisms, appears to be associated with WM damage in areas extending beyond the pure lesion sites. In fact, a study that focused on the degeneration of the cerebellum in MS found that decreased *FA* in cerebellar normal appearing WM negatively correlated with WM lesion volume and WM/GM ratio [78]. Moreover, detrimental effects of active lesions have been reported to impact also brain morphology since their presence was associated with loss of neural tissue volume in nearby and even functionally related regions [79]. Hence, these convergent findings seem to suggest that lesions due to MS represent a visible sign of complex pathological processes that involve networks of structurally related brain areas.

As MS is a disease characterized by a high degree of variability and, especially in the RRMS phenotype, by alternating phases of demyelination and remyelination of changeable duration, attempts have been made to clarify the evolution of damage in structural connectivity. Haung *et al* [80] compared patients with clinically isolated syndrome and MS to age- and gender-matched healthy controls and found that changes in DTI indices compatible with WM microstructural damage (decreased *FA* and increased diffusivity) can be detected in several tracts in the early stages of the disease (clinically isolated syndrome). Similar alterations were more severe and widespread in the MS group. However, inconsistent findings emerged from longitudinal studies: although Raz *et al* [81] reported no changes in DTI measures in the year following the first relapse in a sample of 33 patients, subsequent studies carried out on larger cohorts and with longer follow-ups reported a significant deterioration of WM microstructural integrity as MS pathology progressed [82, 83].

Neural damage consequent to MS may occur in any brain compartment, however, a recent meta-analysis including 12 studies, for a total of 495 patients with MS and 253 healthy controls, found that peaks of *FA* decrease are more often seen in the corpus callosum, periventricular WM and the fornix [84]. Interestingly, the authors also performed meta-regression analyses to investigate where in the brain damage to structural connections is more strongly associated with specific symptoms, finding only partially overlapping results. Level of physical disability was negatively correlated with *FA* values in the fornix and in posterior sections of some WM tracts, namely the cingulum, the splenium of the corpus callosum and the inferior fronto-occipital fasciculus. Conversely, cognitive impairment appeared to be negatively associated with WM microstructural damage in the genu of the corpus callosum, thalamic WM, the fornix and the posterior cingulum. Therefore, while physical symptoms are more associated with posterior WM degeneration, cognition seems to be impacted more substantially by injury in structural connections in frontal regions.

While MS-related motor dysfunction, such as limb weakness, has been consistently linked with degeneration of the corticospinal tracts [85–87], the neural correlates of fatigue remain still poorly understood, despite the frequency of this symptom in MS. Pardini *et al* [88], using a voxel-wise correlational approach, found that the level of perceived fatigue correlated significantly with lower *FA* only in a cluster of WM in the left frontal lobe comprising fibers of different tracts: inferior fronto-occipital fasciculus, anterior limb of the internal capsule, anterior thalamic radiations and the anterior cingulum. More recently, instead, findings point either at the involvement of a single WM tract, i.e. the cingulum [89], or at a much more extended network including WM clusters also in the corona radiata and brainstem [90]. Variability in findings may be partially due to discrepancies in the measures used to evaluate this symptom in these studies and, therefore, currently a definite neural signature for fatigue due to MS has not been identified yet.

For cognition, a longitudinal study showed that generalized degradation of WM microstructural integrity predicts cognitive impairment in early phases of MS, while in the progressive forms of this disease cognitive impairment seems driven mainly by GM atrophy, the main hallmark of neurodegeneration [91]. Indeed, people with RRMS and cognitive deficits show extensively lower degrees of WM microstructural integrity than healthy controls [92]. In line with the findings from Walton *et al* [84], a recent review showed that there is a trend towards an association between decline in speed of information processing, a distinctive symptom experienced by people with MS, and disruption in structural connections in frontal regions [93]. It cannot be ruled out, however, that impairment in different cognitive domains may be due to damage in alternative structural networks. To date, further investigations appear to be needed in order to associate clearly breakdowns in specific WM tracts caused by MS pathological processes and one or more cognitive symptoms.

10.3.1.2 Tractography

Alongside the study of microstructural properties of structural cerebral connections, diffusion MRI also offers the possibility to study the morphology of WM tracts that link different GM areas using tractography. The first studies to use such technique in rat [94] and human brains [95] date back to only 20 years ago. Tractography allows *in vivo* tri-dimensional reconstruction of WM tracts by exploiting the directionality of diffusion of water molecules, i.e. *FA* values derived from diffusion-weighted MRI (figure 10.2). Therefore, after setting one or two 'seed' regions known to be crossed or connected by a specific WM tract, fibers are tracked by following the preferred diffusion direction in each voxel starting from the seeds [96]. Indeed, tractography algorithms infer that diffusion directionality is similar in adjacent voxels assumed to be part of the same WM tract. Different types of information can be investigated, such as total WM tract volume, total count of tracked lines (not indicative of the actual number of axons) and diffusivity properties in the tract.

One of the main challenges concerning the application of tractography to the study of brains affected by MS is due to the presence of lesions. In fact, discrepancy in *FA* values has been observed between demyelinating lesions and the surrounding normal appearing WM [76]. The presence of abrupt changes in *FA* across adjacent voxels may be interpreted by tracking algorithms as the termination of a WM tract and, in turn, hamper the process of tract reconstruction. However, it is possible to overcome this issue by reconstructing a given tract in a sample of healthy subjects to create a probability map and use this to derive diffusivity metrics in tracts of patients with MS [98, 99].

Being a recent methodology, tractography is still under development and there has been limited application to MS. Indeed, this technique mainly relies on time-consuming and labor intensive manual procedures that may be partially dependent on individual neuroanatomical knowledge and lead to variable results. For this reason, the outcome of conventional (manual) versus automated reconstruction methodologies has been compared for some WM tracts most commonly affected by MS pathology: corpus callosum, corticospinal tracts, optic radiations and tracts. Automated tractography performed similarly to conventional reconstruction and

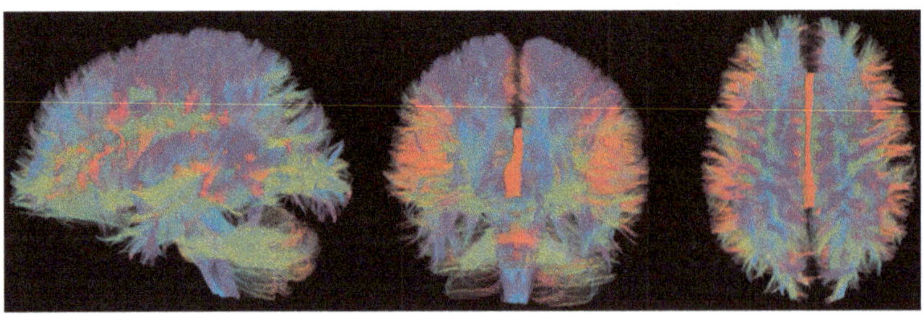

Figure 10.2. Whole brain tractography for reconstruction of WM fibers color-coded according to their directionality: blue for dorsal–ventral, red for left–right, green for anterior-posterior. Adapted from Tax *et al* [97] and used under the Creative Commons Attribution License.

was not affected by lesions. Diffusivity indices obtained with the two approaches were moderately to highly correlated except for those of the optic tracts [100].

Performance of different tractography algorithms was also assessed by contrasting deterministic and probabilistic reconstruction of WM tracts. The deterministic approach was the first to be developed based on the assumption that WM fibers in each voxel are parallel to the prominent diffusion direction, therefore leading to the reconstruction of a single path from the seed. Probabilistic tractography, instead, assumes that different fiber orientations may be possible, thus tracing multiple paths from the seed region and subsequently identifying the most likely direction from a distribution of different alternative orientations [101]. In a study carried out on 28 people affected by RRMS and 28 age-matched healthy controls both procedures found consistent results: reduction in tracked lines and fiber density that were negatively associated with disability levels in MS patients [102].

More recently, a new analytical framework, named profilometry, has been proposed with the aim of investigating how combinations of different MRI parameters along reconstructed WM tracts were affected by MS [103]. In particular, the authors integrated RD, associated with both inflammation and myelin status, and myelin water fraction, i.e. an index that is considered an estimate of the amount of myelin in each voxel [104]. Both measures of structural integrity were found altered, especially in lesion sites and in the forceps minor, but myelin water fraction discriminated between patients and healthy controls better than RD. Although this new method appears interesting for the possibility to visualize different measures along reconstructed tracts, the authors suggest its use is best suited to large cohorts of patients with MS characterized by more consistent lesion location.

Indications that structural brain connectivity is affected by MS pathology appear clearly, although the complex interactions between lesion formation, disruption of WM tract and GM atrophy are still a matter of debate. In fact, a significant relationship between lesion location and WM tract atrophy was not found by a study that observed uniform damage throughout most tracts, explained by the authors as a consequence of widespread neural inflammation [105]. However, disruption in different WM tracts may be associated with the presence of lesions [106]. Moreover, the same study observed that volume loss in frontal callosal fibers as well as in the inferior fronto-occipital and longitudinal fasciculus were linked to GM atrophy in cortical regions connected by such tracts. Consistently, it has been suggested that structural disconnection could drive GM volume loss [107], but could also occur consequently to MS-related GM damage [108]. Therefore, these findings suggest the existence of mutual influences between atrophy in WM tracts and in GM areas connected by them and these abnormalities are thought to underlie the clinical manifestations typical of MS. In fact, correlations have been consistently found between disability level [109], specific sensory [110] and cognitive deficits [111, 112] and atrophy in relevant WM tracts.

The field of neuroimaging analysis has recently seen also the application of a novel mathematical approach based on graph theory to the study of the so-called *connectome*: term coined to describe the complex of all the cerebral connections [113] that has attracted a great deal of interest in neuroscience [114]. Several studies have used graph theory to investigate both functional (resting-state MRI and neurophysiological signal) and structural connections (diffusion MRI and tractography) in healthy and diseased brains [115]. This technique is based on the generation of a theoretical representation of the brain as a set of distinct regions, called nodes, connected by edges [116] (figure 10.3).

The identification of the nodes may vary across neuroimaging modalities, but for MRI data are usually based on the anatomical parcellation of the brain into a given number of areas. Pairwise associations across all nodes is consequently calculated and based, for example, on connection probability for diffusion MRI or inter-regional correlations between resting-state MRI signals. An *adjacency matrix* is then compiled with data on the pairwise associations and graph-based network parameters derived by this for statistical analyses. Several different graph-based measures have been used to investigate the topographical properties of the brain leading to consistent observations, especially about its modular and small-world organization [115, 117].

This theoretical framework has also been proficiently used with the aim of characterizing brain-wise and network-specific alterations due to MS [118]. Indeed, the ubiquitous distribution of demyelinating lesions makes this approach particularly interesting to study metrics of structural disconnection across the whole brain. The most commonly investigated index of global structural connectivity is *efficiency*, defined as the inverse of the average shortest path length, i.e. the average of the minimum number of edges to go from one node to any other in the brain. In particular, efficiency appears decreased across several networks in people with MS and correlated with WM lesion load and disability status [119]. Loss of network efficiency has also been associated with markers of neural tissue damage, such as myoinositol and *N*-acetylaspartate, and may explain severity of cognitive impairment [120, 121]. Such changes have been consistently reported to occur from the clinically isolated syndrome stage and shown to worsen later with progression of the disease [122–124]. Convergent findings show that disruptions affect structural connections between different networks [122] and are believed to cause increased brain modularization and clustering: MS pathology causes the brain to reorganize in networks segregated from one another but with more intra-networks connections [123].

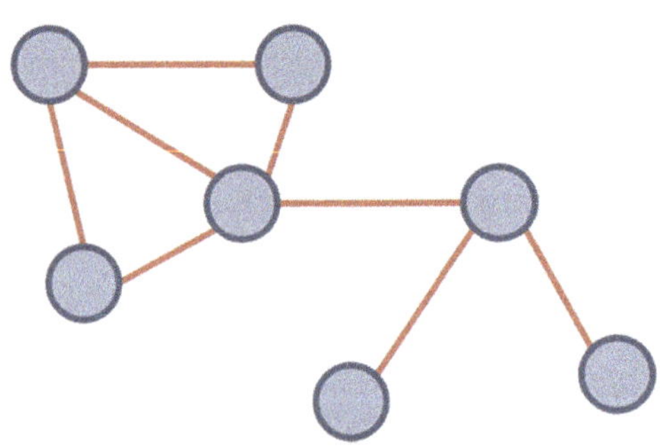

Figure 10.3. Simple representation of a network as a graph made of nodes (blue dots) and edges (red connections).

This loss of connectivity, in turn, leads to hampered communications in between nodes belonging to different networks. Frontal, hippocampal, precentral and occipital areas appear particularly susceptible as patients, compared to healthy controls, show decreased *network communicability*, a measure of how efficiently information may spread across networks [125]. This index is calculated as the total number of paths connecting each couple of nodes scaled by their length, so that longer paths have less weight than shorter (and more direct) ones. However, for the patient sample the authors also reported increases in communicability in subcortical structures (thalamus and putamen) interpreted as compensatory adaptations.

The emerging picture is that of extensive structural disconnections occurring as a consequence of the demyelinating lesions that characterize MS and associated, on one hand, with loss of neural tissue and, on the other, with clinical symptomatology. Structural damage appears to exert wide effects by driving reorganizational changes in brain architecture that encompass both structural and functional levels. The next section will focus, therefore, on studies that have investigated disconnection in terms of alterations in brain functioning at rest and during active performance.

10.3.2 Functional connectivity

Repercussions of lesion sprouting due to MS have been extensively investigated by means of several different MRI methodologies to ascertain cerebral changes, both global and localized. In particular, positron emission tomography studies have shown how metabolic demands are altered by MS pathology [126]. In fact, by injecting radioligands, i.e. radioactive biologically active substances, glucose metabolism appears significantly increased within active WM lesions [127]. In contrast, global metabolic rates of both glucose [128] and oxygen [129] have been consistently observed to decrease across different brain areas in people affected by MS. These changes were inversely correlated with the amount of lesional WM [129] and atrophy of the corpus callosum seems to drive metabolic reductions, especially in the left hemisphere [130].

Parallel and similar findings have also been highlighted for cerebral blood perfusion changes, mainly by using arterial spin labeling [131]. This technique allows the quantification of brain-wise perfusion by acquiring two images, one with and one without magnetically labeling arterial blood water directed to the brain. Labeling is achieved by delivering a radio frequency pulse before the blood accesses the brain in order to invert the blood water magnetization and by acquiring an image after a set delay time. Since the amount of labeled blood water is proportional to the amount of cerebral blood flow, the resulting difference image provides a quantification of cerebral perfusion across the brain [132]. In MS, increases in perfusion have been detected in normal appearing WM prior to lesion enhancement [133]. However, lesion accumulation appears to affect negatively global cerebral perfusion [134], which occurs throughout the whole brain well before GM atrophy can be detected [135].

Additionally, one study also reported changes in resting-state functional connectivity of the left precuneus that became more connected with its homologous after the emergence of lesions in its proximity [136]. Taken together, all these findings suggest that MS pathology, in addition to damaging WM structural connections, also generates a cascade of alterations in brain functioning, the nature and the clinical relevance of which will be further discussed in the next sections with reference to different applications of functional MRI.

10.3.2.1 Resting-state functional MRI

Brain functioning can be assessed in two different but related modes: at rest and during performance of a task. Together these methodologies fall under the name of functional MRI because they quantify brain activity by measuring the so-called blood-oxygen-level-dependent (BOLD) signal [137]. This signal originates from activation-related changes in the concentration of deoxyhemoglobin that causes disruption of the MRI signal due to its paramagnetic properties. In fact, when a specific brain area activates, a localized increase of cerebral blood flow higher than the cerebral metabolic rate of oxygen is triggered [138]. As a consequence, the amount of oxyhemoglobin (which, differently from deoxyhemoglobin, is diamagnetic) grows and generates a transient increment in the local magnetic field followed by a return to baseline values after brain activity terminates.

The series of changes in local blood supply inherently associated with brain activity (and the BOLD signal) are named hemodynamic response [139]. This process has been extensively studied with the aim of localizing brain activation associated with task performance by comparing the BOLD signal generated in different experimental conditions [140]. However, the needs for deeper understanding of the neurophysiological origins of the BOLD signal led to the development of resting-state functional MRI (RS-fMRI), used to assess human brain activity of people not actively engaged in any task. In particular, this technique enables the measurement of low-frequency fluctuations in the BOLD signal (<0.1 Hz) the time course of which is highly correlated in networks of anatomically distinct but functionally related areas [141].

The most famous and widely investigated network is the default mode network (DMN) (figure 10.4), that comprises the ventromedial prefrontal cortex, the posterior cingulate cortex (PCC), the precuneus, part of the inferior parietal lobule and the hippocampus [142, 143]. A series of other networks have also been described, namely somatosensory (SMN), visual, auditory, executive control (ECN), salience, left and right fronto-parietal (FPN), basal ganglia and cerebellar.

However, the number, the composition and the functions of these and other potential networks have not been definitely identified, since this research field has emerged only in the past two decades. Indeed, several studies have been carried out to characterize such resting-state networks not only in healthy individuals, but also in people affected by several medical conditions such as MS [57]. RS-fMRI appears especially suitable for all clinical populations because it has the advantage of offering a window on the functional architecture of the brain without the cognitive, motor and even emotional demands posed by task performance inside the scanner.

Functional coupling of different brain networks at rest appears to be variably affected by RRMS. In general, decreased connectivity in the DMN has been

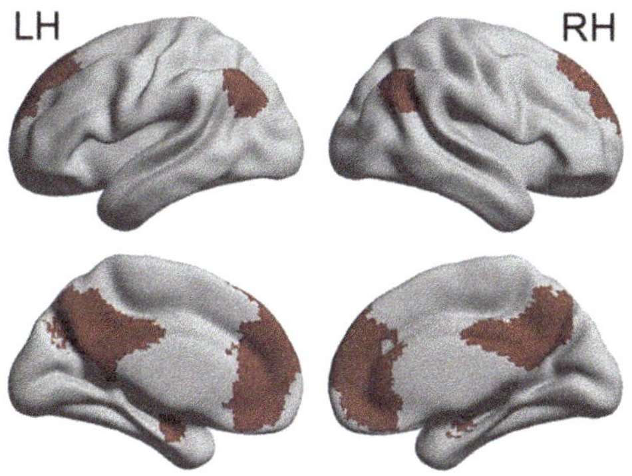

Figure 10.4. DMN areas extending in the left (LH) and right hemisphere (RH). Adapted from Zhou *et al* [144] and used under the Creative Commons Attribution License.

detected by several studies [145–148] with few exceptions [149]. This network undergoes a reorganization by expanding in posterior occipital areas [145] and decreasing its interactions with the ECN [148]. In contrast, connectivity between the DMN and the FPN appears stable in this MS phenotype [147]. Alterations that occur in the DMN after patients transition to SPMS are still not well characterized, since both decreases [150] and increases [151] in functional connectivity have been reported.

Unclear findings also emerge from the investigation of other networks, possibly due to the fact that only a few have been thoroughly studied in association with brain pathology and phenotypic expression. Connectivity of the visual and sensorimotor networks, in fact, has been observed to decrease [146, 148] but also increase across MS phenotypes [149, 151] compared to that of healthy controls. Similarly, the ECN and the FPN were found functionally intact by Janssen *et al* [149], but altered by other studies [147, 148].

More consistent, instead, are the observations about changes in functional connectivity of mediotemporal and subcortical structures. The hippocampus appears disconnected from a wide range of other GM structures because of its atrophy, even in the absence of memory deficits [152]. In particular, Gao *et al* [153] found that this structure is also less functionally integrated in the DMN. Thalamic nuclei have also been found to have stronger connectivity within the two thalami and weaker connectivity with other GM structures [154]. However, such functional alterations appear more complex, probably because of the numerous connections of the thalamus, and characterized both by over-expression, especially with the left insula [155], and down-regulation of connectivity [156, 157]. The resting-state activity of the basal ganglia, instead, appears to be more strongly coupled in MS patients with the SMN [158], the dorsolateral prefrontal cortex [159] and with a group of subcortical nuclei as well [160]. All these changes appear to be related to more severe symptomatology and, in fact, these have been found to worsen in SPMS [160].

Functional connectivity alterations subsequent to MS onset, therefore, do not necessarily follow a univocal trajectory, but rather appear to show fluctuations in both directions within and between networks. The engine promoting these processes is intuitively identified in the spreading of structural damage [136] and a few studies have attempted to clarify such a hypothesis. WM lesion volume has been linked to multiple functional alterations: connectivity decreases have been observed across several predominantly cognitive and cortical networks, namely DMN, ECN, FPNs and salience network [148]; but increases in connectivity have also been detected for the thalamus and the hippocampus–amygdala complex [161, 162]. Consistently, also the degree of WM microstructural damage appears to induce a strengthening of connectivity between DMN areas [144] and to be associated with decreased connectivity in the auditory and cerebellar networks [163]. Hence, disruption to structural connections causes a breakdown in communication across brain areas and triggers the reshaping of the brain functional organization.

Considerable rearrangements in brain functional architecture are highly likely to be accompanied by symptomatic manifestations. In particular, great attention has been drawn to cognitive decline experienced by a large proportion of patients: decreases in functional connectivity have been observed in patients with MS across a range of networks associated with different cognitive functions [164]. Global cognitive impairment has been associated with several different alterations, namely the reorganization of the posterior DMN [145], disconnection between the anterior and posterior hubs of the DMN [165], increased thalamic connectivity [157, 166] and increased resting-state coupling between the right caudate and the orbitofrontal cortex [167]. Moreover, deficits within the memory domain emerged especially as a consequence of depleted connectivity of the DMN [168] and, more specifically, of both increases [169, 170] and decreases [171] in hippocampal connectivity.

Less clear are the neural correlates of fatigue, although most findings point towards some sort of involvement of movement-related structures. Bisecco *et al* [172] found that fatigued patients, compared to non-fatigued ones, show increased connectivity of the posterior cingulate of the DMN and of the primary and supplementary motor areas of the SMN, while resting-state activity of the anterior cingulate appeared decreased. Severity of fatigue has been, instead, associated with: decreased coupling between the supplementary motor area and the primary motor cortex [173]; lower connectivity between the basal ganglia and midline cortices belonging to the DMN [174]; higher thalamic connectivity with different networks [175]; weak connectivity between the caudate/ventral striatum and sensorimotor cortices, and strong coupling between the dorsolateral prefrontal cortex and sensorimotor cortices [176]. Such a variety of results may be explained by the fact that fatigue itself is a symptom poorly understood that entails both objective and subjective factors in its manifestation.

Finally, graph theory analysis has also revealed how decreased connectivity, especially between the two hemispheres, discriminates patients from controls and is correlated with total WM lesion load [177]. Rocca *et al* [178] found that brains affected by MS undergo a general reconfiguration of network hubs and modifications in the strength of connections between nodes, that were associated with cognitive decline. Moreover, longitudinal investigations found that patients with MS compared to healthy controls experience a general increase in connection density that may represent a compensatory adaptation, since its decrease over time was reported to be associated with worsening of disability [179]. A similar time-dependent decline has also been observed in the average number of connections for a given node and in *betweenness centrality*, an index that measures how central a node is within a network, but not in global efficiency [180]. Similarly, no differences in efficiency were found between healthy people and patients with clinically isolated syndrome, thus suggesting that this graph-based measure is preserved in functional networks in the early phases of the disease [122].

MS-related changes occurring in resting-state brain activity appear multifaceted and have an impact potentially on the whole brain architecture. Currently, the widespread preference for investigations of the DMN has led to the accumulation of little knowledge about what dysfunctions may interest other networks, e.g. the salience network. However, it appears clearly that damage to structural connections drives a series of adaptations in brain functioning that are probably clinically relevant and dynamic throughout the disease course.

10.3.2.2 Task-based functional MRI

Similarly to RS-fMRI, the use of experimental tasks to study alterations in the hemodynamic response has also offered insights into brain activity associated with performance maintenance or failure in patients with MS. Two main areas have been explored: motor execution and cognitive functioning.

Studies on motor function mainly used a simple experimental paradigm declined in a range of similar tasks of finger flexion–extension with either the dominant hand or both hands. A consistent finding highlighted across studies is that patients with MS usually show enhanced task-related activation [181–186]. In particular, this phenomenon appears to unfold in two different ways as over-activation of areas usually active also in healthy controls and as recruitment of additional areas, especially the controlateral homologous cortices [183–185] and the dorsolateral prefrontal cortex [182, 186]. Such changes have been observed similarly in patients with so-called benign MS [183], defined as having an Expanded Disability Status Scale score $\leqslant 3$ after 15 years of disease, as well as in PPMS [181] and in SPMS [185].

Pantano *et al* [184] investigated movement-related brain activation in a longitudinal study and found that, at follow-up (that occurred over a variable period of time of about 1–2 years), patients showed declining over-recruitment of the right cerebellum and of the left sensorimotor cortices. Hence, this result suggests that higher brain activity might represent a compensatory mechanism in response to MS pathology that supports task performance. In fact, the majority of studies found that different measures of GM [186] and WM microstructural pathology [181] and WM total lesion volume [183–185] correlate with the observed increases in brain activation. Moreover, both WM lesion volume at baseline and its increase at follow-up correlated with decline in activation of different over-recruited areas [184].

Additionally, in right-handed patients communication during performance of motor tasks was also altered between sensorimotor cortices associated with the dominant hand and different frontal and parietal areas. Indeed, when compared to healthy controls, people with PPMS showed increased connectivity between the left primary sensorimotor cortex and the right cuneus, but lower connectivity between the left primary sensorimotor cortex and the left inferior frontal gyrus [181]. Similarly, a multicenter study also found that functional connectivity of the left sensorimotor cortex with right precentral gyrus, right middle frontal gyrus and bilateral postcentral gyri was enhanced in people affected by MS [187].

In constrast, studies of brain activation associated with cognitive performance appear more variegated, in terms of both domains investigated and tasks used. However, despite the presence of variability, it is striking to observe how increased activity in the prefrontal cortex of patients during task performance emerges as a distinctive finding, independently of the cognitive function assessed.

A considerable number of studies used the Paced Auditory Serial Addition Test (PASAT), a test commonly used in the cognitive assessment of people with MS [188], and its visual equivalent. Patients without cognitive deficits generally over-activate frontal and parietal areas compared to controls [189–191]. In particular, these increases appeared negatively correlated with total lesion volume [190] and with microstructural damage to the superior longitudinal fasciculus [189]. Only Baltruschat *et al* [192] found no significant differences in PASAT-related activations between patients and controls. However, they observed greater functional connectivity between the left posterior cingulate/precuneus and the left middle temporal gyrus and cerebellum. Additionally, connectivity between left posterior cingulate/precuneus and left cerebellum was negatively correlated with brain parenchymal fraction.

Using a simple button-press task Hubbard *et al* [193] found that patients with MS showed reduced BOLD hemodynamic response peak amplitude in two regions of interest, namely the primary visual and motor cortices. This reduction was directly correlated with normal appearing WM microstructural integrity, but not with total lesion volume. Instead, comparing experimental conditions differing for levels of difficulty, both in tasks of working memory [194] and response inhibition [195], it was shown that frontal activation was depleted in patients in the more challenging conditions and associated with a drop in performance. Moreover, Cader *et al* [194] observed that activation of the two prefrontal cortices was highly correlated only in patients, hence suggesting a need for additional neural resources to support task performance. In contrast, a study carried out on patients with executive deficits in planning abilities found no voxel-wise differences in task-related activation, but a post hoc region-of-interest analysis revealed that, among the involved areas, only the cerebellum was significantly more activated in patients [196].

Finally, neural activity supporting episodic memory encoding was also found enhanced in patients with preserved performance. Mainero *et al* [190] detected larger activation during recall of words in fronto-temporal and basal ganglia areas and was correlated with total WM volume. Similarly, hippocampal activation was also found to be elicited to a greater extent than in controls by a visual episodic memory task [170].

It is worth noting that similar findings about increased functional activation and connectivity in relation to performance of several different cognitive and motor tasks has also been documented by means of a different neuroimaging technique developed over the past three decades: functional near-infrared spectroscopy (fNIRS) [197]. This technique of optical imaging allows the quantification of changes in the hemodynamic response thanks to the fact that human tissues are transparent to near-infrared (650–100 nm) light which, in turn, can scatter within them and be absorbed by chromophores, i.e. pigmented compounds of red blood cells: oxyhemoglobin and deoxyhemoglobin. The concentration of both chromophores and their sum can be assessed by placing a series of optodes, i.e. optical fibers, that deliver near-infrared light of different wavelengths to the scalp and detect the photons reemerging from it. Despite the low spatial resolution, fNIRS is less prone to motion artifacts and this makes it particularly suitable for investigating brain activity in naturalistic environments [198].

A handful of fNIRS studies have been carried out to shed light on functional reorganization due to MS. Stojanovic-Radic *et al* [199] investigated brain activity dynamic over the prefrontal cortex while patients and healthy controls were performing a verbal working memory task. They found increased levels of oxyhemoglobin (i.e. activation) in the patient group in the left superior frontal gyrus for the less demanding experimental conditions. However, activation in the same area significantly dropped in the difficult conditions, thus suggesting that the compensation needed by patients to support performance could not be sustained when the task became too challenging.

Alterations have also been reported for motor-related activity, since Jimenez *et al* [200] found that, when compared to controls, patients showed smaller increases in total and oxyhemoglobin, and reduced frequency coherence for total hemoglobin between the two primary motor cortices during performance of a finger tapping task. The authors interpreted these changes as reduced interhemispheric communication between areas involved in movement execution. Moreover, a simple walking task, compared to the standing condition, was also found to induce an increase in oxyhemoglobin levels in the right premotor cortex of patients that was significantly higher than in controls [201]. When normal walking was compared with a dual task (walking while listing alternate letters of the alphabet starting from B), clear stronger increases of oxyhemoglobin were detected over the prefrontal cortex during the dual task condition in patients with MS than in controls in the absence of performance deficits [202].

Therefore, convergent findings suggest that structural damage in MS drives functional reorganizations at rest and during task performance that are thought to represent, at least in the early stages of the disease, compensatory processes to overcome the manifestation of deficits across different domains. In particular, brain activation and functional connectivity related to task performance appear enhanced in people with MS who are able to perform as well as healthy matched controls. Such adaptive changes, however, undergo a weakening process over time and appear to be depleted both in challenging experimental task conditions and in more advanced disease phases.

10.4 Conclusions and future developments

The increasing knowledge about the sequelae of neural processes triggered by MS pathology is showing the existence of intertwined factors that underlie the multiplicity of symptoms associated with this disease. Microstructural damage in normal appearing neural tissue and global macrostructural lesion volume appear associated with reorganizational changes that have been reported in both structural and functional connectivity (figure 10.5). Brains affected by MS are more modularized than healthy ones, i.e. areas and clusters of areas that are mainly involved in a set of specific processes become more isolated due to disruption in WM tracts. As a consequence, communication between connected networks is weakened and different bits of information requested to perform the majority of the tasks each one of us encounters in daily life are integrated with more effort. Such effort is evident in the recurrent observation that patients, in order to perform as well as healthy people in both motor and cognitive tasks, need increases in cerebral activation spreading to prefrontal areas that would not normally be active in those tasks. Nonetheless, in more demanding task conditions such compensatory brain activity drops (as well as performance accuracy), thus strengthening the hypothesis of a depletion in neural capacity. Consistently, longitudinal studies have found a similar decline in brain activation in parallel to disease progression.

The complex scenario that characterizes the neural and clinical manifestations associated with MS and the need for a deeper and more comprehensive understanding of these has recently led to the increasing application of novel analytical approaches to neuroimaging data from this clinical population [203–205]. In particular, advancements in mathematical and statistical methods applied to neuroimaging have started to emerge with the aim of supporting human abilities in making sense of all the current findings: computational modeling and machine learning. Computational modeling refers to computer-generated simulations of biological and neuroimaging-derived features of MS that account for the variety

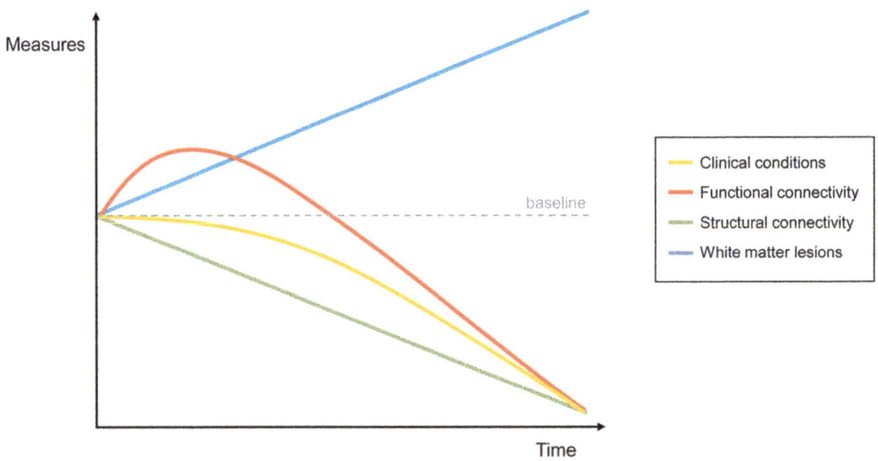

Figure 10.5. Simple representation of neural and clinical changes associated with MS.

of observed phenotypes. Machine learning, instead, consists of a group of analytical methods used to detect patterns and regularities in a sample dataset with the aim of creating a mathematical model of it that could enable automatized predictions and decision making.

Computational models have mainly tried to reproduce the dynamic combinations of pathological factors that may help explaining the manifestation of different MS phenotypes. Kannan *et al* [206] created a model incorporating CNS capacity against neurodegeneration and two immune components: one pro-inflammatory, that can be influenced by fluctuations in environmental factors and influences the CNS component, and one anti-inflammatory, that together form a negative loop. Interactions between these components explain the alternation of relapses and remissions, while strong disregulation of inflammation leads to general worsening of conditions characteristic of progressive MS phenotypes.

Additionally, other models have been able to reproduce the dynamics of CNS damage and disease courses by either combining multiple factors, such as myelinated and demyelinated axons, remyelination capacity and axon degeneration [207], or applying a chaos model to explain the non-linear variations in pathogenic immunity strength [208].

Moreover, further insights emerged about the relationship between structural damage and functional reorganization that are in line with findings currently available in the literature. In fact, Patel *et al* [209] created a computational model of resting-state functional connectivity across pairs of brain areas in the absence of damage to structural connections. Modifying tractography-derived values of structural connectivity on the basis of those obtained from individuals with MS, the model produced increases in functional connectivity consistent with those observed in patients. Similarly, in a functional model of the thalamo-cortical system constrained by diffusion MRI data, WM damage was reported to induce an initial increase in functional connectivity followed by a decrease, while GM damage (both thalamic and cortical) induced only increases [210].

Among the different approaches developed in the field of machine learning, instead, unsupervised and supervised learning methods represent the main ones. Unsupervised learning methodologies are aimed at detecting patterns in a given dataset without prior knowledge of its organization. In contrast, supervised learning is based on two sequential steps: first, a so-called 'training dataset' is processed with the aim of mapping it onto a series of categories defined *a priori*; second, the results of this step are used to create a function for classification of completely new data. This approach appears the most commonly used in applications to both neurological and psychiatric conditions [211].

In this field, most efforts have been dedicated to the discrimination of patients from controls, or even between different MS phenotypes, on the basis of different neural features. Saccà *et al* [212] compared the performance of different machine learning algorithms in classifying early RRMS and healthy controls by using average functional connectivity of 15 brain networks. Decreases in connectivity within the SMN was the best feature that enabled accurate discrimination between patients and controls, especially by using random forest and support vector machine approaches. Conversion from clinically isolated syndrome to RRMS, instead, was predicted by a random forest classifier on the basis of lesion shape parameters [213]. Moreover, Kocevar *et al* [214] used support vector machine to classify different MS phenotypes by combining several graph-theory-based features. For patients with SPMS specifically, accurate discrimination from those with either RRMS or PPMS was achieved by considering just brain modularity.

Additionally, applications were also tested to classify patients with specific MS-related symptoms. In fact, patients with and without upper limb motor impairments were distinguished by a combination of widespread GM atrophy, increased functional connectivity between areas in the left hemisphere and decreases in connectivity across the whole brain [215]. Similarly, cognitively impaired patients were accurately classified on the basis of different sets of features: increased *FA* in several thalamic areas, more atrophy in anterior thalamic regions and altered DTI indices in all thalamic WM tracts [216]; but also reduced volume in the left thalamus, right hippocampus, parietal GM and posterior WM regions and widespread alterations in WM diffusivity [217].

Currently, from the published literature it appears that different approaches to the analysis of neuroimaging data in MS have yielded consistent findings about the presence and the effects of widespread neural disconnections. In particular, recent interesting results and a deeper understanding of disease mechanisms emerging from the application of new increasingly more sophisticated imaging and analytic techniques may potentially lead to the discovery of new treatments for such a debilitating disease.

References

[1] Compston A and Coles A 2008 Multiple sclerosis *Lancet* **372** 1502–17

[2] Browne P *et al* 2014 Atlas of multiple sclerosis 2013: A growing global problem with widespread inequity *Neurology* **83** 1022–4

[3] Compston A *et al* 2006 *McAlpine's Multiple Sclerosis* 4th edn (London: Churchill Livingstone/Elsevier) pp 1–946

[4] Milo R and Kahana E 2010 Multiple sclerosis: Geoepidemiology, genetics and the environment *Autoimmun. Rev.* **9** A387–94

[5] Goodin D S 2016 The epidemiology of multiple sclerosis: Insights to a causal cascade *Handb. Clin. Neurol.* **138** 173–206

[6] Zivadinov R *et al* 2009 Gene-environment interactions between HLA B7/A2, EBV antibodies are associated with MRI injury in multiple sclerosis *J. Neuroimmunol.* **209** 123–30

[7] Mallucci G, Peruzzotti-Jametti L, Bernstock J D and Pluchino S 2015 The role of immune cells, glia and neurons in white and gray matter pathology in multiple sclerosis *Prog. Neurobiol.* **127–8** 1–22

[8] Elong Ngono A *et al* 2012 Frequency of circulating autoreactive T cells committed to myelin determinants in relapsing-remitting multiple sclerosis patients *Clin. Immunol.* **144** 117–26

[9] Hellings N *et al* 2001 T-cell reactivity to multiple myelin antigens in multiple sclerosis patients and healthy controls *J. Neurosci. Res.* **63** 290–302

[10] Johnson A J, Suidan G L, McDole J and Pirko I 2007 The CD8 T cell in multiple sclerosis: Suppressor cell or mediator of neuropathology? *Int. Rev. Neurobiol.* **79** 73–97
[11] Hauser S L and Oksenberg J R 2006 The neurobiology of multiple sclerosis: Genes, inflammation, and neurodegeneration *Neuron* **52** 61–76
[12] Mahad D H, Trapp B D and Lassmann H 2015 Pathological mechanisms in progressive multiple sclerosis *Lancet Neurol.* **14** 183–93
[13] Stadelmann C, Wegner C and Brück W 2011 Inflammation, demyelination, and degeneration—recent insights from MS pathology *Biochim. Biophys. Acta* **1812** 275–82
[14] Lublin F D *et al* 2014 Defining the clinical course of multiple sclerosis: The 2013 revisions *Neurology* **83** 278–86
[15] Howard J, Trevick S and Younger D S 2016 Epidemiology of multiple sclerosis *Neurol. Clin.* **34** 919–39
[16] Rovaris M, Confavreux C, Furlan R, Kappos L, Comi G and Filippi M 2006 Secondary progressive multiple sclerosis: Current knowledge and future challenges *Lancet Neurol.* **5** 343–54
[17] Koch M, Kingwell E, Rieckmann P and Tremlett H 2009 The natural history of primary progressive multiple sclerosis *Neurology* **73** 1996–2002
[18] Miller D H and Leary S M 2007 Primary-progressive multiple sclerosis *Lancet Neurol.* **6** 903–12
[19] Ontaneda D, Thompson A J, Fox R J and Cohen J A 2017 Progressive multiple sclerosis: Prospects for disease therapy, repair, and restoration of function *Lancet* **389** 1357–66
[20] Amato M P, Ponziani G, Rossi F, Liedl C L, Stefanile C and Rossi L 2001 Quality of life in multiple sclerosis: The impact of depression, fatigue and disability *Mult. Scler.* **7** 340–4
[21] Kluger B M, Krupp L B and Enoka R M 2013 Fatigue and fatigability in neurologic illnesses: Proposal for a unified taxonomy *Neurology* **80** 409–16
[22] Lerdal A, Celius E G, Krupp L and Dahl A A 2007 A prospective study of patterns of fatigue in multiple sclerosis *Eur. J. Neurol.* **14** 1338–43
[23] Toosy A T, Mason D F and Miller D H 2013 Optic neuritis *Lancet Neurol.* **13** 83–99
[24] Rae-Grant A D, Eckert N J, Bartz S and Reed J F 1999 Sensory symptoms of multiple sclerosis: A hidden reservoir of morbidity *Mult. Scler.* **5** 179–83
[25] Chiaravalloti N D and DeLuca J 2008 Cognitive impairment in multiple sclerosis *Lancet Neurol.* **7** 1139–51
[26] Boeschoten R E *et al* 2016 Prevalence of depression and anxiety in multiple sclerosis: A systematic review and meta-analysis *J. Neurol. Sci.* **372** 331–41
[27] Polman C H *et al* 2010 Diagnostic criteria for multiple sclerosis: 2010 revisions to the McDonald criteria *Ann. Neurol.* **69** 292–302
[28] Montalban X *et al* 2010 MRI criteria for MS in patients with clinically isolated syndromes *Neurology* **74** 427–34
[29] Rovira A *et al* 2009 A single, early magnetic resonance imaging study in the diagnosis of multiple sclerosis *Arch. Neurol.* **66** 587–92
[30] Filippi M *et al* 2016 MRI criteria for the diagnosis of multiple sclerosis: MAGNIMS consensus guidelines *Lancet Neurol.* **15** 292–303
[31] Dalton C M *et al* 2011 Brain lesion location and clinical status 20 years after a diagnosis of clinically isolated syndrome suggestive of multiple sclerosis *Mult. Scler.* **18** 322–8
[32] Filli L *et al* 2012 Spatiotemporal distribution of white matter lesions in relapsing-remitting and secondary progressive multiple sclerosis *Mult. Scler.* **18** 1577–84

[33] Haider L *et al* 2016 The topograpy of demyelination and neurodegeneration in the multiple sclerosis brain *Brain* **139** 807–15

[34] Kuhlmann T, Ludwin S, Prat A, Antel J, Bruck W and Lassmann H 2016 An updated histological classification system for multiple sclerosis lesions *Acta Neuropathol.* **133** 13–24

[35] Franklin R J and Ffrench-Constant C 2008 Remyelination in the CNS: From biology to therapy *Nat. Rev. Neurosci.* **9** 839–55

[36] Patrikios P *et al* 2006 Remyelination is extensive in a subset of multiple sclerosis patients *Brain* **129** 3165–72

[37] Bramow S *et al* 2010 Demyelination versus remyelination in progressive multiple sclerosis *Brain* **133** 2983–98

[38] Kearney H, Miller D H and Ciccarelli O 2015 Spinal cord MRI in multiple sclerosis--diagnostic, prognostic and clinical value *Nat. Rev. Neurol.* **11** 327–38

[39] Sethi V *et al* 2015 A longitudinal study of cortical grey matter lesion subtypes in relapse-onset multiple sclerosis *J. Neurol. Neurosurg. Psychiatry* **87** 750–3

[40] Klaver R, De Vries H E, Schenk G J and Geurts J J 2013 Grey matter damage in multiple sclerosis: A pathology perspective *Prion* **7** 66–75

[41] Calabrese M, Favaretto A, Martini V and Gallo P 2013 Grey matter lesions in MS: from histology to clinical implications *Prion* **7** 20–7

[42] Geurts J J, Pouwels P J, Uitdehaag B M, Polman C H, Barkhof F and Castelijns J A 2005 Intracortical lesions in multiple sclerosis: improved detection with 3D double inversion-recovery MR imaging *Radiology* **236** 254–60

[43] Nelson F, Poonawalla A, Hou P, Wolinsky J S and Narayana P A 2008 3D MPRAGE improves classification of cortical lesions in multiple sclerosis *Mult. Scler.* **14** 1214–9

[44] Sethi V *et al* 2012 Improved detection of cortical MS lesions with phase-sensitive inversion recovery MRI *J. Neurol. Neurosurg. Psychiatry* **83** 877–82

[45] Calabrese M, Magliozzi R, Ciccarelli O, Geurts J J, Reynolds R and Martin R 2015 Exploring the origins of grey matter damage in multiple sclerosis *Nat. Rev. Neurosci.* **16** 147–58

[46] Vollmer T *et al* 2015 The natural history of brain volume loss among patients with multiple sclerosis: A systematic literature review and meta-analysis *J. Neurol. Sci.* **357** 8–18

[47] Azevedo C J *et al* 2015 Early CNS neurodegeneration in radiologically isolated syndrome *Neurol. Neuroimmunol. Neuroinflamm.* **2** e102

[48] Lansley J, Mataix-Cols D, Grau M, Radua J and Sastre-Garriga J 2013 Localized grey matter atrophy in multiple sclerosis: A meta-analysis of voxel-based morphometry studies and associations with functional disability *Neurosci. Biobehav. Rev.* **37** 819–30

[49] Grothe M, Lotze M, Langner S and Dressel A 2016 The role of global and regional gray matter volume decrease in multiple sclerosis *J. Neurol.* **263** 1137–45

[50] Ontaneda D and Fox R J 2017 Imaging as an outcome measure in multiple sclerosis *Neurotherapeutics* **14** 24–34

[51] Altermatt A *et al* 2018 Clinical correlations of brain lesion location in multiple sclerosis: Voxel-based analysis of a large clinical trial dataset *Brain Topogr.* **31** 886–94

[52] Preziosa P *et al* 2017 Progression of regional atrophy in the left hemisphere contributes to clinical and cognitive deterioration in multiple sclerosis: A 5-year study *Hum. Brain Mapp.* **38** 5648–65

[53] Lindeboom J and ter Horst R 1988 Interhemispheric disconnection effects in multiple sclerosis *J. Neurol. Neurosurg. Psychiatry* **51** 1445–7

[54] Rao S M, Bernardin L, Leo G J, Ellington L, Ryan S B and Burg L S 1989 Cerebral disconnection in multiple sclerosis. Relationship to atrophy of the corpus callosum *Arch. Neurol.* **46** 918–20

[55] Calabrese P and Penner I K 2007 Cognitive dysfunctions in multiple sclerosis—a multiple disconnection syndrome? *J. Neurol.* **254** II18–21

[56] Filley C M 2010 White matter: organization and functional relevance *Neuropsychol. Rev.* **20** 158–73

[57] Sbardella E, Petsas N, Tona F and Pantano P 2015 Resting-state fMRI in MS: general concepts and brief overview of its application *Biomed. Res. Int.* **2015** 212693

[58] Le Bihan D, Breton E, Lallemand D, Grenier P, Cabanis E and Laval-Jeantet M 1986 MR imaging of intravoxel incoherent motions: application to diffusion and perfusion in neurologic disorders *Radiology* **161** 401–7

[59] Basser P J, Mattiello J and LeBihan D 1994 MR diffusion tensor spectroscopy and imaging *Biophys. J.* **66** 259–67

[60] Le Bihan D *et al* 2001 Diffusion tensor imaging: Concepts and applications *J. Magn. Reson. Imaging* **13** 534–46

[61] Pierpaoli C and Basser P J 1996 Toward a quantitative assessment of diffusion anisotropy *Magn. Reson. Med.* **36** 893–906

[62] Frank L R 2001 Anisotropy in high angular resolution diffusion-weighted MRI *Magn. Reson. Med.* **45** 935–9

[63] Tuch D S, Reese T G, Wiegell M R, Makris N, Belliveau J W and Wedeen V J 2002 High angular resolution diffusion imaging reveals intravoxel white matter fiber heterogeneity *Magn. Reson. Med.* **48** 577–82

[64] Dell'Acqua F, Rizzo G, Scifo P, Clarke R A, Scotti G and Fazio F 2007 A model-based deconvolution approach to solve fiber crossing in diffusion-weighted MR imaging *IEEE Trans. Bio-med. Eng.* **54** 462–72

[65] Cory D G and Garroway A N 1990 Measurement of translational displacement probabilities by NMR: an indicator of compartmentation *Magn. Reson. Med.* **14** 435–44

[66] Assaf Y and Cohen Y 1999 Structural information in neuronal tissue as revealed by q-space diffusion NMR spectroscopy of metabolites in bovine optic nerve *NMR Biomed.* **12** 335–44

[67] Cercignani M and Wheeler-Kingshott C G 2019 From micro- to macro-structures in multiple sclerosis: what is the added value of diffusion imaging *NMR Biomed.* **32** e3888

[68] Ferizi U *et al* 2013 A ranking of diffusion MRI compartment models with *in vivo* human brain data *Magn. Reson. Med.* **72** 1785–92

[69] Panagiotaki E, Schneider T, Siow B, Hall M G, Lythgoe M F and Alexander D C 2011 Compartment models of the diffusion MR signal in brain white matter: a taxonomy and comparison *NeuroImage* **59** 2241–54

[70] Zhang H, Schneider T, Wheeler-Kingshott C A and Alexander D C 2012 NODDI: Practical *in vivo* neurite orientation dispersion and density imaging of the human brain *NeuroImage* **61** 1000–16

[71] Enzinger C *et al* 2015 Nonconventional MRI and microstructural cerebral changes in multiple sclerosis *Nat. Rev. Neurol.* **11** 676–86

[72] Mahajan K R and Ontaneda D 2017 The role of advanced magnetic resonance imaging techniques in multiple sclerosis clinical trials *Neurotherapeutics* **14** 905–23

[73] Barkhof F 2002 The clinico-radiological paradox in multiple sclerosis revisited *Curr. Opin. Neurol.* **15** 239–45

[74] Ontaneda D *et al* 2014 Identifying the start of multiple sclerosis injury: A serial DTI study *J. Neuroimaging* **24** 569–76

[75] Filippi M, Rocca M A, Martino G, Horsfield M A and Comi G 1998 Magnetization transfer changes in the normal appearing white matter precede the appearance of enhancing lesions in patients with multiple sclerosis *Ann. Neurol.* **43** 809–14

[76] Droby A *et al* 2015 The impact of isolated lesions on white-matter fiber tracts in multiple sclerosis patients *Neuroimage Clin.* **8** 110–6

[77] Chiang G C, Pinto S, Comunale J P and Gauthier S A 2016 Gadolinium-enhancing lesions lead to decreases in white matter tract fractional anisotropy in multiple sclerosis *J. Neuroimaging* **26** 289–95

[78] Deppe M *et al* 2015 Evidence for early, non-lesional cerebellar damage in patients with multiple sclerosis: DTI measures correlate with disability, atrophy, and disease duration *Mult. Scler.* **22** 73–84

[79] Fox J *et al* 2016 Individual assessment of brain tissue changes in MS and the effect of focal lesions on short-term focal atrophy development in MS: A voxel-guided morphometry study *Int. J. Mol. Sci.* **17** 489

[80] Huang J *et al* 2018 White matter microstructural alterations in clinically isolated syndrome and multiple sclerosis *J. Clin. Neurosci.* **53** 27–33

[81] Raz E *et al* 2010 Gray- and white-matter changes 1 year after first clinical episode of multiple sclerosis: MR imaging *Radiology* **257** 448–54

[82] Harrison D M *et al* 2011 Longitudinal changes in diffusion tensor-based quantitative MRI in multiple sclerosis *Neurology* **76** 179–86

[83] Rocca M A *et al* 2016 Clinically isolated syndrome suggestive of multiple sclerosis: Dynamic patterns of gray and white matter changes-A 2-year MR imaging study *Radiology* **278** 841–53

[84] Welton T, Kent D, Constantinescu C S, Auer D P and Dineen R A 2015 Functionally relevant white matter degradation in multiple sclerosis: A tract-based spatial meta-analysis *Radiology* **275** 89–96

[85] Baird J F, Hubbard E A, Sutton B P and Motl R W 2018 The relationship between corticospinal tract integrity and lower-extremity strength is attenuated when controlling for age and sex in multiple sclerosis *Brain Res.* **1701** 171–6

[86] Reich D S *et al* 2008 Corticospinal tract abnormalities are associated with weakness in multiple sclerosis *AJNR Am. J. Neuroradiol.* **29** 333–9

[87] Tovar-Moll F *et al* 2014 Diffuse and focal corticospinal tract disease and its impact on patient disability in multiple sclerosis *J. Neuroimaging* **25** 200–6

[88] Pardini M, Bonzano L, Mancardi G L and Roccatagliata L 2010 Frontal networks play a role in fatigue perception in multiple sclerosis *Behav. Neurosci.* **124** 329–36

[89] Pardini M *et al* 2015 Cingulum bundle alterations underlie subjective fatigue in multiple sclerosis *Mult. Scler.* **21** 442–7

[90] Bisecco A *et al* 2016 Fatigue in multiple sclerosis: The contribution of occult white matter damage *Mult. Scler.* **22** 1676–84

[91] Eijlers A J C *et al* 2018 Predicting cognitive decline in multiple sclerosis: a 5-year follow-up study *Brain* **141** 2605–18

[92] Zhang X *et al* 2017 Contribution of gray and white matter abnormalities to cognitive impairment in multiple sclerosis *Int. J. Mol. Sci.* **18** E46

[93] Manca R, Sharrack B, Paling D, Wilkinson I D and Venneri A 2018 Brain connectivity and cognitive processing speed in multiple sclerosis: A systematic review *J. Neurol. Sci.* **388** 115–27
[94] Mori S, Crain B J, Chacko V P and van Zijl P C 1999 Three-dimensional tracking of axonal projections in the brain by magnetic resonance imaging *Ann. Neurol.* **45** 265–9
[95] Jones D K, Simmons A, Williams S C and Horsfield M A 1999 Non-invasive assessment of axonal fiber connectivity in the human brain via diffusion tensor MRI *Magn. Reson. Med.* **42** 37–41
[96] Ciccarelli O, Catani M, Johansen-Berg H, Clark C and Thompson A 2008 Diffusion-based tractography in neurological disorders: concepts, applications, and future developments *Lancet Neurol.* **7** 715–27
[97] Tax C M *et al* 2015 Seeing more by showing less: Orientation-dependent transparency rendering for fiber tractography visualization *PLoS One* **10** e0139434
[98] Lin F, Yu C, Jiang T, Li K and Chan P 2007 Diffusion tensor tractography-based group mapping of the pyramidal tract in relapsing-remitting multiple sclerosis patients *AJNR Am. J. Neuroradiol.* **28** 278–82
[99] Pagani E, Filippi M, Rocca M A and Horsfield M A 2005 A method for obtaining tract-specific diffusion tensor MRI measurements in the presence of disease: application to patients with clinically isolated syndromes suggestive of multiple sclerosis *Neuroimage* **26** 258–65
[100] Reich D S, Ozturk A, Calabresi P A and Mori S 2010 Automated vs. conventional tractography in multiple sclerosis: variability and correlation with disability *Neuroimage* **49** 3047–56
[101] Parker G J and Alexander D C 2005 Probabilistic anatomical connectivity derived from the microscopic persistent angular structure of cerebral tissue *Philos. Trans. R. Soc. Lond. B. Biol. Sci.* **360** 893–902
[102] Hu B *et al* 2011 Quantitative diffusion tensor deterministic and probabilistic fiber tractography in relapsing-remitting multiple sclerosis *Eur. J. Radiol.* **79** 101–7
[103] Dayan M *et al* 2016 Profilometry: A new statistical framework for the characterization of white matter pathways, with application to multiple sclerosis *Hum. Brain Mapp.* **37** 989–1004
[104] Raj A, Pandya S, Shen X, LoCastro E, Nguyen T D and Gauthier S A 2014 Multi-compartment T2 relaxometry using a spatially constrained multi-Gaussian model *PLoS One* **9** e98391
[105] Kezele I B, Arnold D L and Collins D L 2008 Atrophy in white matter fiber tracts in multiple sclerosis is not dependent on tract length or local white matter lesions *Mult. Scler.* **14** 779–85
[106] Jehna M *et al* 2013 An exploratory study on the spatial relationship between regional cortical volume changes and white matter integrity in multiple sclerosis *Brain Connect.* **3** 255–64
[107] Steenwijk M D *et al* 2015 Unraveling the relationship between regional gray matter atrophy and pathology in connected white matter tracts in long-standing multiple sclerosis *Hum. Brain Mapp.* **36** 1796–807
[108] Mangeat G *et al* 2018 Changes in structural network are associated with cortical demyelination in early multiple sclerosis *Hum. Brain Mapp.* **39** 2133–46
[109] Gorgoraptis N *et al* 2010 Combining tractography and cortical measures to test system-specific hypotheses in multiple sclerosis *Mult. Scler.* **16** 555–65
[110] Kacar K *et al* 2011 Overcoming the clinical-MR imaging paradox of multiple sclerosis: MR imaging data assessed with a random forest approach *AJNR Am. J. Neuroradiol.* **32** 2098–102

[111] Audoin B *et al* 2007 Structure of WM bundles constituting the working memory system in early multiple sclerosis: a quantitative DTI tractography study *Neuroimage* **36** 1324–30
[112] Llufriu S *et al* 2017 Structural networks involved in attention and executive functions in multiple sclerosis *Neuroimage Clin.* **13** 288–96
[113] Sporns O, Tononi G and Kötter R 2005 The human connectome: A structural description of the human brain *PLoS Comput. Biol.* **1** e42
[114] Catani M, Thiebaut de Schotten M, Slater D and Dell'Acqua F 2013 Connectomic approaches before the connectome *Neuroimage* **80** 2–13
[115] Bullmore E T and Bassett D S 2011 Brain graphs: graphical models of the human brain connectome *Annu. Rev. Clin. Psychol.* **7** 113–40
[116] Bullmore E and Sporns O 2009 Complex brain networks: graph theoretical analysis of structural and functional systems *Nat. Rev. Neurosci.* **10** 186–98
[117] Bassett D S and Bullmore E 2006 Small-world brain networks *Neuroscientist* **12** 512–23
[118] Fleischer V *et al* 2017 Graph theoretical framework of brain networks in multiple sclerosis: A review of concepts *Neuroscience* **403** 35–53
[119] Shu N *et al* 2011 Diffusion tensor tractography reveals disrupted topological efficiency in white matter structural networks in multiple sclerosis *Cereb. Cortex* **21** 2565–77
[120] Llufriu S *et al* 2018 Hippocampal-related memory network in multiple sclerosis: A structural connectivity analysis *Mult. Scler.* 1352458518771838
[121] Solana E *et al* 2018 Magnetic resonance markers of tissue damage related to connectivity disruption in multiple sclerosis *Neuroimage Clin.* **20** 161–8
[122] Liu Y, Duan Y, Dong H, Barkhof F, Li K and Shu N 2018 Disrupted module efficiency of structural and functional brain connectomes in clinically isolated syndrome and multiple sclerosis *Front. Hum. Neurosci.* **12** 138
[123] Muthuraman M, Fleischer V, Kolber P, Luessi F, Zipp F and Groppa S 2016 Structural brain network characteristics can differentiate CIS from early RRMS *Front. Neurosci.* **10** 14
[124] Shu N *et al* 2016 Disrupted topological organization of structural and functional brain connectomes in clinically isolated syndrome and multiple sclerosis *Sci. Rep.* **6** 29383
[125] Li Y *et al* 2013 Diffusion tensor imaging based network analysis detects alterations of neuroconnectivity in patients with clinically early relapsing-remitting multiple sclerosis *Hum. Brain Mapp.* **34** 3376–91
[126] Niccolini F, Su P and Politis M 2015 PET in multiple sclerosis *Clin. Nucl. Med.* **40** e46–52
[127] Schiepers C *et al* 1997 Positron emission tomography, magnetic resonance imaging and proton NMR spectroscopy of white matter in multiple sclerosis *Mult. Scler.* **3** 8–17
[128] Bakshi R, Miletich R S, Kinkel P R, Emmet M L and Kinkel W R 1998 High-resolution fluorodeoxyglucose positron emission tomography shows both global and regional cerebral hypometabolism in multiple sclerosis *J. Neuroimaging* **8** 228–34
[129] Sun X, Tanaka M, Kondo S, Okamoto K and Hirai S 1998 Clinical significance of reduced cerebral metabolism in multiple sclerosis: a combined PET and MRI study *Ann. Nucl. Med.* **12** 89–94
[130] Pozzilli C *et al* 1992 Relationship between corpus callosum atrophy and cerebral metabolic asymmetries in multiple sclerosis *J. Neurol. Sci.* **112** 51–7
[131] Lapointe E, Li D K B, Traboulsee A L and Rauscher A 2018 What have we learned from perfusion MRI in multiple sclerosis? *AJNR Am. J. Neuroradiol.* **39** 994–1000
[132] Williams D S, Detre J A, Leigh J S and Koretsky A P 1992 Magnetic resonance imaging of perfusion using spin inversion of arterial water *Proc. Natl. Acad. Sci. U. S. A.* **89** 212–6

[133] Wuerfel J *et al* 2004 Changes in cerebral perfusion precede plaque formation in multiple sclerosis: a longitudinal perfusion MRI study *Brain* **127** 111–9
[134] Amann M *et al* 2012 3D GRASE arterial spin labelling reveals an inverse correlation of cortical perfusion with the white matter lesion volume in MS *Mult. Scler.* **18** 1570–6
[135] Debernard L *et al* 2014 Reduced grey matter perfusion without volume loss in early relapsing-remitting multiple sclerosis *J. Neurol. Neurosurg. Psychiatry* **85** 544–51
[136] Droby A *et al* 2016 Changes in brain functional connectivity patterns are driven by an individual lesion in MS: a resting-state fMRI study *Brain Imaging Behav.* **10** 1117–26
[137] Ogawa S and Lee T M 1990 Magnetic resonance imaging of blood vessels at high fields: *in vivo* and *in vitro* measurements and image simulation *Magn. Reson. Med.* **16** 9–18
[138] Fox P T and Raichle M E 1986 Focal physiological uncoupling of cerebral blood flow and oxidative metabolism during somatosensory stimulation in human subjects *Proc. Natl. Acad. Sci. U. S. A.* **83** 1140–4
[139] Buxton R B, Uludağ K, Dubowitz D J and Liu T T 2004 Modeling the hemodynamic response to brain activation *Neuroimage* **23** S220–33
[140] Bandettini P A, Wong E C, Hinks R S, Tikofsky R S and Hyde J S 1992 Time course EPI of human brain function during task activation *Magn. Reson. Med.* **25** 390–7
[141] Biswal B, Yetkin F Z, Haughton V M and Hyde J S 1995 Functional connectivity in the motor cortex of resting human brain using echo-planar MRI *Magn. Reson. Med.* **34** 537–41
[142] Raichle M E, MacLeod A M, Snyder A Z, Powers W J, Gusnard D A and Shulman G L 2001 A default mode of brain function *Proc. Natl. Acad. Sci. U. S. A.* **98** 676–82
[143] Buckner R L, Andrews-Hanna J R and Schacter D L 2008 The brain's default network: anatomy, function, and relevance to disease *Ann. N. Y. Acad. Sci.* **1124** 1–38
[144] Zhou F *et al* 2014 Altered inter-subregion connectivity of the default mode network in relapsing remitting multiple sclerosis: a functional and structural connectivity study *PLoS One* **9** e101198
[145] Bonavita S *et al* 2011 Distributed changes in default-mode resting-state connectivity in multiple sclerosis *Mult. Scler.* **17** 411–22
[146] Castellazzi G *et al* 2018 Functional connectivity alterations reveal complex mechanisms based on clinical and radiological status in mild relapsing remitting multiple sclerosis *Front. Neurol.* **9** 690
[147] Huang M *et al* 2018 Synchronization within, and interactions between, the default mode and dorsal attention networks in relapsing-remitting multiple sclerosis *Neuropsychiatr. Dis. Treat.* **14** 1241–52
[148] Rocca M A *et al* 2012 Large-scale neuronal network dysfunction in relapsing-remitting multiple sclerosis *Neurology* **79** 1449–57
[149] Janssen A L, Boster A, Patterson B A, Abduljalil A and Prakash R S 2013 Resting-state functional connectivity in multiple sclerosis: an examination of group differences and individual differences *Neuropsychologia* **51** 2918–29
[150] Rocca M A *et al* 2010 Default-mode network dysfunction and cognitive impairment in progressive MS *Neurology* **74** 1252–9
[151] Basile B *et al* 2014 Functional connectivity changes within specific networks parallel the clinical evolution of multiple sclerosis *Mult. Scler.* **20** 1050–7
[152] Roosendaal S D *et al* 2010 Structural and functional hippocampal changes in multiple sclerosis patients with intact memory function *Radiology* **255** 595–604

[153] Gao F *et al* 2018 Altered hippocampal GABA and glutamate levels and uncoupling from functional connectivity in multiple sclerosis *Hippocampus* **28** 813–23

[154] Liu Y *et al* 2015 Altered thalamic functional connectivity in multiple sclerosis *Eur. J. Radiol.* **84** 703–8

[155] d'Ambrosio A *et al* 2017 Structural connectivity-defined thalamic subregions have different functional connectivity abnormalities in multiple sclerosis patients: Implications for clinical correlations *Hum. Brain Mapp.* **38** 6005–18

[156] Lin F *et al* 2018 Altered nuclei-specific thalamic functional connectivity patterns in multiple sclerosis and their associations with fatigue and cognition *Mult. Scler.* 1352458518788218

[157] Tona F *et al* 2014 Multiple sclerosis: altered thalamic resting-state functional connectivity and its effect on cognitive function *Radiology* **271** 814–21

[158] Dogonowski A M *et al* 2013 Expanded functional coupling of subcortical nuclei with the motor resting-state network in multiple sclerosis *Mult. Scler.* **19** 559–66

[159] Cui F *et al* 2017 Altered functional connectivity of striatal subregions in patients with multiple sclerosis *Front. Neurol.* **8** 129

[160] Meijer K A, Eijlers A J C, Geurts J J G and Schoonheim M M 2018 Staging of cortical and deep grey matter functional connectivity changes in multiple sclerosis *J. Neurol. Neurosurg. Psychiatry* **89** 205–10

[161] Zhou F *et al* 2015 Disconnection of the hippocampus and amygdala associated with lesion load in relapsing-remitting multiple sclerosis: a structural and functional connectivity study *Neuropsychiatr. Dis. Treat.* **11** 1749–65

[162] Zhou F *et al* 2016 Intrinsic functional plasticity of the thalamocortical system in minimally disabled patients with relapsing-remitting multiple sclerosis *Front. Hum. Neurosci.* **10** 2

[163] Sbardella E *et al* 2015 Functional connectivity changes and their relationship with clinical disability and white matter integrity in patients with relapsing-remitting multiple sclerosis *Mult. Scler.* **21** 1681–92

[164] Nejad-Davarani S P *et al* 2016 Resting state fMRI connectivity analysis as a tool for detection of abnormalities in five different cognitive networks of the brain in Multiple Sclerosis patients *Clin. Case Rep. Rev.* **2** 464–71

[165] Louapre C *et al* 2014 Brain networks disconnection in early multiple sclerosis cognitive deficits: an anatomofunctional study *Hum. Brain Mapp.* **35** 4706–17

[166] Schoonheim M M *et al* 2015 Thalamus structure and function determine severity of cognitive impairment in multiple sclerosis *Neurology* **84** 776–83

[167] Cruz-Gómez Á J, Aguirre N, Sanchis-Segura C, Ávila C and Forn C 2018 Subcortical grey matter structures in multiple sclerosis: what is their role in cognition? *Neuroreport* **29** 547–52

[168] Leavitt V M, Paxton J and Sumowski J F 2014 Default network connectivity is linked to memory status in multiple sclerosis *J. Int. Neuropsychol. Soc.* **20** 937–44

[169] González Torre J A, Cruz-Gómez Á J, Belenguer A, Sanchis-Segura C, Ávila C and Forn C 2017 Hippocampal dysfunction is associated with memory impairment in multiple sclerosis: A volumetric and functional connectivity study *Mult. Scler.* **23** 1854–63

[170] Hulst H E, Schoonheim M M, Van Geest Q, Uitdehaag B M, Barkhof F and Geurts J J 2015 Memory impairment in multiple sclerosis: Relevance of hippocampal activation and hippocampal connectivity *Mult. Scler.* **21** 1705–12

[171] Karavasilis E *et al* 2018 Hippocampal structural and functional integrity in multiple sclerosis patients with or without memory impairment: a multimodal neuroimaging study *Brain Imaging Behav.* **13** 1049–59

[172] Bisecco A *et al* 2018 Fatigue in multiple sclerosis: The contribution of resting-state functional connectivity reorganization *Mult. Scler.* **24** 1696–705
[173] Cruz Gómez Á J, Ventura Campos N, Belenguer A, Ávila C and Forn C 2013 Regional brain atrophy and functional connectivity changes related to fatigue in multiple sclerosis *PLoS One* **8** e77914
[174] Finke C *et al* 2015 Altered basal ganglia functional connectivity in multiple sclerosis patients with fatigue *Mult. Scler.* **21** 925–34
[175] Hidalgo de la Cruz M *et al* 2018 Abnormal functional connectivity of thalamic sub-regions contributes to fatigue in multiple sclerosis *Mult. Scler.* **24** 1183–95
[176] Jaeger S *et al* 2018 Multiple sclerosis-related fatigue: Altered resting-state functional connectivity of the ventral striatum and dorsolateral prefrontal cortex *Mult. Scler.* 1352458518758911
[177] Richiardi J *et al* 2012 Classifying minimally disabled multiple sclerosis patients from resting state functional connectivity *Neuroimage* **62** 2021–33
[178] Rocca M A, Valsasina P, Meani A, Falini A, Comi G and Filippi M 2016 Impaired functional integration in multiple sclerosis: a graph theory study *Brain Struct. Funct.* **221** 115–31
[179] Faivre A *et al* 2016 Depletion of brain functional connectivity enhancement leads to disability progression in multiple sclerosis: A longitudinal resting-state fMRI study *Mult. Scler.* **22** 1695–708
[180] Koubiyr I *et al* 2018 Longitudinal study of functional brain network reorganization in clinically isolated syndrome *Mult. Scler.* 1352458518813108
[181] Ceccarelli A *et al* 2010 Structural and functional magnetic resonance imaging correlates of motor network dysfunction in primary progressive multiple sclerosis *Eur. J. Neurosci.* **31** 1273–80
[182] Faivre A *et al* 2015 Brain functional plasticity at rest and during action in multiple sclerosis patients *J. Clin. Neurosci.* **22** 1438–43
[183] Giorgio A *et al* 2010 Cortical functional reorganization and its relationship with brain structural damage in patients with benign multiple sclerosis *Mult. Scler.* **16** 1326–34
[184] Pantano P *et al* 2005 A longitudinal fMRI study on motor activity in patients with multiple sclerosis *Brain* **128** 2146–53
[185] Petsas N *et al* 2013 Evidence of impaired brain activity balance after passive sensorimotor stimulation in multiple sclerosis *PLoS One* **8** e65315
[186] Rocca M A *et al* 2003 Functional cortical changes in patients with multiple sclerosis and nonspecific findings on conventional magnetic resonance imaging scans of the brain *Neuroimage* **19** 826–36
[187] Valsasina P *et al* 2011 A multicentre study of motor functional connectivity changes in patients with multiple sclerosis *Eur. J. Neurosci.* **33** 1256–63
[188] Gronwall D M 1977 Paced auditory serial-addition task: a measure of recovery from concussion *Percept. Mot. Skills* **44** 367–73
[189] Bonzano L, Pardini M, Mancardi G L, Pizzorno M and Roccatagliata L 2009 Structural connectivity influences brain activation during PVSAT in Multiple Sclerosis *Neuroimage* **44** 9–15
[190] Mainero C *et al* 2004 fMRI evidence of brain reorganization during attention and memory tasks in multiple sclerosis *Neuroimage* **21** 858–67

[191] Staffen W *et al* 2002 Cognitive function and fMRI in patients with multiple sclerosis: evidence for compensatory cortical activation during an attention task *Brain* **125** 1275–82
[192] Baltruschat S A, Ventura-Campos N, Cruz-Gómez Á J, Belenguer A and Forn C 2015 Gray matter atrophy is associated with functional connectivity reorganization during the Paced Auditory Serial Addition Test (PASAT) execution in Multiple Sclerosis (MS) *J. Neuroradiol.* **42** 141–9
[193] Hubbard N A *et al* 2016 Multiple sclerosis-related white matter microstructural change alters the BOLD hemodynamic response *J. Cereb. Blood Flow Metab.* **36** 1872–84
[194] Cader S, Cifelli A, Abu-Omar Y, Palace J and Matthews P M 2006 Reduced brain functional reserve and altered functional connectivity in patients with multiple sclerosis *Brain* **129** 527–37
[195] Bonnet M C, Allard M, Dilharreguy B, Deloire M, Petry K G and Brochet B 2010 Cognitive compensation failure in multiple sclerosis *Neurology* **75** 1241–8
[196] Lazeron R H, Rombouts S A, Scheltens P, Polman C H and Barkhof F 2004 An fMRI study of planning-related brain activity in patients with moderately advanced multiple sclerosis *Mult. Scler.* **10** 549–55
[197] Ferrari M and Quaresima V 2012 A brief review on the history of human functional near-infrared spectroscopy (fNIRS) development and fields of application *Neuroimage* **63** 921–35
[198] Pinti P *et al* 2018 The present and future use of functional near-infrared spectroscopy (fNIRS) for cognitive neuroscience *Ann. N. Y. Acad. Sci.* doi: 10.1111/nyas.13948
[199] Stojanovic-Radic J, Wylie G, Voelbel G, Chiaravalloti N and DeLuca J 2015 Neuroimaging and cognition using functional near infrared spectroscopy (fNIRS) in multiple sclerosis *Brain Imaging Behav.* **9** 302–11
[200] Jimenez J J *et al* 2014 Detection of reduced interhemispheric cortical communication during task execution in multiple sclerosis patients using functional near-infrared spectroscopy *J. Biomed. Opt.* **19** 076008
[201] Saleh S *et al* 2018 Supra-spinal modulation of walking in healthy individuals and persons with multiple sclerosis: A fNIRS mobile imaging study *Conf. Proc. IEEE Eng. Med. Biol. Soc.* **2018** 3156–9
[202] Hernandez M E *et al* 2016 Brain activation changes during locomotion in middle-aged to older adults with multiple sclerosis *J. Neurol. Sci.* **370** 277–83
[203] Goodwin S J 2016 Multiple sclerosis: integration of modeling with biology, clinical and imaging measures to provide better monitoring of disease progression and prediction of outcome *Neural Regen. Res.* **11** 1900–3
[204] Pappalardo F, Rajput A M and Motta S 2018 Computational modeling of brain pathologies: the case of multiple sclerosis *Brief Bioinform.* **19** 318–24
[205] Sakai K and Yamada K 2019 Machine learning studies on major brain diseases: 5-year trends of 2014–2018 *Jpn. J. Radiol.* **37** 34–72
[206] Kannan V, Kiani N A, Piehl F and Tegner J 2017 A minimal unified model of disease trajectories captures hallmarks of multiple sclerosis *Math. Biosci.* **289** 1–8
[207] Kotelnikova E *et al* 2017 Dynamics and heterogeneity of brain damage in multiple sclerosis *PLoS Comput. Biol.* **13** e1005757
[208] Akaishi T, Takahashi T and Nakashima I 2018 Chaos theory for clinical manifestations in multiple sclerosis *Med. Hypotheses* **115** 87–93

[209] Patel K R, Tobyne S, Porter D, Bireley J D, Smith V and Klawiter E 2018 Structural disconnection is responsible for increased functional connectivity in multiple sclerosis *Brain Struct. Funct.* **223** 2519–26

[210] Tewarie P *et al* 2018 Explaining the heterogeneity of functional connectivity findings in multiple sclerosis: An empirically informed modeling study *Hum. Brain Mapp.* **39** 2541–8

[211] Orrù G, Pettersson-Yeo W, Marquand A F, Sartori G and Mechelli A 2012 Using support vector machine to identify imaging biomarkers of neurological and psychiatric disease: a critical review *Neurosci. Biobehav. Rev.* **36** 1140–52

[212] Saccà V *et al* 2018 Evaluation of machine learning algorithms performance for the prediction of early multiple sclerosis from resting-state FMRI connectivity data *Brain Imaging Behav.* **13** 1103–14

[213] Zhang H *et al* 2019 Predicting conversion from clinically isolated syndrome to multiple sclerosis-An imaging-based machine learning approach *Neuroimage Clin.* **21** 101593

[214] Kocevar G *et al* 2016 Graph theory-based brain connectivity for automatic classification of multiple sclerosis clinical courses *Front. Neurosci.* **10** 478

[215] Zhong J, Chen D Q, Nantes J C, Holmes S A, Hodaie M and Koski L 2017 Combined structural and functional patterns discriminating upper limb motor disability in multiple sclerosis using multivariate approaches *Brain Imaging Behav.* **11** 754–68

[216] Bisecco A *et al* 2015 Connectivity-based parcellation of the thalamus in multiple sclerosis and its implications for cognitive impairment: A multicenter study *Hum. Brain Mapp.* **36** 2809–25

[217] Preziosa P *et al* 2016 Structural MRI correlates of cognitive impairment in patients with multiple sclerosis: A Multicenter Study *Hum. Brain Mapp.* **37** 1627–44

IOP Publishing

Neurological Disorders and Imaging Physics, Volume 2
Engineering and clinical perspectives of multiple sclerosis
Ayman El-Baz and Jasjit S Suri

Chapter 11

Gait analyses in multiple sclerosis; and time series

Hilal Keklicek and Sezer Ulukaya

Multiple sclerosis (MS) is a progressive neurodegenerative disease and leads to gait problems. In order to understand the gait deviations in MS and to use gait analysis as a diagnostic and a monitoring tool, it is necessary to understand the nature of the walk. The walking pattern of an individual who is healthy depends upon the healthy activity of all body system functions. The multifaceted nature of gait is one of the important subjects of health-related mechanics, and has been studied by different professional groups over the years. There are various gait analysis methods to evaluate and/or detect deviations from normal. Gait consists of both peripheral movements of the body and neural system outputs. The human walk is shaped by personalized features and is accommodated to environmental factors. The complex nature of MS leads to difficulties in the analyzing the central nervous system-rooted causes of gait deviations. Almost all gait analysis methods give an opinion on the musculoskeletal deviations of the gait in individuals with MS. But, there is still not a gold standard to detect MS at the early stage and/or determine the risk of MS. Therefore, the important point of gait analyses of individuals with MS is choosing the right analyzing method. This chapter was written to give clinicians and engineers an insight about the principles of clinical reasoning of individuals with MS.

11.1 Introduction

MS is a common, progressive neurodegenerative disease. Gait disturbance in MS is one of the common symptoms and may be caused by many reasons. In individuals with MS, it is important to recognize the symptoms that may cause deviations in walking, and to choose the correct walking analysis method. In order to understand gait disorders in MS, to evaluate with appropriate methods and to compare with healthy individuals, it is necessary to examine the health related nature of gait. In this section, the parameters which constitute walking as a starting point will be mentioned and then deviations specific to MS will be discussed.

doi:10.1088/978-0-7503-1762-7ch11

The multifaceted nature of the human walk
Walk; it is one of the basic functions of the individual and plays an important role in achieving many purposes. Our walk represents our physical skills, how our neuromotor system is organized and even our emotional state. The walking pattern exhibited by an individual who is healthy in all system functions and the gait of an individual living any failure in her/his system is different. In our different emotional states such as happiness, excitement, being in a rush, tension, self-confidence, sadness, our walk becomes unique. To understand the nature of the gait, it is important to examine in detail all the factors that affect the gait.

The gait, which is one of the important subjects of health-related mechanics, has been studied by different professional groups over the years. Characteristics of the nature of the walk have been defined and these characteristics have been accepted as guidelines for clinical interpretations.

It is necessary to understand the parts of the walking puzzle to interpret the gait deviations in an individual with MS and to use gait analysis as both a diagnostic and a monitoring tool. Thus, it may be possible to choose the appropriate method in the walking analysis of the individual with MS.

11.2 Determinants of gait

In terms of kinesiology, human gait has some biomechanical characteristics and these traits are named as determinants of gait [1]. In the past, while walking analyzes are still at the basic level, these characteristics are still valid today. However, progress in technology has shown that the gait contains a more complex set of events than can be seen.

Outlined below are six major biomechanical determinants of gait. Other musculoskeletal events are shaped around these determinants [2, 3].

- Vertical displacement of the gravity center;
- Lateral displacement of the gravity center;
- Pelvic rotation;
- Pelvic tilt;
- Foot motion;
- Ankle motion.

The determinants of gait play an important role in effective walking with minimal center of gravity displacement on the support surface [2]. The gravity center of the body corresponds to the front of the sacral 2 vertebrae while standing. In order to minimize the change of the gravity center during the walk and thus perform effective walking by spending less energy, the lower extremity performs a limited range of motion changes. The key points are pelvis, knee, ankle and feet [2, 4].

The angular rotation of the pelvis in the transverse plane is limited to about 5°. This movement extends the length of the limb relatively by limiting the downward movement of the gravity center. On the side of the swinging limb, the pelvic displaces 5° laterally and 5° vertically. The rotation center is the hip joint of the leg in the stance phase. The movement of the gravity center to the vertical is limited by the lateral movement and depression of the pelvis, where the gluteus medius muscle plays a major role in the stance phase. However, this displacement also limits the free area of the foot on the swinging side. Angular movements controlled by pelvic tilt in other joints—in particular knee flexion—give enough clarity for the foot movements [5, 6].

The plantar flexion of the ankle is the focal point of the foot and ankle movements. Basically, the plantar flexion movement starts immediately after the initial contact and continues until the terminal stance. This plantar flexion movement at the beginning of the stance phase allows plantigrade contact and limits the rise of the gravity center. Plantar flexion at the end of the stance phase ensures heel rise and prevents the rapid tibial progression and prevents a sudden drop of the gravity center [7, 8].

11.3 Kinetic and kinematics of gait

The kinetic and kinematic terms of gait are used to describe the properties of a single-cell walking cycle in the musculoskeletal system. In a simple sense, a gait cycle begins with the contact of the heel to the ground and continues until the same heel contacts the ground again. At different moments during this cycle, the interaction of all elements of the musculoskeletal system is examined. The term kinematic refers to the angular values during the cycle; the term kinetic includes the concepts of muscular and temporal. A gait cycle consists of two phases, outlined: the stance phase and the swing phase. Kinetic and kinematic events are examined in these phases [9, 10].

The walking phases are performed in the same order in both extremities, but at different times. Coordinated rhythmic movement is very important in order to perform the walking phases properly.

11.4 Phases of the gait cycle

The walking cycle is simply divided into two as the stance phase and the swing phase [11] (figure 11.1(a) and (b)).

11.4.1 Stance phase

The stance phase refers to all the events that begin immediately after the first contact of the limb and the period during which the limb is in contact with the ground.

- The *initial contact* is not a functional element of the stance phase. It is accepted that it corresponds to 0% of the gait.
- The *loading response* begins immediately after the first contact and continues until the opposite limb is removed.
- The *double support period* is a term that covers all the times when both limbs are in contact with the ground at the same time.

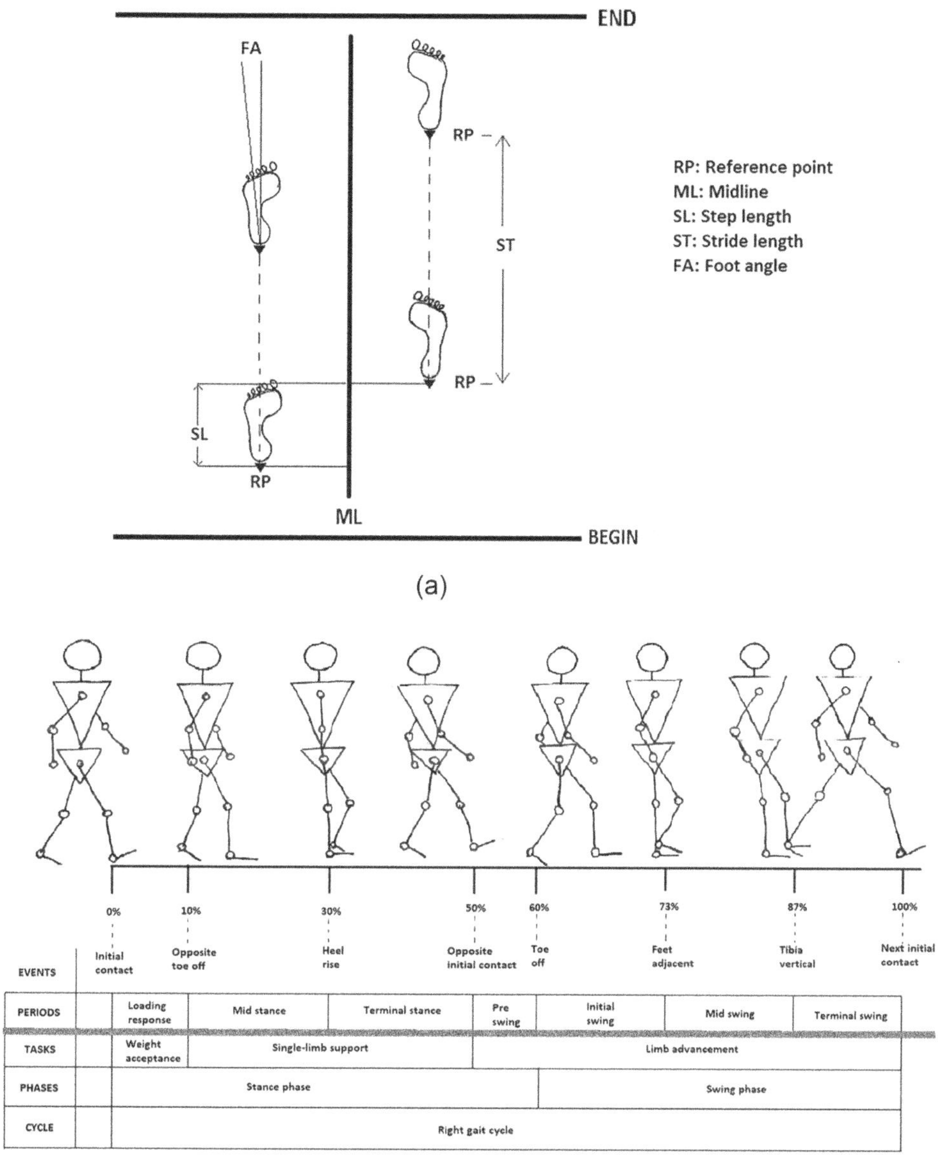

Figure 11.1. (a) Gait in graph. (b) Phases of gait.

- The *midstance phase* starts with the interruption of contact of the opposite side limb and the same side continues until the heel rises from the ground. The body weight is transferred to the front in the middle posture phase. In the *midstance phase*, the opposite limb is in the swing phase.
- The *terminal stance* starts with the heel rise from the ground and ends when the other heel makes the initial contact with the ground. In the terminal

stance phase, body weight continues to be forward. Terminal stance corresponds to the second half of the single support period.
- *Preswing* occurs when the limb is lifted off the ground. At this time, the opposing limb contacts the ground. In this phase, the limb is displaced to the front significantly.

11.4.2 Swing phase

Swing phase consists of three sections and covers 60%–100% of the gait cycle.
- The *initial swing* refers to the period during the foot rises from the ground until the level of the opposite ankle. Proper execution of this phase is important to prevent obstacles.
- The *midswing phase* lasts until the tibia becomes perpendicular to the ground. The extremity is accelerating within the midswing phase.
- In the terminal swing phase, the verticality of the tibia is reduced. The extremity has completed acceleration.

During the phases of the gait, the foot and ankle complex serve as a pivot point.

11.5 Temporal–spatial features of gait

The temporal–spatial features of gait consist of basic characteristics of gait. The term *stride* refers to the whole of events between two movements, which begin with the first contact of a limb and make the first contact again. One stride corresponds to the complete gait cycle (0%–100%).
- The distance between the strides is expressed as *stride length.*
- The time until stride is defined as *stride time.*
- *A step length* is performed between the first contact of the limb and the first contact of the opposite limb.
- The time between them is called as *step time.*
- The *step width* is the distance between the two heels during the double support period and shows the support surface width.
- *Cadance* is a total count of repeated steps during a comfortable walk in one minute. It is expected to be between 90–120 per minute.
- *Velocity* refers to the distance received within a specified period [10].

Holistic movements of the musculoskeletal system are important in the realization of the basic features of the gait. These are grouped under kinetics and kinematics [12–14].

11.6 Kinetics of gait

The forces applied to the ground by the foot are known as foot forces. The forces applied by the ground to the feet are known as ground reaction forces. These forces are equal and opposite (Law of Newton III). Ground reaction forces are named according to Cartesian coordinate systems: vertical, anterior–posterior, medial–lateral (figure 11.2). The vector sum of these forces is expressed by a single force

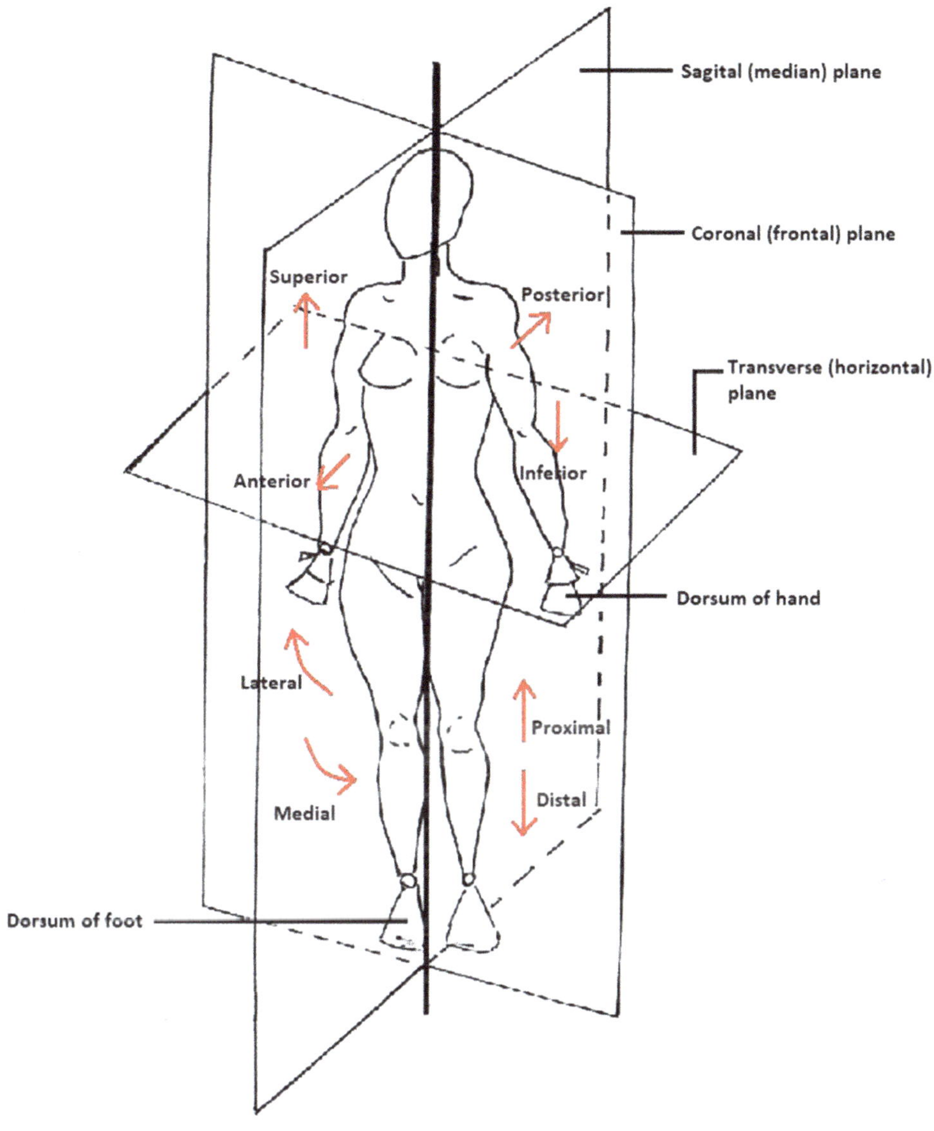

Figure 11.2. Cartesian coordinate systems of the body.

between the foot and the ground. The sum of the components of the anterior–posterior forces and vertical forces is observed as the classical butterfly sign [10, 14].

11.6.1 Vertical forces

The vertical forces are exposed around the support surface. The peak force in the vertical direction is observed twice on the walk.

The loading response and the forces during the last load are slightly greater than the body weight. The ground reaction forces are slightly less than the body weight during the midstance. This slight fluctuation occurs due to the vertical acceleration of the center of mass (CoM) ($F = ma$). In the loading response the CoM moves down. In the mid-stance, the ground reaction forces are less than the body weight because of the relatively low load. This reduction occurs with the upward momentum of the body in the early phase of the stance. At the end of the stance phase, a higher reaction force is released. This increase is due to the movement of the plantar flexor and the transition to the swing phase.

11.6.2 Anterior–posterior forces

Friction force occurs on the support surface in the anterior posterior direction. Ground reaction force is in the posterior direction during heel contact. At the same time, sufficient friction between the foot and the floor prevents sliding forward. The ground reaction force increases in long steps. The friction force is less effective in walking with short steps.

The ground reaction force is accurate to the anterior at the end of the stance phase and before the swing phase. The foot, allows the body to move forward by applying force in the posterior direction. In the meantime, due to insufficient friction, the foot slides without taking the body forward. The peak anterior–posterior reaction force is 20% of the total body weight.

A large part of the friction force depends on whether the body is in the anterior or posterior. A bigger step width and higher friction force result from the increased angle between the lower extremity and the ground. Structural properties of the body, such as momentum, cause antero-posterior reaction forces. The ground reaction forces in the posterior direction of the heel contact control the forward movement of the body. Conversely, the forward acceleration movement at the toe-off is the product of the ground reaction forces in the anterior direction.

At a constant speed, the forward thrust occurs at the end of the stance phase and the breaking force occurs at the early phases of the stance. These forces are almost equal and inverse, so that the balance is achieved when the body weight is passed from one step to the other. Deceleration requires a greater amount of breaking force than the thrust force. Acceleration is the opposite.

11.6.3 Medial–lateral forces

The size of the ground reaction force is relatively low in the mediolateral direction and it varies from person to person. As with the anteroposterior friction, the mediolateral frictional force also depends on the position of the CoM relative to the foot. Although mediolateral ground reaction forces are hardly felt during walking, they are noticeable when walking with very wide steps. The peak mediolateral location reaction force is often observed in individuals walking with wide steps.

11.7 Joint torques and forces/kinematics

Joint surfaces, ligaments and tendons are subjects of tension, compression and friction forces. These forces cannot be measured directly. They are mostly measured indirectly by biomechanical analysis and modeling. Also, these powers can be surprisingly large.

Information on the horizontal kinematics of the lower limb is limited. In order to improve the accuracy of the measurements, researchers developed some materials placed on the tibia femur. Markers enable the use of video systems to measure bone movements. Joint rotational movements are less in the frontal plane compared to sagittal plan movements. Rotations are especially important in hip and subtalar joints.

It is necessary to stand in front of or behind the individual to observe the frontal plan movements in the best way. Hip movements play an important role in minimizing vertical displacement of the body center of gravity.

The foot becomes flexible and can adapt to the ground with rapid pronation after heel contact. At the end of the stance phase-between the heel-off and the toe-off, the inversion of the foot is ensured. Also, this movement enables the foot to move into the rigid structure and take the position to move forward. At the heel contact, center of pressure is located at the slight lateral of the heel. At a time until the mid-stance, the pressure line runs to the lateral of the middle foot [10, 13].

11.7.1 Muscle activity

During the gait cycle, many muscles of the lower limb produce one or two shorter explosive forces. Specialized roles of the muscles determine when muscles are active in walking. Clinicians, who know the function of muscles, better interpret walking anomalies. The activity of lower extremity muscles can be studied with electromyography (EMG).

The role of muscle structures in the trunk during the walk is underestimated. Based on the evolution of the vertebral spine, Gracovetsky proposed the 'spinal engine' theory for the first time with the motion of the spine [15]. Future research should take into account the hypothesis that the spine plays an important role in walking. The movements of the erector spina and rectus abdominis muscles control the forward momentum of the trunk in the heel contact. The activity of the body flexors also corresponds to the time that hip flexors actively flexed the hip.

Body control is important to achieve the intended movement of the limbs. In body control, the postural stability is provided by the central nervous system and activates the deep trunk muscles while we are still thinking about the movement. This initial activation continues with repeated fluctuations during the continuation of the movement. This ensures a stable and rhythmic trunk movement. In other words, maintaining postural stability is the basis for a good walking function [9, 12].

11.8 The layout of the gait function in chaos AND the complexity of the gait function in order

As in all fields, walking analysis methods have been diversified along with the developing technology in the field of kinesiology and biomechanics. The analyses have started to be detailed, in-depth and processed from a wide perspective. Beyond the determinants of the gait, concepts related to holistic and system functions are now on the agenda, with gait stability based on these concepts.

Current gait analysis methods, along with the main determinants of the walk, have provided new knowledge such as 'variability', 'autocorrelation' and 'fractal structure'. In the light of all this information, researches are starting to give an idea about the nature of the gait.

11.8.1 The ability of variability at walk: the two-edged knife

When viewed with long loops, it was seen that the determinant parameters of the gait did not repeat each other [16]. It was realized that the events occurring in each step cycle showed changes within certain limits. The definition of gait variability was born here.

When the gait cycle of the individual is divided into step cycles and divided into sub-steps, it can be seen that the revealed steps are similar but not identical. In this way, the individual can walk in her/his neuro-biomechanical infrastructure with varying step lengths, step widths, acceleration and/or deceleration. The variable nature of the gait is part of the nature of life, so, walking is no longer mechanical and becomes specific to the living being.

The ability to change on a walk is necessary for the person to adapt to different surfaces, speeds, environmental conditions and his or her own bio-social status [16]. At the same time, this variability must take place within certain limits. When the other conditions are fixed, if the boundaries of variability are not balanced, it is considered that the systems associated with gait are in a disruption [17]. When we examine a single step cycle, the steps may be symmetrical, but this does not mean that the walk is normal. Likewise, in an asymmetrical gait, variability may be kept within reasonable limits. In order to be able to talk about the variability, it is necessary to collect a certain number of step cycles.

The fluctuations in the walk in previous years were considered as nonessential variables and the step cycles that caused the differences were removed from the evaluations [17]. It has been realized that fluctuations are an important source of understanding the nature of the walk and the prediction and/or severity of abnormalities occurring in body systems.

It is known that there is a strong link between variability and fall risk. Although the descriptive parameters of gait may be normal or symmetrical, the increased variability in gait is directly and strongly associated with the risk of fall [18]. Gait variability provides deeper and more valuable information about locomotor system functions than appears.

Long-range gait analysis may be appropriate to achieve realistic results of variability in a walk. Long-range gait analysis can be examined by the atomic structure of gait; steps and step time (ST). The studies in the literature are generally concentrated on 512 steps [19–23]. After each step is recorded in time series, the average step time (AST) is calculated. The fluctuation magnitude is then calculated using the coefficient of variation [19–23];

$$\text{(CoV) CoV} = (\text{Standard Deviation}/\text{AST})*100$$

11.8.2 Fractal organization of gait; structure of variability

Fractal is the common name given to complex geometric shapes that are self-resembling. The repetitive and infinitely shrinking shapes are an expression used to understand a whole of small pieces that resemble oneself, and the components of this whole [24]. It is necessary to understand the nature of variability in order to determine the possible role of gait variability in pathologies. Using the average of various sub-parameters is not sufficient to provide real information about the general nature of gait.

Each step is the 'final' output of a multidimensional neuromuscular control system, and is influenced by many factors, both internal and external. With this feature, the steps can be compared to each heart beat which is the final output of the autonomic system. Timing of heel strokes, times between steps etc, all sub-elements of the rhythmically repeating gait may meet regular strokes such as a clock showing the operation of the locomotor system (figure 11.3) [17].

Theoretically, fractal structure provides information about the organization, regulation, interactions and stability of the locomotor system [25]. Researches conducted on these hypotheses were carried out to determine whether there is fractal structuring which is the expression of naturalness in the walk [17, 25]. In order to find out if the walk shows a fractal structure, autocorrelation should be examined in long gait cycles. Analyzes with a small number of time series may not be sufficient to determine the fractal structure of gait. Patterns that create the walking cycle must proceed according to a rule. Using a few repetitions may be insufficient to identify the pattern. In addition, the exposed pattern must be able to grow or shrink [21, 26–28]. For these reasons, it is more meaningful to use a large number of data,

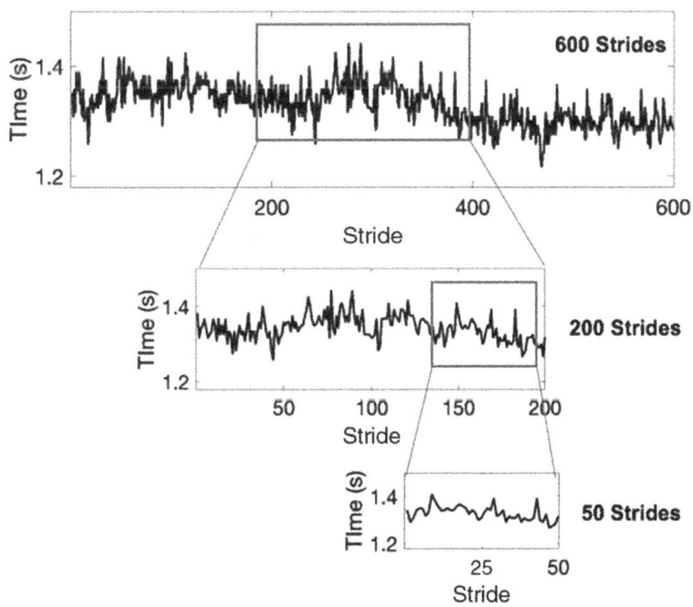

Figure 11.3. Self similarity of locomotor stride times. Reprinted with permission from [25].

including long walking cycles, in order to be able to talk about the autocorrelation of gait. It is more meaningful to use a large number of data—long walking cycles—in order to be able to talk about the autocorrelation of gait [16, 25, 27, 29].

The term autocorrelation is, conceptually, the relationship between the different values of the signal or value of a series at any time. It expresses the relationship between consecutive values in the series. The presence of autocorrelation indicates that the deviations in the series are not random [16, 17]. Autocorrelation in walking shows consistency and similarity in repeated fluctuations. Studies on long gait cycles have shown that the existing variability of gait is not actually random, it repeats itself systematically and resembles the whole of gait. In healthy individuals, each parameter of walking is related to each other. These parameters show fractal properties at different speeds and running [16, 17, 25]. When the *X* series is taken as a process, the autocorrelation relationship ($R(s, t)$) between *s* and *t* times is explained by the following formula.

$$R(s, t) = E\{(X_t - \mu_t)(X_s - \mu_s)\}/\sigma_t * \sigma_s,$$

where 'E' is the mean value finder, 'μ' is the mean, and 'σ' is the standard deviation.

According to researches, cognition-conscious control has a direct effect on autocorrelation and fractal structuring characteristics of walking. In other words, the cognitive level is very important in maintaining the natural structuring of gait during the double tasks performed at walk (speech, etc). As the cognitive skill weakens, the internal organization of gait deteriorates. Similarly, when the conditioned walk was performed (rhythmic auditor stimulation, etc), the increase in symmetry in the walk and the decrease in the variability have been shown to lead to disruption in the fractal nature of the walk [30–35]. The results of these studies led to the re-discussion of the automatic process in the organization of gait. The walk is a set of long-term and detailed systematic patterns, its organization is more related to upper centers and is linked to system functions.

Many methods have been used to describe the autocorrelation and fractal nature of gait. To calculate the Hurst exponential in literature, rescaled range analysis [20–22, 36, 37], detrended fluctuation analysis [22, 23, 28, 33, 36, 38, 39], power spectral density [19–23, 36, 37], multi-scale entropy, entropy analysis [19, 40, 41] and fractal analysis [22, 42–44] methods were used. It has been found that these methods can give incorrect results when used alone. Therefore, re-scaled range analysis and power spectral density were used together. [20, 21]. Detrended fluctuation analysis (DFA) and power spectral density are the two most commonly used methods.

An $x(t)$ time series signal provided by DFA is expressed as;

$$Y(k) = \sum(X_i - X_{\text{mean}}), \quad i = 1, \ldots, k$$

Then $Y(k)$ is divided into equal 'n' intervals and every line is tried to fit a line. Fluctuation changes are also calculated by;

$$F = \sqrt{1/N \sum[X(k) - X_n(k)]^2}$$

11.8.3 Gait dynamics and postural instability: fall risk

Falling is an important socioeconomic constraint and brings along secondary problems. It is an independent cause of death in elderly individuals [45]. Even if there are no identified clinical findings; increased variability, decreased autocorrelation, and the relationship between fractal configuration and the risk of falls are shown directly [46]. It has been shown that not only falling individuals but also potential candidates who are under risk, present gait with increased variability. Gait variability provides important information about the individual's fall risk.

It has been reported that individuals who have no observed fall and no defined neuromotor diseases but have increased gait variability have experienced a fall in the follow-up years even if all other walking parameters or musculoskeletal health tests have normal features [46]. Evidence-based studies to date have benefited from the gait assessment to serve many purposes, such as the response of diseases to treatment, the examination of clinical conditions, the discovery of differences in health conditions, the objective determination of mobility and functional status etc [47–51]. The multidimensional nature of gait led to the development of research in a descriptive manner. Gait is worth examining not only for the analysis of existing conditions but also for the purpose of identifying the risks involved in the lives of individuals. The results to date have shown that gait is a combination of highly complex processes and contains many questions that need to be answered.

The discovery that the variable configuration of gait is the systemic parts of a whole has led researchers to look at the whole picture. To measure the quality of the walk, to determine its similarity with the natural and to provide important information about the functions of the whole body system, it is necessary to search for the determinants of gait in the cross-sectional analysis and internal harmony of gait. Recently, gait stability is adopted as an important concept that gives direction to gait-related studies. As mentioned, gait is a multifaceted concept and requires the optimal functioning of all body systems.

Even if no deviations are observed in the determinants and/or basic characteristics of the walk, deterioration in the general organization of the walk can be detected early. This early awareness is very important in identifying individuals at risk and predicting disease progression. For this reason, in addition to peripheral musculoskeletal damage, it is necessary to examine whether the gait is stable especially for the foresight of the neural system disorders.

While the main characteristics of the lower extremities were prominent in previous years, the use of autocorrelation and fractal analyses eliminated the dependence of gait analysis on extremities. It is possible to reach a general judgment by evaluating the successive signals collected from many regions (head, body, pelvis, etc) during which a rhythmic movement is observed during walking. Understanding the stable nature of gait is important for detection before symptomatic decay in central nervous system diseases such as MS.

11.8.4 Biometric features of gait

Studies are still ongoing in order to examine the biometric characteristics of gait. In order to determine the biometric feature of the walk, it is necessary record the gait of an individual in the long term and at different conditions in the natural area of the person. Thus, the person does not need to cooperate with the test. However, the ethical aspect of this method is controversial [52].

11.9 Gait analysis methods

The methods of gait analysis can simply be classified as follows:

- visual methods;
- sensor based methods;
- angular measurement methods;
- medical imaging techniques;
- machine learning.

11.9.1 Visual methods

Markers can be used in methods where visualization is used, or indirect methods may be tried. In systems where markers are used, optoelectronic systems using active or passive markers are prominent. In other visual oriented analyzes; image-based, model-based or hybrid approaches are used. Images taken with analogue or digital cameras are processed. In these methods, the main output is the detection of segmental events and phases. This is especially useful in kinematic analysis. They are used as real-time image-based analysis. Optoelectronic systems convert light signals into electrical signals and work on the principle that light reflected from the markers. The cameras used in these systems send infrared signals. Thus, the position of the marker can be determined. Although there are some advantages of these methods, cables, markers, cameras etc prevent the person from exhibiting a natural walk. It is widely used in two-dimensional and three-dimensional analysis. As the number of cameras increases, the movement plan that can be observed increases. Markers are not used in indirect methods. The image at any time is selected and analysis is performed on this selected image. It is a clinically practical method. It is suitable for examining the phase-based extremity-trunk responses. It can be used to see the effects of a symptom in other regions at a given time. However, it provides limited information and is highly dependent on individual errors [52–56].

11.9.2 Sensor based methods

Sensor-based approaches include sensors on the individual or on the ground. The sensors may be specialized for collecting many different types of signal. EMG is placed on the individual to monitor muscle response. It is especially used for evaluating the action potential of the motor unit. Each electrode acts for a muscle group. Analysis with EMG still needs to be developed. Because the collected EMG signals are likely to be affected by relative muscle tension and the activity of other muscles [57, 58].

In the inertial systems, the resistance to change of motion is evaluated. The accelerators measure the inertia and the gyroscopes measure the segmental orientation. Combination of these two materials may be useful in reaching information on kinematics.

It is possible to determine ground reaction force, force pattern, base pressure distribution, step and stride phases in measurements made with sensors placed on the floor. Ground reaction force is the reactive counterpart of the body-induced load. This force is measured by transducers. The force is converted into electrical signals and allows the determination of the pressure center. These orthogonal elements define the movement of the individual. Pressure sensors measure the load directly. When mechanical strain occurs, these piezoelectric based sensors produce electrical signals. But the system has spatial limitations. The individual tries to place his foot on the force platform while he is walking, which distorts the naturalness of the walk considerably. On the other hand, pressure sensors can also be placed in shoes [57, 58].

11.9.3 Angular measurement methods

Electrogoniometers can be used to determine the change of joint angles during walking [57, 59]. It must be calibrated before each measurement to obtain the correct data. Electrogoniometers do not provide timing-based measurements.

11.9.4 Medical imaging techniques

Neuroimaging of gait is difficult. MRI findings are exacerbated with the increase in the severity of the disease. And, if the walk is disrupted, there is probably widespread damage in the central nervous system. Technically, utilizing neuroimaging techniques during movement (fMRI, electroencephalography, positron emission tomography, etc) cannot be very useful. In this type of imaging, immobility is essential.

fMRI can be used to identify the central representative area of some distal limb movements (for example, wrist, ankle movement). However, during a combined motion such as gait, the MRI does not yet produce a clear result. Generally, gait-related brain activity responses are sought by simulating a specific ratio of reality. There are studies using mental walking imagery or walking video images to determine the gait specific central area. With this method, it is possible to examine the sections related to motor planning in the brain. When we look at healthy individuals, the relationship of the gait with certain regions seems to be determined by functional neuroimaging. Nevertheless, it is not possible to distinguish whether the responses revealed during the actual movement are related to the isolated gait function or to the sensorial input. All these other factors cause movement artefacts [60].

Neuroimaging can be performed during real walking with the methods as follows: near-infrared spectrographic imaging (NIRS) [61], transcranial magnetic techniques (TMS) [62], single photon emission tomography (SPECT) [63], electroencephalography (EEG) [64], fMRI [65], H215O-PET [66], f-fluorodeoxyglucose positron emission tomography (FDG-PET) [67] can be examples. While NIRS, FDG-PET, SPECT and TMS provide imaging during gait function, EEG, fMRI, H215O-PET can provide imaging during walk planning or repetitive foot movements. Each of the methods has its own disadvantages [60]. There is still a need for a gold standard data processing process in central imaging methods.

According to researches, the mental imaging of the movement and the cortical activity revealed during the real movement are similar. However, it is known that activity in the premotor area is affected by individual differences. Although individuals exhibit almost the same gait, the mental imaging processes can have distinct differences. Therefore, it is not yet possible to determine the cortical functions associated with gait by the mental imaging method completely [68–74].

The results of neuroimaging methods in which the gait is executed as a real-motor function or processed by the mental imaging technique show some similarities and differences [71, 75–78]. Previously, some studies have been carried out on whether the activity of the cortical representation area of the gait can be measured with ankle movements or not. In the light of the findings, it was concluded that ankle movements would not be sufficient [73, 79, 80]. When the gait-related brain activity was examined by mental imaging methods, it was determined that the cortical activity increased in some areas. In general, there is an increase in activity in the supplementary motor area, precentral gyrus, left dorsal premotor area and cingulate motor area [71]. Excessive activity increase in the bilateral sensorimotor cortex was detected in studies using active motor motion. In the studies, utilized with the mental imaging method, a relatively limited activity increase was observed in bilateral precentral gyrus. It has been shown that more anterior zones of the medial sensorimotor areas are activated in gait imagination and the actual walk. In this context, the increase in precentral gyrus activity can be considered as more closely related to gait-specific activities. During the mental imaging, the pre-supplementary motor field was more active than the supplementary motor area. While the pre-supplementary area is more active during the activation phase, the supplementary motor area engine operates prominently during movement. For this reason, it can be concluded that pre-supplementary motor area and supplementary motor area are activated together in the actual movement while the pre-supplementary area is prominent in the mental imaging process. In other words, caudal supplementary motor area functions to express movement [73, 81, 82].

In addition, the activity of the mesencephalic locomotor area, the basal ganglia, the cerebellum, mirror neurons and the hipcampo-limbic arch are undeniable in gait function.

11.9.5 Machine learning

Machine learning techniques or deep learning techniques include many singular or mixed methods. If the problem is linear, it can be used as a good measurement. However, while it may be preferable to indicate the classification or recognition of the groups, it may not be an efficient method in the clinical follow-up of individuals [83, 84].

11.10 Gait problems and cortical involvement in multiple sclerosis: choosing the right analysis method

It is very important to select the appropriate gait analysis method for effective clinical applications. Walking can be evaluated in many ways, but the data may not measure the information sought. In terms of multiple sclerosis, it may be appropriate to select kinetic–kinematic gait analysis to determine the effective clinical approaches in the treatment of the peripheral aberrations. Evaluating signal processing methods and methods of sequential information can be considered more appropriate to determine fall risk, predict disease progression and investigate the postural control skills. In addition, it will not be possible to obtain the answer to questions such as how the additional symptoms (e.g. cortical fatigue) affect the gait by using cross-sectional kinetic–kinematic analyses. Therefore, instead of cross-sectional analyses, it would be appropriate to examine features such as stability in walking, which gives insight into the central organization of the walk.

The rate of gait disturbance was reported higher than 60% in individuals with MS [85]. These individuals stated that their most important complaint was deterioration in gait [86]. In individuals with MS, more than 50% of falls occur during walking [87–89]. In addition, individuals with MS spend intensive effort organizing their walks [90]. In MS, the deviations of walking vary depending on the pyramidal, extrapyramidal or mixed involvement (table 11.1 indicating the gait problems according to the affected neural system in individuals with MS; and also showing the gait features of MS). Deviations in gait are usually caused by loss of strength, sensory disorders, fatigue, ataxia, visual impairment, tone disorder and pain [91, 92].

Kinetic deviations

Individuals with MS exhibit slower walking than healthy individuals. The slower speed is observed for both the fast walk and the preferred walking speed. Stride lengths are shortened. Step lengths are shortened. Swing phase times are prolonged. Even if they increase walking speeds, the situation does not change. Also, the double support periods are prolonged. These features are the most common deviations in the clinic. The step widths and stride times of individuals with MS increase. These problems are relatively less observed. The least difference is revealed in cadences. When individuals with MS were forced to increase their speed, deviations of the parameters increase too [93–100].

Muscle impairment and gait

The abduction force of the hip muscles, the endurance of the plantar flexor muscles, the endurance of the trunk flexor muscles are directly related to the walking speed and gait endurance in individuals with MS. Hip abductor muscles and trunk flexors show their effectiveness by providing postural stabilization through proximal joints. Thus, it is easier to produce a repetitive alternative rhythmic movement. Plantar flexors should be particularly active at the end of the stop phase, especially during the initiation of the forward displacement process. The effective activity of plantar flexors at this stage is necessary to achieve maximal velocity. The strength of the

Table 11.1. Gait impairments in individuals with MS.

Kinetic Deviations	• Gait speed—decreased • Stride lengths—shortened • Step lengths—shortened • Cadance—decreased • Swing phase times—increased • Double support periods—increased • The step widths—increased • Stride times—increased
Muscle impairment	• The abduction force of the hip muscles—decreased • the endurance of the plantar flexor muscles—decreased • the endurance of the trunk flexor muscles—decreased • knee flexor force—decreased • Push off power—decreased • repetitive alternative rhythmic movement—decreased • maximal velocity—decreased
Postural instability and gait	• Gait variability—increased • The risk of falling and falling rate—increased
Pyramidal and Extrapyramidal impairment and gait	• Ataxia—increased • Postural control—decreased • Variability and deterioration of the kinetic and kinematic values at the stance phase and the swing phase—increased
Ground reaction forces and gait	• Initially contact with the anterior parts of the foot • A delay between heel contact and full loading the heel • The load progression is located in the lateral regions of the foot • the accelerated forward transmission of the load
Fatigue and gait	• Difficulty in performing the long gait
Cognitive impairment and gait	• intensive effort to organize the gait

knee flexors in individuals with MS is also an important determinant of the velocity. Effective use of the knee flexor muscles, especially in the swing phase, enables rapid activity. The concentric contraction of the knee flexor muscles governs the acceleration process in the knee joint and the eccentric contraction controls the deceleration [91, 101, 102].

Postural instability and gait: Long-range organization of gait

The variability in the walk due to the deterioration of postural control was determined in almost every measured parameter in individuals with MS. Many time–distance characteristics (joint angles, muscle activation patterns of the lower extremity, torque and power generation in the lower extremity, ground reaction forces, body angular velocities and acceleration values) were found to increase in variability. As the variability increases, the risk of falling and falling rate increase. It has been shown that walking variability increases even in MS patients with minimal clinical findings [94, 103–107].

It was observed that speed-related commands given to individuals with MS completely disrupt the walk. It has been shown that the cognitive dual task causes deterioration in the phases of speed, cadence and double support periods of individuals with MS. However, it is also reported that the mental effort in order to control the gait is significantly high in individuals with MS [108, 109]. The issue that should be considered is that it is not enough to look at the walking of MS patients only in terms of musculoskeletal system analysis. For focused intervention approaches, peripheral information taken at a certain time will be useful. For example, as suitable orthosis designs, etc. However, if the peripheral reflections of the neuromotor organization of the individual and the response to the stimuli are to be tested, the methods of processing the signals to be collected with long-range data will be appropriate. It may not be possible to say that the walking characteristics of MS patients at any cross-sectional moment completely reflect their general condition. Because individuals with MS are not able to perform a walk with quality, consistency, durability, the multiple data collection methods that require continuity are largely dependent on the motorized treadmill. Therefore, multi-signal processing methods can be negatively affected, especially in terms of speed and timing factors. Ideally, the instrument used should be able to adapt to the spontaneous speed–time changes of the person. Nevertheless, it is also possible to have an idea about the whole event with a limited number of data by using appropriate formulations.

Pyramidal or/and extrapyramidal impairment and gait

If MS is characterized by the extrapyramidal system, the most commonly seen walking disorder is ataxia [110]. Ataxia can be considered as trunk ataxia and/or limb ataxia. Individuals have difficulty in stabilizing their bodies due to the influence of the neurophysiological arch which is responsible for providing postural control. Individuals may have oscillations in varying amplitudes at standing and during walking. If trunk ataxia is prominent, gait disturbances will occur in both the stance phase and the swing phase. If extremity ataxia is prominent, swing phase findings will be more observed [111, 112]. In the early stages of the MS, when the findings of the trunk and/or extremities are limited, the postural stability and gait stability can be interpreted by using the body angular acceleration values. In other words, consecutive data collection methods are more appropriate. However, if ataxia symptoms are clearly visible, it would be more useful to determine kinetic and kinematic values by cross-sectional analysis.

If individuals with MS have pyramidal system involvement, the long-range autocorrelation and the variability of gait can be examined in detail to predict the progression of the pathology in the early stage of the disease and to determine the risk of fall. However, when symptoms begin to become more apparent (especially in mild-moderate disease severity), almost any pathway used in gait analysis may be preferred. Because of pyramidal involvement, the rate of onset of various symptoms such as peripheral weakness, loss of sensation and tonus increase is high in isolated muscle groups. In advanced stages of the disease, cross-sectional kinetic–kinematic analyses will be more meaningful.

Cortical impairment and gait

It is a well-known fact that deep brain structures in cortex and especially white matter are affected in gait disorders and especially in MS. However, due to the complex nature of the MS, the distinctive areas specific to the walk have not yet been revealed. If the central damage is noticeable before clinical symptoms are revealed, interaction between multiple sclerosis and the dynamic configuration of gait can be illuminated. However, very early diagnosis usually cannot be made before the revealing of clinical findings. Therefore, central differences associated with gait in MS cannot be clearly defined. Changes in the macro and microstructure of the central nervous system in relation to gait disorders of individuals with MS have not been clarified yet. For this reason, fMRI usage comes to the fore for identification purposes. It has been shown that step time variability was associated with left hippocampal and left putamen volumes in fallers with MS [113]. Also, the supplementary motor area interhemispheric tract may have a role in dual-task performance during walking in individuals with MS and MS patients have greater variability in spatiotemporal parameters and higher activity in the interhemispheric supplementary motor area, axial diffusivity, radial diffusivity indicating lower white matter integrity. The supplementary motor area tract may be more related to dual-task while walking in individuals with MS, rather than a function of damaged corpus callosum [114]. A study also demonstrated that the activity of the right premotor cortex activities were higher than the left premotor and bilateral supplementary motor areas in the MS. However, healthy individuals had higher activity level in these areas. Results of the study confirmed the role of the premotor cortices in movement planning and in modulating walking activities. Also, the results showed that individuals with mild MS have a similar premotor control strategy to healthy controls while walking with the same task [65]. It has also been shown that while right premotor cortex activation was recruited more in the healthy group during walking with a dual task, right premotor cortex and bilateral supplementary motor area activity were higher in individuals with MS while standing with a dual task [115]. Another study indicated that the left parahippocampal gyrus and transverse temporal gyrus, and the right fusiform gyrus, inferior temporal gyrus, lingual gyrus, pericalcarine cortex, superior temporal gyrus, and transverse temporal gyrus were significantly associated with the timed-25 foot walk test [116].

Although there were some studies that examined the brain activity during actual walking in individuals with MS, MS specific gait-related brain damage has not yet been illuminated.

Ground reaction and gait

Plantar pressure analysis can be useful in examining the deviations of gait due to hypertonia [117]. The ground reaction forces are evaluated as pressure based by creating the map of the foot. Individuals with MS have a different plantar pressure map than healthy individuals due to the severity of increased hypertonicity observed in the lower extremity muscles, especially plantar flexors [118]. Healthy individuals touch the ground with the posterolateral area of heel at initial contact. Then, gradual pronation occurs in the subtalar joint with the controlled plantar flexion movement. In this way, plantigrade contact is provided at the stance phase. The loading intensity draws a line from the post-lateral portion of the foot towards the mid-medial of the foot. After the stance phase is terminated, the subtalar joint is supine during the heel-rise period, and serves as a rigid lever. With strong plantar flexor activity, approximately 60% of the load is transferred to the direction of the first metatarsal head and the push-off phase of the gait is performed. Active-contact areas of the foot in healthy individuals in stance phase are the heel (mostly heel lateral), foot laterally, metatarsal head. However, there is a certain amount of load bearing on the other contact areas (such as middle feet and fingers etc). The load is transferred rhythmically from the back of the foot to the front and the timing is done in accordance with the gait phases [118, 119]. In MS patients, the first contact phase is usually inaccurate. Depending on the severity of the hypertonicity in the plantar flexors, the individual makes the initial contact with the anterior parts of the foot. If the individual can transfer any amount of the load to the foot, he/she can make a certain amount of heel contact while passing from the initial contact to the loading phase. But in individuals with MS, there is a delay between heel contact and fully loading the heel. In healthy individuals, the load progression line that moves from the lateral to the medial is located in the lateral regions of the foot in individuals with MS. In addition, since the controlled plantar flexion movement cannot be performed accurately, the forward transmission of the load to the fore-foot is accelerated. In other words, early heel-rise occurs [118]. This movement combines with early knee flexion. Consequently, both the timing factors, the presence of symmetry, and the pressure mapping of ground forces acting on the foot can be examined by pressure analysis methods. However, changes in the proximal joints cannot be determined by this method. In addition, it is not possible to determine the swing phase problems in patients with ataxia symptoms by pressure analysis methods. However, as the movement changes in the subtalar joint are significantly reflected in the plantar pressure, an idea about the ability to stabilize the subtalar joint at the stance phase can be obtained. The amount of the fluctuation in the subtalar joint movements may provide good knowledge of the neuromuscular control over the peripheral joints and the co-contraction capabilities of the muscles. In the plantar pressure analysis, multi-signal processing methods can give distinctive findings. In particular, the variability in the load transfer timing can provide good predictions about postural control.

Fatigue and gait

An important issue that should be considered while carrying out the gait analysis process in MS is fatigue [120, 121]. Central, peripheral and/or mixed fatigue patterns make it difficult to analyze the gait with multiple data. An individual with MS should perform long-term performance to use direct signal processing methods which require more than 500 steps from individuals. Individuals suffered from higher fatigue-related symptoms probably cannot perform such a long gait. In this case, ways to look at the whole with fewer data can be tried.

Cognitive impairment and gait
It is known that individuals with MS have difficulties with cognitive processes. However, it can be observed at different rates in the early stages of the disease [122]. Whether the cognitive effect is of such a magnitude as to influence the walking stability and fractal-like nature of the gait can be examined by gait analysis. But it is more meaningful to do this type of analysis in the earliest phase of the disease, because the complex nature of MS makes it difficult to determine the origin of the deviations in walking in the progressive stages of the disease.

Table 11.2 is a sample for optimally analyzing methods for certain aims.

11.11 Conclusion

The complex nature of MS complicates gait analysis. It is still quite difficult to determine the central damage characteristics of gait disorders in MS. It is necessary to measure the searched properties in terms of clinical and engineering science with the correct method. The correct evaluation of the results obtained is only possible by understanding the order of the natural walk in chaotic structure. In the future, there will still be a strong need for hybrid gait analysis methods that can detect MS at the early stage and/or determine its risk.

Acknowledgments

The authors thank Mesude Asimoglu, Physical Therapist, for preparing the drawings.

Gait terminology:

- Determinants of gait: basic characteristics of gait.
- Gait cycle: the period of time from one event of one foot to the following occurrence of the same event with the same foot.
- Stance phase: the period of time when the foot is in contact with the ground.
- Swing phase: the period of time when the foot is not in contact with the ground.
- Initial contact: the point in the gait cycle when the foot initially makes contact with the ground.
- Heel contact: the term describing the initial contact made with the heel.
- Loading response: the initial double support stance period which is defined from initial contact.
- Double support: the period of time when both feet are in contact with the ground.
- Single support: the period of time when only one foot is in contact with the ground.
- Midstance: the first half of the single support period.

Table 11.2. Target focused gait analysis.

Target	Data	Method	Cross-sectional	Multi-signal processing
Musculoskeletal system responses	• Spatiotemporal parameters	• Marker based systems • Optoelectronic systems • Sensor based systems	√	
Postural/Gait stability	• Spatiotemporal parameters • Muscle activity • Angular motions • Ground reaction forces • Fall risk • Prediction of the disease progression	• Marker based systems • Optoelectronic systems • Sensor based systems • Force plates		√
Effects of Cognition	• Spatiotemporal parameters • Muscle activity • Angular motions • Ground reaction forces • Fall risk	• Marker based systems • Optoelectronic systems • Sensor based systems • Force plates	√	√
Brain Map	• Prediction of the disease progression • Definition of the disease-specific brain area sensitive to the motion	• Neuroimaging techniques with hybrid system		√
Fatigue	• Spatiotemporal parameters • Muscle activity • Angular motions • Ground reaction forces	• Marker based systems • Optoelectronic systems • Sensor based systems • Force plates	√	√

- Terminal stance: the time from heel rise until the other limb makes contact with the floor.
- Preswing: the final double support stance period which is defined from the time of initial contact with the contralateral limb to ipsilateral toe-off.

- Initial swing: The initial third of the swing phase, is defined from toe-off to when the swing limb foot is opposite the stance limb.
- Midswing: the middle third of the swing phase, defined from the time the swing foot is opposite the stance limb to when the tibia is vertical.
- Terminal swing: the final third of the swing phase, defined from the time when the tibia is vertical to initial contact
- Stride: the distance from initial contact of one foot to the following initial contact of the same foot.
- Stride length: the distance from initial contact of one foot to the following initial contact of the same foot.
- Stride time: the period of time from initial contact of one foot to the following initial contact of the same foot.
- Step length: the distance from a point of contact with the ground of one foot to the following occurrence of the same point of contact with the other foot.
- Step time: the period of time taken for one step is measured from an event of one foot to the following occurrence of the same event with the other foot.
- Step width: the distance between two lines cutting feet equal halves.
- Cadance: steps per minute.
- Toe-off: when terminal contact is made with the toe.
- Heel-rise: the point in time in stance phase when the heel leaves the ground.
- Push-off: the period in time in late stance.

Abbreviations

- MS: multiple sclerosis
- CoM: center of mass
- EMG: electromyography
- ST: step time
- AST: average step time
- CoV: coefficient of variation
- DFA: detrended fluctuation analysis
- fMRI: functional magnetic resonance imaging
- NIRS: near-infrared spectrographic imaging
- TMS: transcranial magnetic techniques
- SPECT: single photon emission tomography
- EEG: electroencephalography
- FDG-PET: f-fluorodeoxyglucose positron emission tomography

References

[1] Saunders J B, Inman V T and Eberhart H D 1953 The major determinants in normal and pathological gait *J. Bone Joint Surg. Am.* **35-A** 543–58

[2] Della Croce U, Riley P O, Lelas J L and Kerrigan D C 2001 A refined view of the determinants of gait *Gait Posture* **14** 79–84

[3] Perry J and Burnfield J M 2010 Gait analysis: normal and pathological function *J. Sports Sci. Med.* **9** 353

[4] Webster J B and Darter B J 2019 Principles of normal and pathologic gait *Atlas of Orthoses and Assistive Devices* 5th edn ed J B Webster and D P Murphy (Philadelphia, PA: Elsevier) ch 4 pp 49–62

[5] Gard S A and Childress D S 1997 The effect of pelvic list on the vertical displacement of the trunk during normal walking *Gait Posture* **5** 233–8

[6] Kerrigan D C, Riley P O, Lelas J L and Della Croce U 2001 Quantification of pelvic rotation as a determinant of gait *Arch. Phys. Med. Rehabil.* **82** 217–20

[7] Błażkiewicz M, Wiszomirska I, Kaczmarczyk K, Naemi R and Wit A 2017 Inter-individual similarities and variations in muscle forces acting on the ankle joint during gait *Gait Posture* **58** 166–70

[8] Kitaoka H B, Crevoisier X M, Hansen D, Katajarvi B, Harbst K and Kaufman K R 2006 Foot and ankle kinematics and ground reaction forces during ambulation *Foot Ankle Int.* **27** 808–13

[9] Neumann D 2017 *Kinesiology of the Musculoskeletal System: Foundations for Rehabilitation* 3rd edn (St Louis, MO: Mosby Elsevier) 350–68

[10] Paul Jackson Mansfield M, Neumann D A and Fapta P P 2019 *Essentials of Kinesiology for the Physical Therapist Assistant* (St Louis, MO: Mosby)

[11] Perry J and Davids J R 1992 Gait analysis: normal and pathological function *J. Pediatr. Orthop.* **12** 815

[12] Sutherland D H 2001 The evolution of clinical gait analysis Part l: kinesiological EMG *Gait Posture* **14** 61–70

[13] Sutherland D H 2002 The evolution of clinical gait analysis. Part II: kinematics *Gait Posture* **16** 159–79

[14] Sutherland D H 2005 The evolution of clinical gait analysis Part III: kinetics and energy assessment *Gait Posture* **21** 447–61

[15] Gracovetsky S 1997 Linking the spinal engine with the legs *Movement, Stability and Low Back Pain-The Essential Role of the Pelvis* ed A Vleeming (New York: Churchill Livingstone)

[16] Hausdorff J M, Peng C, Ladin Z, Wei J Y and Goldberger A L 1995 Is walking a random walk? Evidence for long-range correlations in stride interval of human gait *J. Appl. Physiol.* **78** 349–58

[17] Hausdorff J M 2005 Gait variability: methods, modeling and meaning *J. Neuroeng. Rehabil.* **2** 19

[18] Hausdorff J M, Lertratanakul A, Cudkowicz M E, Peterson A L, Kaliton D and Goldberger A L 2000 Dynamic markers of altered gait rhythm in amyotrophic lateral sclerosis *J. Appl. Physiol.* **88** 2045–53

[19] Bollens B, Crevecoeur F, Detrembleur C, Guillery E and Lejeune T 2012 Effects of age and walking speed on long-range autocorrelations and fluctuation magnitude of stride duration *Neuroscience* **210** 234–42

[20] Bollens B, Crevecoeur F, Detrembleur C, Warlop T and Lejeune T M 2014 Variability of human gait: effect of backward walking and dual-tasking on the presence of long-range autocorrelations *Ann. Biomed. Eng.* **42** 742–50

[21] Bollens B, Crevecoeur F, Nguyen V, Detrembleur C and Lejeune T 2010 Does human gait exhibit comparable and reproducible long-range autocorrelations on level ground and on treadmill? *Gait Posture* **32** 369–73
[22] Delignieres D, Ramdani S, Lemoine L, Torre K, Fortes M and Ninot G 2006 Fractal analyses for 'short'time series: a re-assessment of classical methods *J. Math. Psychol.* **50** 525–44
[23] Warlop T, Detrembleur C, Stoquart G, Lejeune T and Jeanjean A 2018 Gait complexity and regularity are differently modulated by treadmill walking in parkinson's disease and healthy population *Front. Physiol.* **9** 68
[24] Riley Ebma V A N and Orden G 2005 *Tutorials in Contemporary Nonlinear Methods* (Arlington, VA: National Science Foundation)
[25] Ducharme S W and van Emmerik R E 2018 Fractal dynamics, variability, and coordination in human locomotion *Kinesiol. Rev.* **7** 26–35
[26] Crevecoeur F, Bollens B, Detrembleur C and Lejeune T 2010 Towards a 'gold-standard' approach to address the presence of long-range auto-correlation in physiological time series *J. Neurosci. Methods* **192** 163–72
[27] Goldberger A L, Amaral L A, Hausdorff J M, Ivanov P, Peng C K and Stanley H E 2002 Fractal dynamics in physiology: alterations with disease and aging *Proc. Natl. Acad. Sci. U.S.A.* **99** 2466–72
[28] Hausdorff J M 2007 Gait dynamics, fractals and falls: finding meaning in the stride-to-stride fluctuations of human walking *Hum. Mov. Sci.* **26** 555–89
[29] Ducharme S W and van Emmerik R E A 2019 Multifractality of unperturbed and asymmetric locomotion *J. Mot. Behav.* **51** 394–405
[30] Fino P C, Mancini M, Curtze C, Nutt J G and Horak F B 2018 Gait stability has phase-dependent dual-task costs in Parkinson's disease *Front. Neurol.* **9** 373
[31] Hausdorff J M, Zemany L, Peng C and Goldberger A L 1999 Maturation of gait dynamics: stride-to-stride variability and its temporal organization in children *J. Appl. Physiol.* **86** 1040–7
[32] Hausdorff J M, Lowenthal J, Herman T, Gruendlinger L, Peretz C and Giladi N 2007 Rhythmic auditory stimulation modulates gait variability in Parkinson's disease *Eur. J. Neurosci.* **26** 2369–75
[33] Hausdorff J M, Mitchell S L, Firtion R, Peng C-K, Cudkowicz M E, Wei J Y and Goldberger A L 1997 Altered fractal dynamics of gait: reduced stride-interval correlations with aging and Huntington's disease *J. Appl. Physiol.* **82** 262–9
[34] Kikkert L H, Vuillerme N, van Campen J P, Appels B A, Hortobágyi T and Lamoth C J 2018 The relationship between gait dynamics and future cognitive decline: a prospective pilot study in geriatric patients *Int. Psychogeriatr.* **30** 1301–9
[35] Krasovsky T, Weiss P L and Kizony R 2018 Older adults pay an additional cost when texting and walking: effects of age, environment, and use of mixed reality on dual-task performance *Phys. Ther.* **98** 549–59
[36] Warlop T B, Bollens B, Detrembleur C, Stoquart G, Lejeune T and Crevecoeur F 2017 Impact of series length on statistical precision and sensitivity of autocorrelation assessment in human locomotion *Hum. Mov. Sci.* **55** 31–42
[37] Warlop T B, Bollens B, Crevecoeur F, Detrembleur C and Lejeune T M 2013 Dynamics of revolution time variability in cycling pattern: Voluntary intent can alter the long-range autocorrelations *Ann. Biomed. Eng.* **41** 1604–12

[38] Choi J-S, Kang D-W, Seo J-W and Tack G-R 2015 Reliability of the walking speed and gait dynamics variables while walking on a feedback-controlled treadmill *J. Biomech.* **48** 1336–9
[39] González I, Fontecha J and Bravo J 2017 Relationship between stride interval variability and aging: Use of linear and non-linear estimators for gait variability assessment in assisted living environments *J. Ambient Intell. Humaniz. Comput.* **10** 2095–109
[40] Costa M, Peng C-K, Goldberger A L and Hausdorff J M 2003 Multiscale entropy analysis of human gait dynamics *Physica* A **330** 53–60
[41] Riva F, Bisi M C and Stagni R 2014 Gait variability and stability measures: minimum number of strides and within-session reliability *Comput. Biol. Med.* **50** 9–13
[42] Dierick F, Nivard A L, White O and Buisseret F 2017 Fractal analyses reveal independent complexity and predictability of gait *PLoS One* **12** e0188711
[43] Hausdorff J M, Ashkenazy Y, Peng C-K, Ivanov P C, Stanley H E and Goldberger A L 2001 When human walking becomes random walking: fractal analysis and modeling of gait rhythm fluctuations *Physica* A **302** 138–47
[44] Sekine M, Tamura T, Akay M, Fujimoto T, Togawa T and Fukui Y 2002 Discrimination of walking patterns using wavelet-based fractal analysis *IEEE Trans. Neural Syst. Rehabil. Eng.* **10** 188–96
[45] Guideline for the prevention of falls in older persons. American Geriatrics Society, British Geriatrics Society, and American Academy of Orthopaedic Surgeons Panel on Falls Prevention 2001 *J. Am. Geriatr. Soc.* **49** 664–72
[46] Hausdorff J M, Rios D A and Edelberg H K 2001 Gait variability and fall risk in community-living older adults: a 1-year prospective study *Arch. Phys. Med. Rehabil.* **82** 1050–6
[47] Benson L C, Clermont C A, Bošnjak E and Ferber R 2018 The use of wearable devices for walking and running gait analysis outside of the lab: A systematic review *Gait Posture* **63** 124–38
[48] Jarchi D, Pope J, Lee T K M, Tamjidi L, Mirzaei A and Sanei S 2018 A review on accelerometry-based gait analysis and emerging clinical applications *IEEE Rev. Biomed. Eng.* **11** 177–94
[49] Peel N M, Alapatt L J, Jones L V and Hubbard R E 2019 The association between gait speed and cognitive status in community-dwelling older people: A systematic review and meta-analysis *J. Gerontol. Ser.* A **74** 943–8
[50] Van Criekinge T, Saeys W, Blanckaert K, Maebe Z, van der Waal C, Vink M, De Hertogh W and Truijen S 2018 The effect of trunk training on trunk control, standing balance and gait: a systematic review and meta-analysis *Int. Conf. on Neuro Rehabilitation* (Berlin: Springer)
[51] Zago M, Sforza C, Bonardi D R, Guffanti E E and Galli M 2018 Gait analysis in patients with chronic obstructive pulmonary disease: a systematic review *Gait Posture* **61** 408–15
[52] De Marsico M, Fartade E G and Mecca A 2018 Feature-based analysis of gait signals for biometric recognition *Proc. of the 7th Int. Conf. on Pattern Recognition Applications and Methods (ICPRAM 2018)* 630–7
[53] Ortells J, Herrero-Ezquerro M T and Mollineda R A 2018 Vision-based gait impairment analysis for aided diagnosis *Med. Biol. Eng. Comput.* **56** 1553–64
[54] Prakash C, Kumar R, Mittal N and Raj G 2018 Vision based identification of joint coordinates for marker-less gait analysis *Proc. Comput. Sci.* **132** 68–75

[55] Wang J, She M, Nahavandi S and Kouzani A 2010 A review of vision-based gait recognition methods for human identification *2010 IEEE Int. Conf. on Digital Image Computing: Techniques and Applications (DICTA)*
[56] Whittle M W 2014 *Gait Analysis: An Introduction* (Oxford: Butterworth-Heinemann)
[57] Prakash C, Kumar R and Mittal N 2018 Recent developments in human gait research: parameters, approaches, applications, machine learning techniques, datasets and challenges *Artif. Intell. Rev.* **49** 1–40
[58] Qiu S, Wang Z, Zhao H, Liu L, Li J, Jiang Y and Fortino G 2018 Body sensor network based robust gait analysis: toward clinical and at home use *IEEE Sens. J.* doi: 10.1109/JSEN.2018.2860938
[59] Agostini V, Gastaldi L, Rosso V, Knaflitz M and Tadano S 2017 A wearable magneto-inertial system for gait analysis (H-Gait): validation on normal weight and overweight/obese young healthy adults *Sensors* **17** 2406
[60] Bakker M, Verstappen C C, Bloem B R and Toni I 2007 Recent advances in functional neuroimaging of gait *J. Neural Transm.* **114** 1323–31
[61] Schneider S, Christensen A, Häußinger F B, Fallgatter A J, Giese M A and Ehlis A-C 2014 Show me how you walk and I tell you how you feel—a functional near-infrared spectroscopy study on emotion perception based on human gait *Neuroimage* **85** 380–90
[62] Camus M, Pailhous J and Bonnard M 2006 On-line flexibility of the cognitive tuning of corticospinal excitability: a TMS study in human gait *Brain Res.* **1076** 144–9
[63] Matsui H, Udaka F, Miyoshi T, Hara N, Tamaura A, Oda M, Kubori T, Nishinaka K and Kameyama M 2005 Three-dimensional stereotactic surface projection study of freezing of gait and brain perfusion image in Parkinson's disease *Mov. Disord.* **20** 1272–7
[64] De Tommaso M, Vecchio E, Ricci K, Montemurno A, De Venuto D and Annese V 2015 Combined EEG/EMG evaluation during a novel dual task paradigm for gait analysis *2015 6th IEEE Int. Workshop on Advances in Sensors and Interfaces (IWASI) (IEEE, Piscataway, NJ)* pp 181–6
[65] Sandroff B M, Owoeye O, Vitiello T, Hoxha A, Yue G and DeLuca J 2018 Supra-spinal modulation of walking in healthy individuals and persons with multiple sclerosis: a fnirs mobile imaging study *2018 40th Annual Int. Conf. of the IEEE Engineering in Medicine and Biology Society (EMBC) (IEEE, Piscataway, NJ)* pp 3156–9
[66] de Jong B M, Leenders K L and Paans A M 2002 Right parieto-premotor activation related to limb-independent antiphase movement *Cereb. Cortex* **12** 1213–7
[67] Bartels A L, de Jong B M, Giladi N, Schaafsma J D, Maguire R P, Veenma L, Pruim J, Balash Y, Youdim M B and Leenders K L 2006 Striatal dopa and glucose metabolism in PD patients with freezing of gait *Mov. Disord.* **21** 1326–32
[68] Groff B R, Antonellis P, Schmid K K, Knarr B A and Stergiou N 2019 Stride-time variability is related to sensorimotor cortical activation during forward and backward walking *Neurosci. Lett.* **692** 150–8
[69] Jahn K, Deutschlander A, Stephan T, Strupp M, Wiesmann M and Brandt T 2004 Brain activation patterns during imagined stance and locomotion in functional magnetic resonance imaging *Neuroimage* **22** 1722–31
[70] Labriffe M, Annweiler C, Amirova L E, Gauquelin-Koch G, Ter Minassian A, Leiber L M, Beauchet O, Custaud M A and Dinomais M 2017 Brain activity during mental imagery of

gait versus gait-like plantar stimulation: a novel combined functional MRI paradigm to better understand cerebral gait control *Front. Hum. Neurosci.* **11** 106

[71] Miyai I, Tanabe H C, Sase I, Eda H, Oda I, Konishi I, Tsunazawa Y, Suzuki T, Yanagida T and Kubota K 2001 Cortical mapping of gait in humans: a near-infrared spectroscopic topography study *Neuroimage* **14** 1186–92

[72] Sirigu A and Duhamel J 2001 Motor and visual imagery as two complementary but neurally dissociable mental processes *J. Cogn. Neurosci.* **13** 910–9

[73] Wang C, Wai Y, Kuo B, Yeh Y Y and Wang J 2008 Cortical control of gait in healthy humans: an fMRI study *J. Neural Transm.* **115** 1149–58

[74] Yuan J, Blumen H M, Verghese J and Holtzer R 2015 Functional connectivity associated with gait velocity during walking and walking-while-talking in aging: a resting-state fMRI study *Hum. Brain Mapp.* **36** 1484–93

[75] Jeannerod M 2001 Neural simulation of action: a unifying mechanism for motor cognition *Neuroimage* **14** S103–9

[76] Jeannerod M 2006 *Motor Cognition: What Actions Tell the Self* (Oxford: Oxford University Press)

[77] Munzert J, Lorey B and Zentgraf K 2009 Cognitive motor processes: the role of motor imagery in the study of motor representations *Brain Res. Rev.* **60** 306–26

[78] Sacco K, Cauda F, Cerliani L, Mate D, Duca S and Geminiani G 2006 Motor imagery of walking following training in locomotor attention. The effect of 'the tango lesson' *Neuroimage* **32** 1441–9

[79] Dobkin B H, Firestine A, West M, Saremi K and Woods R 2004 Ankle dorsiflexion as an fMRI paradigm to assay motor control for walking during rehabilitation *Neuroimage* **23** 370–81

[80] Kapreli E, Athanasopoulos S, Papathanasiou M, Van Hecke P, Strimpakos N, Gouliamos A, Peeters R and Sunaert S 2006 Lateralization of brain activity during lower limb joints movement. An fMRI study *Neuroimage* **32** 1709–21

[81] Cunnington R, Windischberger C, Robinson S and Moser E 2006 The selection of intended actions and the observation of others' actions: a time-resolved fMRI study *Neuroimage* **29** 1294–302

[82] Malouin F, Richards C L, Jackson P L, Dumas F and Doyon J 2003 Brain activations during motor imagery of locomotor-related tasks: a PET study *Hum. Brain Mapp.* **19** 47–62

[83] Begg R and Kamruzzaman J 2005 A machine learning approach for automated recognition of movement patterns using basic, kinetic and kinematic gait data *J. Biomech.* **38** 401–8

[84] Sacca V *et al* 2019 Evaluation of machine learning algorithms performance for the prediction of early multiple sclerosis from resting-state fMRI connectivity data *Brain Imaging Behav.* **13** 1103–14

[85] Larocca N G 2011 Impact of walking impairment in multiple sclerosis: perspectives of patients and care partners *Patient* **4** 189–201

[86] Heesen C, Böhm J, Reich C, Kasper J, Goebel M and Gold S 2008 Patient perception of bodily functions in multiple sclerosis: gait and visual function are the most valuable *Mult. Scler. J.* **14** 988–91

[87] Comber L, Galvin R and Coote S 2015 The causes, context and consequences of falls in people with multiple sclerosis: preliminary results from an irish cross-sectional study *Int. J. MS Care* **17** 9–10

[88] Matsuda P N, Shumway-Cook A, Bamer A M, Johnson S L, Amtmann D and Kraft G H 2011 Falls in multiple sclerosis *PM&R* **3** 624–32

[89] Nilsagård Y E, von Koch L K, Nilsson M and Forsberg A S 2014 Balance exercise program reduced falls in people with multiple sclerosis: a single-group, pretest-posttest trial *Arch. Phys. Med. Rehabil.* **95** 2428–34

[90] Postigo-Alonso B, Galvao-Carmona A, Benitez I, Conde-Gavilan C, Jover A, Molina S, Pena-Toledo M A and Aguera E 2018 Cognitive-motor interference during gait in patients with Multiple Sclerosis: a mixed methods systematic review *Neurosci. Biobehav. Rev.* **94** 126–48

[91] Armutlu K, Fil Balkan A, Salci Y, Cetin B, Karanfil E, Ceren A and Karabudak R 2018 *Nörolojik Hastalıklarda Görülen Yürüyüş Bozuklukları* (Ankara: Hipokrat Kitabevi)

[92] Bethoux F 2013 Gait disorders in multiple sclerosis *Continuum (Minneap Minn)* **19** 1007–22

[93] Comber L, Galvin R and Coote S 2017 Gait deficits in people with multiple sclerosis: A systematic review and meta-analysis *Gait Posture* **51** 25–35

[94] Denommé L T, Mandalfino P and Cinelli M E 2014 Strategies used by individuals with multiple sclerosis and with mild disability to maintain dynamic stability during a steering task *Exp. Brain Res.* **232** 1811–22

[95] Kalron A, Dvir Z and Achiron A 2010 Walking while talking—difficulties incurred during the initial stages of multiple sclerosis disease process *Gait Posture* **32** 332–5

[96] Preiningerova J L, Novotna K, Rusz J, Sucha L, Ruzicka E and Havrdova E 2015 Spatial and temporal characteristics of gait as outcome measures in multiple sclerosis (EDSS 0 to 6.5) *J. Neuroeng. Rehabil.* **12** 14

[97] Remelius J G, Jones S L, House J D, Busa M A, Averill J L, Sugumaran K, Kent-Braun J A and Van Emmerik R E 2012 Gait impairments in persons with multiple sclerosis across preferred and fixed walking speeds *Arch. Phys. Med. Rehabil.* **93** 1637–42

[98] Socie M J, Motl R W and Sosnoff J J 2014 Examination of spatiotemporal gait parameters during the 6-min walk in individuals with multiple sclerosis *Int. J. Rehabil. Res.* **37** 311–6

[99] Sosnoff J J, Sandroff B M and Motl R W 2012 Quantifying gait abnormalities in persons with multiple sclerosis with minimal disability *Gait Posture* **36** 154–6

[100] Spain R, George R S, Salarian A, Mancini M, Wagner J, Horak F and Bourdette D 2012 Body-worn motion sensors detect balance and gait deficits in people with multiple sclerosis who have normal walking speed *Gait Posture* **35** 573–8

[101] Kalron A, Achiron A and Dvir Z 2011 Muscular and gait abnormalities in persons with early onset multiple sclerosis *J. Neurol. Phys. Ther.* **35** 164–9

[102] Mañago M M, Hebert J R, Kittelson J and Schenkman M 2018 Contributions of ankle, knee, hip, and trunk muscle function to gait performance in people with multiple sclerosis: a cross-sectional analysis *Phys. Ther.* **98** 595–604

[103] Gianni C, Prosperini L, Jonsdottir J and Cattaneo D 2014 A systematic review of factors associated with accidental falls in people with multiple sclerosis: a meta-analytic approach *Clin. Rehabil.* **28** 704–16

[104] Huisinga J M, Mancini M, George R J S and Horak F B 2013 Accelerometry reveals differences in gait variability between patients with multiple sclerosis and healthy controls *Ann. Biomed. Eng.* **41** 1670–9

[105] Huisinga J M, Schmid K K, Filipi M L and Stergiou N 2013 Gait mechanics are different between healthy controls and patients with multiple sclerosis *J. Appl. Biomech.* **29** 303–11

[106] Kelleher K J, Spence W, Solomonidis S and Apatsidis D 2010 The characterisation of gait patterns of people with multiple sclerosis *Disabil. Rehabil.* **32** 1242–50

[107] McLoughlin J V, Barr C J, Patritti B, Crotty M, Lord S R and Sturnieks D L 2016 Fatigue induced changes to kinematic and kinetic gait parameters following six minutes of walking in people with multiple sclerosis *Disabil. Rehabil.* **38** 535–43

[108] Butchard-MacDonald E, Paul L and Evans J J 2018 Balancing the demands of two tasks: an investigation of cognitive–motor dual-tasking in relapsing remitting multiple sclerosis *J. Int. Neuropsychol. Soc.* **24** 247–58

[109] Remelius J G, Hamill J, Kent-Braun J and Van Emmerik R E 2008 Gait initiation in multiple sclerosis *Motor Control* **12** 93–108

[110] Salcı Y, Fil A, Armutlu K, Yildiz F G, Kurne A, Aksoy S, Nurlu G and Karabudak R 2017 Effects of different exercise modalities on ataxia in multiple sclerosis patients: a randomized controlled study *Disabil. Rehabil.* **39** 2626–32

[111] Buckley E, Mazza C and McNeill A 2018 A systematic review of the gait characteristics associated with Cerebellar Ataxia *Gait Posture* **60** 154–63

[112] Peebles A T, Reinholdt A, Bruetsch A P, Lynch S G and Huisinga J M 2016 Dynamic margin of stability during gait is altered in persons with multiple sclerosis *J. Biomech.* **49** 3949–55

[113] Kalron A, Allali G and Achiron A 2018 Neural correlates of gait variability in people with multiple sclerosis with fall history *Eur. J. Neurol.* **25** 1243–9

[114] Fritz N E, Kloos A D, Kegelmeyer D A, Kaur P and Nichols-Larsen D S 2019 Supplementary motor area connectivity and dual-task walking variability in multiple sclerosis *J. Neurol. Sci.* **396** 159–64

[115] Saleh S, Sandroff B M, Vitiello T, Owoeye O, Hoxha A, Hake P, Goverover Y, Wylie G, Yue G and DeLuca J 2018 The role of premotor areas in dual tasking in healthy controls and persons with multiple sclerosis: An fNIRS imaging study *Front. Behav. Neurosci.* **12** 296

[116] Bollaert R E, Poe K, Hubbard E A, Motl R W, Pilutti L A, Johnson C L and Sutton B P 2018 Associations of functional connectivity and walking performance in multiple sclerosis *Neuropsychologia* **117** 8–12

[117] Hessert M J, Vyas M, Leach J, Hu K, Lipsitz L A and Novak V 2005 Foot pressure distribution during walking in young and old adults *BMC Geriatr.* **5** 8

[118] Keklicek H, Cetin B, Salci Y, Balkan A F, Altinkaynak U and Armutlu K 2018 Investigating the dynamic plantar pressure distribution and loading pattern in subjects with multiple sclerosis *Mult. Scler. Relat. Disord.* **20** 186–91

[119] Leardini A and Caravaggi P 2018 Kinematic foot models for instrumented gait analysis *Handbook of Human Motion* pp 547–70

[120] Dalgas U, Langeskov-Christensen M, Skjerbæk A, Jensen E, Baert I, Romberg A, Medina C S, Gebara B, de Noordhout B M and Knuts K 2018 Is the impact of fatigue related to walking capacity and perceived ability in persons with multiple sclerosis? A multicenter study *J. Neurol. Sci.* **387** 179–86

[121] Motl R W, Sandroff B M, Suh Y and Sosnoff J J 2012 Energy cost of walking and its association with gait parameters, daily activity, and fatigue in persons with mild multiple sclerosis *Neurorehabil. Neural Repair* **26** 1015–21

[122] Wajda D A, Sandroff B M, Pula J H, Motl R W and Sosnoff J J 2013 Effects of walking direction and cognitive challenges on gait in persons with multiple sclerosis *Mult. Scler. Int.* **2013** 859323

IOP Publishing

Neurological Disorders and Imaging Physics, Volume 2
Engineering and clinical perspectives of multiple sclerosis
Ayman El-Baz and Jasjit S Suri

Chapter 12

A brain–computer interface web browser for multiple sclerosis patients

Víctor Martínez-Cagigal, Eduardo Santamaría-Vázquez, Javier Gomez-Pilar and Roberto Hornero

Brain–computer interfaces (BCIs) have emerged as novel technologies that can bridge the accessibility gap for the disabled by monitoring their brain signals and translating their intentions into application commands. Despite the recent development of the Internet, web browsers are not yet adapted to an assistive context. The objective of this chapter is two-fold: (i) to introduce BCIs as an aid to support the communication of multiple sclerosis (MS) patients; and (ii) to design, develop and test a P300-based BCI web browser that can meet their communication needs. The row–col paradigm is used to generate P300 evoked potentials, which are processed to decode users' intentions. Selected commands are sent to a browser extension that provides visual feedback in real time. Asynchronous management is also implemented in order to avoid selection errors when users want to read a website or watch a video. The system was tested with 5 control subjects and 16 MS patients, reaching average accuracies of 95.75% and 84.14%, respectively. Results suggest that the proposed system allows users to successfully surf the Internet, improving their personal autonomy and quality of life.

12.1 Introduction

Brain–computer interfaces (BCIs) are communication systems aimed to replace, improve, restore, supplement or enhance the neural activity of the user [1]. To that end, BCI systems monitor users' brain activity and translate their intentions into application commands. These features make BCIs specially suited for improving the quality of life of people with motor disabilities, including those caused by neurodegenerative diseases, traumas, muscle disorders, or any illness that impairs the neural pathways that control muscles or the muscles themselves [2, 3]. Although there are several methods to register the brain activity, electroencephalography

doi:10.1088/978-0-7503-1762-7ch12

(EEG) is generally used because of its portability, low-cost and non-invasiveness [2, 3]. Thus, electric brain signals are obtained by placing a set of electrodes over the user's scalp.

MS patients are one of the many groups of subjects that can benefit from this novel technology. MS is the most common autoimmune disorder that affects the central nervous system, causing an inflammation that leads to the demyelination of nerve cells in the brain and spinal cord [4, 5]. This damage reduces the ability of the nervous system to communicate, resulting in a wide range of symptoms, including motor skill problems, cognitive deficits, or even psychiatric disorders [5]. In fact, up to 60% of the MS patients experience motor disabilities twenty years after the onset, hindering their full and effective interaction with the environment and society [4].

In recent decades, the Internet has become an important tool for communication and has been fully integrated into the daily life of our society. This development has led to a world penetration of 53%, reaching 4.021 billion Internet users in 2018 [6]. Notwithstanding the importance of the Internet on a daily basis, web browsers were originally designed for healthy users and thus intended to be used with mouse and keyboard. Currently, their accessibility is still limited when only a small number of input signals are available, restricting the control by motor-disabled users to a great degree [7].

The purpose of this chapter is two-fold: (i) to introduce BCI systems as an aid to support the communication and improve the accessibility for MS patients; and (ii) to design, develop and test an asynchronous BCI web browser that could meet their daily communication needs. Therefore, the book chapter is organized as follows. First, a general background of BCIs is introduced in section 12.2, which includes a discussion about common control signals and types of BCIs, the key aspects that would make a BCI system useful in a real environment, and a state-of-the-art revision related with BCI-based web browsers. Then, the subject database is introduced in section 12.3, followed by the methodology that has been used to design, develop and test the aforementioned BCI web browser in section 12.4. Section 12.5 shows the results of the evaluation under both qualitative and quantitative points of view. Finally, sections 12.6 and 12.7 discuss the experimental outcomes and draw the final conclusions of the study, respectively.

12.2 Background

12.2.1 Types of BCIs

BCIs are defined as communication systems between the brain and the environment that translate users' intentions into application commands in real time [3]. Since these intentions are not directly reflected in the raw EEG signals, BCIs rely on the processing of measurable changes related to cognitive tasks, known as control signals. According to these control signals, BCIs can be categorized as exogenous or endogenous systems [8]. Figure 12.1 depicts four examples of the most commonly used control signals: steady-state visual evoked potentials (SSVEP), P300 evoked potentials, slow cortical potentials (SCP), and sensory-motor rhythms (SMR). In addition, table 12.1 details the advantages and disadvantages of each control signal.

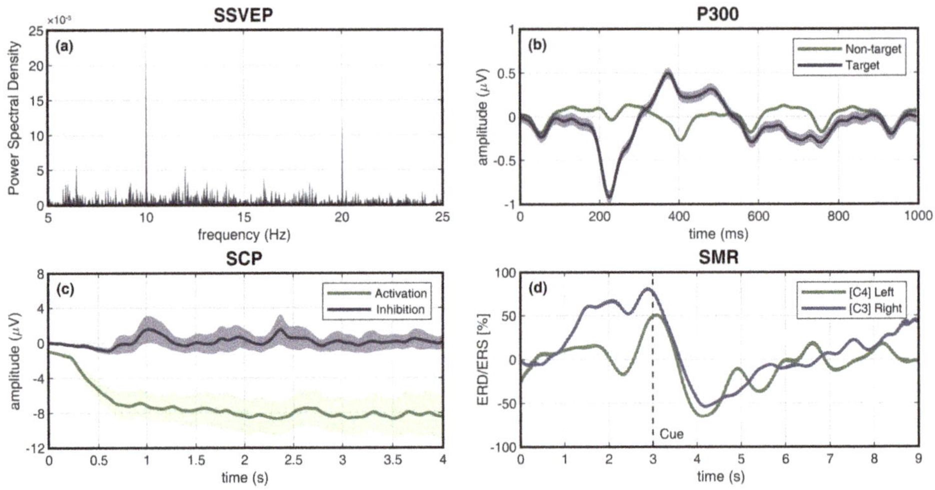

Figure 12.1. Exogenous and endogenous signals that are commonly used to control BCI systems. (a) Steady-state visual evoked potentials (SSVEP), recorded at Oz while a healthy subject looked at a visual stimulus that flickered at 10 Hz [12]. (b) P300 evoked potentials, recorded at Fz while a healthy subject attended to a visual oddball task [13]. Averaged event-related responses of target stimuli are shown in blue, whereas non-target stimuli responses are shown in green. Shaded areas indicate the confidence interval of 95%. (c) Slow cortical potentials (SCP) of a chronic stroke patient at Cz. Solid lines indicate the averaged activity across trials, whereas shaded areas indicate the confidence interval of 95% [14]. (d) Sensory-motor rhythms (SMR) in the μ wave band (i.e. 8–11Hz in motor cortex) of a healthy subject that was asked to imagine left and right hand movements after a cue at $t = 3$ s [15]. SMR averaged responses are shown in relative amplitude units using the event-related desynchronization and synchronization ratio (ERD/ERS). Note that signals are contralateral to the movement: left hand is more prominent at C4 (right hemisphere), whereas right hand is more prominent at C3 (left hemisphere).

Exogenous BCIs are characterized by the use of control signals that are natural responses of our brains to external stimuli. Due to their innate origin, exogenous systems do not require previous training by the user and are able to reach high performances [3, 8]. Among the exogenous control signals, SSVEP and P300 potentials stand out. SSVEPs are produced by a mimetic mechanism. When the retina is excited by visual repetitive stimuli at a specific frequency, the brain generates oscillatory EEG signals at the same frequency [8, 9]. As can be seen in figure 12.1(a), harmonics of the flickering frequency are also visible in the spectrum. A common SSVEP-based setup to spell words is based on displaying a table containing characters that flicker at different frequencies. When the user focuses attention on the desired command, a SSVEP appears in the EEG frequency spectrum and can be identified by the system [3]. Although this arrangement makes possible the selection of a high number of different commands or characters, the most reliable flickering frequencies belongs to the low beta band (i.e. 13–19 Hz), which maximizes the risk of visual fatigue and epileptic seizures [9]. Moreover, the number of possible commands is also slightly restricted by the standardized vertical refreshing rate of LCD screens [10]. Regarding the P300 potentials, they are defined as positive peaks mainly produced in the parietal and occipital cortex as a response

Table 12.1. Summary of the most common BCI control signals.

Name	Phenomena	Type	Number of commands	Training	Advantages	Disadvantages
SSVEP	Oscillatory signals at the same frequency than a flickering visual stimuli	Exogenous	High	No	Very high transmission rates No training required	Possible visual fatigue and epileptic seizures No. of commands limited by the standardized refreshing rate of LCD screens Requires gaze control
P300	Positive peaks in response to unexpected target stimuli	Exogenous	Very high	No	Acceptable transmission rates No training required	Several repetitions of the oddball stimuli are needed in order to records a reliable potential Requires focused attention and gaze control
SCP	Self-regulated slow voltage shifts that reflect cortical activity	Endogenous	Very low (2)	Yes	Do not require focused attention or gaze control High transmission rates	No. of commands limited between 2 (suitable performances) and 4 (poor performances) Intense training
SMR	Modulated frequency rhythms synchronized with kinesthetic activities	Endogenous	Low (2–4)	Yes	Do not require focused attention or gaze control High transmission rates	No. of commands limited up to 4 (poor performances) Intense training

to infrequent and particularly significant stimuli at about 300 ms after their onset [3, 8]. Even though the stimulus may be auditory, tactile or visual, the latter reaches higher performances when applied to BCI systems [3]. The elicitation of the P300 potentials usually relies on the odd-ball paradigm. This paradigm is based on displaying infrequent target stimuli among more frequent distracting stimuli. In general, the lower the probability of the target stimuli, the higher the P300 amplitude [3]. The most common application of oddball paradigm in BCI systems is known as row–col paradigm (RCP). RCP displays a matrix that contains commands or characters, whose rows and columns are randomly flashing. The user just needs to focus attention on the desired command, eliciting a P300 whenever the row and the column that belong to that command are flashed. The desired command can be determined by computing the intersection of the row and the column that produced the potentials [11]. Due to the low signal-to-noise ratio of the P300 responses, stimuli are repeated in order to get a reliable potential. Depending on the subject, 10–15 repetitions (i.e. sequences) are broad enough to reach a maximum accuracy [8]. Note that the P300 potential that is displayed in figure 12.1(b) is an average of the target stimuli EEG samples in a window of 1000 ms. Furthermore, the higher the number of commands, the lower the probability of target stimuli. Therefore, P300-based BCIs favor the inclusion of a high number of different commands. Despite its ability to reach high performances and discriminate among a large number of commands, P300-based BCIs are gaze-dependent. These systems rely on the focused attention and gaze control capabilities of the user.

Endogenous BCIs are based on the self-regulation of brain activity without external stimuli. This can be achieved through neurofeedback training (NFT), which allows users to learn to voluntarily modify their own brain rhythms and potentials [8]. However, intense training is required (from hours to months), and not all users reach enough accuracies to control a practical BCI application [8]. These self-regulated signals can be decoded as SCPs or SMRs. SCPs are slow voltage shifts originated from the upper cortical layer that occur from 0.5–10 s after the onset [3]. The slowness of these potentials makes them appear in low frequency bands of <1 Hz [8]. SCP signals allow users to deliver dichotomous decisions: negative shifts are associated with movement or other functions that involve cortical activation, whereas positive shifts are associated with inhibition or reduced cortical activity [3, 8]. SCP signals of a chronic stroke patient are shown in figure 12.1(c) (blue: inhibition, green: activation). Therefore, SCP-based BCIs usually dissociate the problem-specific range of possible commands into a tree-based selection scheme that allows users to select any command using binary decisions [16–18]. This framework, together with the inherent slow response of the SCPs, produces lower transmission rates in comparison with exogenous BCIs [8]. Training is an essential step, since the quality of the self-regulated signals will affect the subsequent online performance. SCP training through NFT is usually based on displaying a cursor that reflects the amplitude of the SCP shifts in real time, along with visual cues that ask users to activate or inhibit their cortical activity [8, 16]. In contrast to the temporal response of SCPs, SMR signals are measured in the frequency domain. SMR are self-regulated oscillations in the α band (i.e. 8–12 Hz) [3, 8]. Since they are mainly produced in the sensory-motor cortex, they are usually called μ rhythms, which are more prominent at central electrodes [3, 19]. There is evidence that SMR can be also reflected in the β band (i.e. 13–30 Hz), even though most of the activity is associated with harmonics of the μ rhythms [3]. Movement, or even the imagination of the movement, produces a contralateral decrease of μ and β activities, known as event-related desynchronization (ERD) [3, 20]. After the movement or its imagination, μ and β rhythms restore their initial activity during relaxation. This effect is called event-related synchronization (ERS) [3, 20]. Figure 12.1(d) depicts the temporal response of ERD/ERS relative ratio at C4 and C3 when a healthy user imagined left- and right-hand movements, respectively. The fact that SMRs can be self-regulated with the imagination of movement is especially useful for developing BCIs controlled by motor imagery (MI). In order to favor the training of the SMR self-regulation, it has been suggested that users should be asked for empathizing kinesthetic experiences instead of visual representations of movements [8, 21]. Visual feedback that matches the amplitude of the μ band is usually employed as an aid to speed the NFT training. Nevertheless, SMR self-regulation becomes a struggle for most people, and requires a long time to master it [8]. Furthermore, the number of possible commands is still limited. Most of the MI-BCIs discriminate binary decisions (e.g. left versus right hand movements) achieving a suitable control of the system [22]. There are also studies that have employed up to four different MI signals (e.g. left hand, right hand, tongue and feet movements), but reaching poorer performances [8, 22].

12.2.2 Towards a real use of BCIs

BCI studies are generally developed and tested in a laboratory environment, forgetting about the real application of the BCI system. One of the main drawbacks of the BCI literature is that studies usually fail to prove the usability of the proposed applications with end users, who would presumably benefit from them [23]. In fact, most BCI systems are designed to be used by motor-disabled users in order to increment their autonomy and quality of life. Owing to the difficulty in recruiting a motor-disabled population, BCI systems are commonly tested with healthy subjects, or even not tested at all. Nevertheless, care must be taken when generalizing these results, since it has been widely documented that motor-disabled users usually reach lower performances than healthy subjects [24, 25]. Moreover, additional issues arise in a real assessment (e.g. involuntary tremors, nystagmus, poor EEG cap adjustment, insufficient sustained attention, portability). EEG signals also present a high inter-subject variability, which depends on individual factors (e.g. age, motivation), pharmacological aspects (e.g. drugs, medicines) or clinical disorders (e.g. schizophrenia, autism, MS) [26]. Besides these problems, inter-session variability is also noticeably common, requiring an update of the BCI parameters from time to time [27]. According to this rationale, the performance of a BCI system is supposed to vary depending on the subject and thus, channel and feature selection methods, as well as classifiers, must be always optimized for each user. Therefore, an evaluation with end users is essential to assure the feasibility and efficacy of the developed BCI systems in a real environment.

The ultimate goal of a BCI should be to reach an unsupervised use of the system that allows disabled users to attain comprehensive control of an application or external device. However, an unsupervised BCI could not be achieved without a proper asynchrony management. Most BCI applications are synchronous, which means that the system is continuously translating neural signals into commands, even when users do not have any voluntary intention [28]. For instance, the classic RCP constantly displays visual stimuli to the user. The system will make a selection even if the user is not paying attention to the stimulation, which prevents users reading a webpage or pausing the BCI system. Therefore, the synchronous mode is impractical in a real situation [28]. Most BCI studies employ rigid approaches to avoid this issue, such as hiring a supervisor or implementing 'read mode' commands that pause the system for a fixed time [7, 17, 18, 24, 29–31]. Nevertheless, these solutions limit the users' control over the BCI system. In recent years, several efforts have been made to develop methods that can reach a real asynchronous control. Most of them are based on a threshold derived from the classifier's scores [32–37], while others employ frequency features to discriminate between EEG signals of attending (i.e. control state) and ignoring (i.e. non-control state) the stimuli [28, 38–40]. Notwithstanding the importance of an asynchronous control, most studies overlook this step and develop traditional synchronous systems that are able to work in a controlled environment, but will lack autonomy in a real situation.

Portability is another aspect that must be considered. Ubiquitous EEG signal recording can be achieved using wireless headsets or integrating the EEG acquisition equipment in the final environment (e.g. on a wheelchair, workplace) [41]. Development of dry electrodes could also facilitate the use in daily-life, although their performance is still hindered in comparison with wet electrodes [41]. Furthermore, BCI literature is mainly oriented to remove in-lab artifacts (e.g. eye movements), but does not consider other non-expected issues that are usually present in a real environment (e.g. cardiac activity, noise, muscular movements) [41]. Therefore, signal processing methods must be designed to work in a general framework provided that the proposed BCI is intended to have a real application.

12.2.3 Previous approaches

In recent years, the Internet has become an important tool of daily communication in both social and working environments. Therefore, it is not surprising that there have been developed previous attempts to control web browsers using BCI systems. In 2002, Mankoff *et al* established the key aspects to provide web accessibility for motor-disabled users [7]. Furthermore, they proposed a web browser for low bandwidth input that could be controlled using two different frequency-based neural signals. Links were sorted in a list, and users could navigate the list upwards and backwards using a dichotomous neural signal. When the user stopped the cortical activity for 2 s, the currently selected link was then visited [7]. However, no details were given about the nature of these 'neural signals' or the evaluation of the system

[7]. Soon after, Tomori and Moore developed the 'BrainBrowser', an extension of the Mankoff *et al* proposal [29, 30]. 'BrainBrowser' provided a list of general commands (e.g. scrolls, refreshing, printing) and broke up the webpages into segments that prevent the burden of information [29, 30]. To the best of our knowledge, the system was not tested with healthy or disabled subjects and thus, no information about a practical application of the browser is available.

'Descartes', developed by Karim *et al* [17] in 2006, was a further approach that allowed users to write e-mails or visit predefined webpages using a BCI system [17]. SCPs were used to control the system, which constantly dissociated the range of possible selections (e.g. characters, web links) into a tree-based framework of dichotomous decisions [17]. Each subgroup of links or characters was sequentially displayed in a screen for a fixed time. Users were meant to generate a positive SCP when the desired command popped up [17]. 'Descartes' was tested with a locked-in-patient, reaching an average accuracy of 80.00%. However, the web surfing was not comprehensive, since only the browsing within a limited number of webpages was enabled. Non-textual links, such as images or buttons, could also not be selected [17]. In order to overcome these limitations, Bensch *et al* developed an improved version in 2007, known as 'Nessi' [18]. In 'Nessi', SCP or SMR signals were used to control the *Mozilla* web browser. Instead of showing a list of the possible selections, 'Nessi' implemented a graphical interface that put any link in colored frames, allowing the selection of basic graphical items, such as images or buttons [18]. Another tree-based dichotomous strategy was followed, which sequentially divided the total number of current possible selections in two subgroups of items. Item frames were colored either in blue or pink, depending on the group to which they belonged [18]. Feedback in the form of graphical user interface (GUI) was also provided to the user, who could see a cursor that indicated the SMR or SCP cortical activity in real time. The upper part of the GUI was colored in pink, whereas the bottom part was colored in blue; representing the dichotomous decision of selecting pink or blue subgroups [18]. Therefore, users could select any link of the webpage by sequentially generating positive/negative SCPs or right/left hand SMRs until the desired link was left. Nevertheless, there is no supporting evidence that 'Nessi' was tested either with healthy subjects or patients [18].

First approaches, such as 'BrainBrowser', 'Descartes' or 'Nessi'; employed endogenous signals (i.e. SCP and SMR) to control the browsers, requiring an intense training of the users [7, 17, 18, 29, 30]. Moreover, evaluation results are only available in the case of 'Nessi' (1 ALS: 80.00%) and thus, the feasibility of these proposals could be in doubt [18]. Further studies should be carried out in order to assess the practical efficacy of these systems in a real motor-disabled population. In practice, using either SCP or SMR signals implies that the NFT training of the users will take a long time and, in some cases, the reached accuracies could not be suitable for its use in a practical BCI application [8]. In addition, all of them used dichotomous control signals, which led to a tree-based selection strategy that inherently reduced the transmission rate. Besides the slowness of selecting a command, these browsers still needed a supervisor to adjust several parameters (e.g. address book entries, reading speed, fixed pauses) and conduct the experiment

[7, 17, 18, 29, 30]. Most of these limitations were overcome by the proposal of Mugler *et al* in 2010, who developed a P300-based BCI web browser [24]. Due to the exogenous origin of the control signal, the proposed system removed the need to conduct an intense training of users and drastically increased the number of input signals [3, 8]. P300 potentials were generated through an RCP that contained both alphanumeric and application commands. Unique alphanumeric tags that identified each link were placed close to them. Any of these links could be selected by the user if the tag was correctly spelled using the RCP matrix [24]. In order to avoid extra selections when users wanted to read a webpage, the system implemented a 'read mode' command that paused the visual stimulation for a fixed time [24]. The proposed BCI system was tested by 10 healthy subjects and 3 ALS patients, reaching average accuracies of 93.40% and 72.00%, respectively [24]. Sirvent Blasco *et al* also proposed a P300-based BCI web browser in 2012, but used a different approach to select webpage links [31]. Instead of the link tagging, they tried to emulate the movement of the mouse using an RCP matrix. In this way, users could move the cursor a predefined discrete number of pixels following the eight basic directions by means of selecting the matrix commands [31]. A total of three different exchangeable matrices were used: (1) virtual keyboard, intended to spell words and fill forms; (2) virtual mouse, intended to move the cursor around the screen; and (3) motion interval, intended to define the distance jumps [31]. As the proposal of Mugler *et al*, asynchrony management were substituted by a 'read mode' command [24, 31]. The system was tested with four healthy subjects, reaching an average accuracy of 93.00% [31].

More recently, in 2012, Yu *et al* proposed a hybrid BCI web browser that employed both P300 and SMR signals to control the movement of a two-dimensional virtual mouse [42]. Horizontal displacements were controlled using right-/left-hand SMR signals, while vertical displacements and pause commands were handled by P300 potentials. When users desired to select a link, they needed to place the cursor over it, stop the motor imagery and select a 'stop' command with an RCP [42]. In order to isolate the motor imagery and avoid undesirable selections due to the synchronous RCP, an ad hoc threshold for the P300 signals was used. The system was tested with seven healthy subjects, reaching an average accuracy of 93.21% [42].

12.2.4 Our approach

The ultimate goal of this study is to develop a BCI system that allows users to surf the Internet using their own brain signals. In order to assure the efficacy of the system in a real environment and to reach a comprehensive unsupervised control of the web browser, the following aspects must be considered:

1) Ease of use. Since the system will be oriented to work with motor-disabled subjects, it is desirable to minimize the training time and favor the ease of use. Hence, an exogenous BCI is considered. Due to the high number of possible commands that can be included, the P300 evoked potentials are selected as control signals.

2) Item selection. There are two main ways to select web items (i.e. links, buttons, images) using P300 responses: cursor movement and node tagging. The former is based on including an additional RCP matrix intended to move a virtual cursor [31, 42]. However, the speed of the cursor must be adjusted prior to the first session, and the speed of selecting a node is lower than that reached with node tagging [24]. Therefore, web items will be tagged and users could select them by introducing numeric codes.
3) Speed. In order to minimize the required time to select a node, several matrices will be developed: a small navigation matrix, intended to navigate through the web; and a big keyboard matrix, intended to fill out forms, write user names and passwords. Note that the greater number of commands, the greater are the number of flashings required to select them. This approach ensures a quick navigation through the web, using spelling commands only when they are required.
4) Asynchrony. As aforementioned, an asynchrony management is a crucial step to favor the application of the BCI system in a real unsupervised environment. Therefore, our approach must include an asynchronous step that could discern when users are paying attention to the stimuli and when they are not. If the system determines that they are in control state, the selected command must be delivered; otherwise, no command must be selected.
5) Evaluation. The developed BCI system must be evaluated with a population of end users in order to assure its efficacy and make possible the generalization of the results in a real environment. Therefore, the system will be tested with both healthy subjects and MS patients.

12.3 Subject database

A total of sixteen MS patients (42.1 ± 7.5 years; 10 males, 6 females) and five control subjects (26.0 ± 4.6 years; 5 males) were included in the study. Characteristics of the subject population are detailed in table 12.2. MS patients were recruited from the National Reference Centre on Disability and Dependence of León (Spain). All subjects gave their informed consent to participate in the study, which was approved by the local ethics committee prior to the assessment. As can be noticed, the degree of motor disability, cognitive and sustained attention ability is not homogeneous inside the MS population.

12.4 Methods

Figure 12.2 summarizes the general structure of the developed BCI web browser, which can be divided into four main stages: (1) signal acquisition, (2) P300 processing, (3) asynchrony management, and (4) web browser application. These four stages are detailed in depth below.

Table 12.2. Characteristics of the participants.

	Subject	Age	Sex	Degree of motor disability	Degree of cognitive ability	Degree of sustained attention
CS	H01	23	M	N.a.	N.a.	N.a.
	H02	31	M	N.a.	N.a.	N.a.
	H03	23	M	N.a.	N.a.	N.a.
	H04	31	M	N.a.	N.a.	N.a.
	H05	22	M	N.a.	N.a.	N.a.
MS	P01	30	F	Non-existent	Very high	Very high
	P02	31	M	Non-existent	High	Very high
	P03	43	M	Mild	Very high	High
	P04	47	F	Moderate	Normal	High
	P05	56	M	Moderate	Low	Very low
	P06	32	F	Non-existent	Normal	Normal
	P07	35	M	Non-existent	Very high	Very high
	P08	41	M	Non-existent	High	High
	P09	49	F	Non-existent	Normal	Very high
	P10	44	M	Mild	Normal	Low
	P11	41	F	Moderate	Normal	High
	P12	43	M	Moderate	Very high	Normal
	P13	44	M	Non-existent	High	High
	P14	52	M	Moderate	Very high	Normal
	P15	38	F	Non-existent	Normal	High
	P16	47	M	Moderate	Normal	Normal

CS: control subjects, MS: multiple sclerosis patients, M: male, F: female, N.a.: not applicable.

12.4.1 Signal acquisition

The signal acquisition stage was intended to register and monitor the EEG signals of the user. A total of eight electrodes were placed over users' scalps, mainly in the parietal and occipital lobes. According to the International System 10–20, the electrodes were placed on Fz, Cz, Pz, P3, P4, PO7, PO8 and Oz, using Fpz as a ground and the earlobe as reference [43]. Bandpass (0.1–60 Hz), notch (50 Hz) and common average reference (CAR) filters were applied as a pre-processing stage. EEG signals were recorded using g.LADYbird active electrodes and a g.USBamp amplifier, from g.Tec (Austria). The sampling rate of the recording was 256Hz. BCI2000 software was used to process the EEG signals, control the stimuli presentation, record and save data in the laptop (Intel Core i7 @ 2.4 GHz, 8 GB RAM) [44].

12.4.2 P300 processing

The second stage comprises the signal processing of the P300 evoked potentials. This stage is executed in the laptop, which displays the visual stimuli and processes the signal. As aforementioned, these potentials were generated using RCP matrices. The

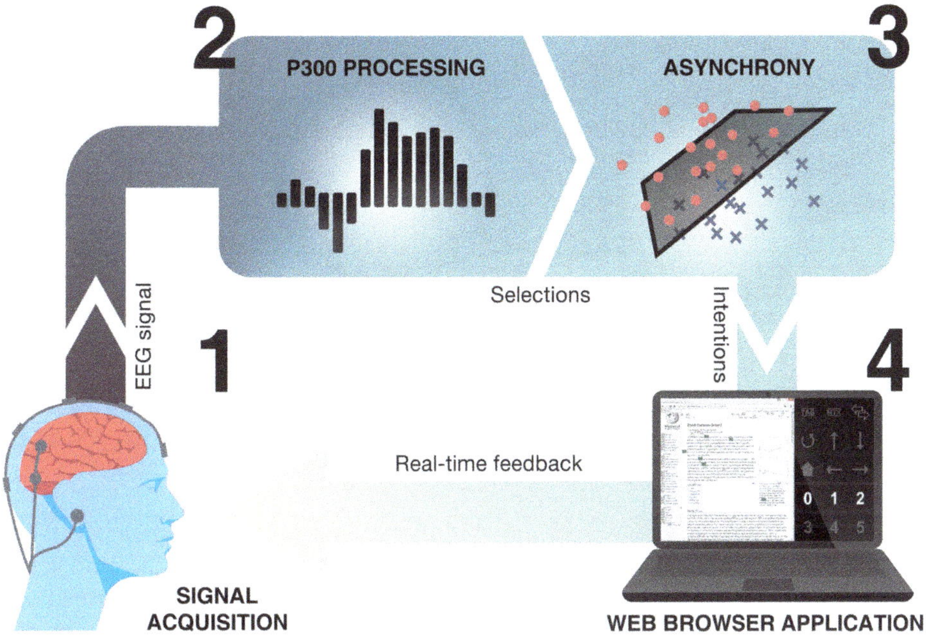

Figure 12.2. General structure of the P300-based BCI web browser, subdivided in the following stages: (1) signal acquisition, intended to register and monitor the EEG signal of the user; (2) P300 processing, intended to apply the required signal processing for determining the commands that the user wants to select; (3) asynchrony, intended to provide a comprehensive unsupervised control of the browser by measuring the level of attention of the user; and (4) web browser application, intended to interpret the received commands and provide feedback in real time to the user.

main flow of the RCP is displayed in figure 12.3. A matrix of commands is displayed in front of the user, who has to attend to the desired command. The rows and the columns of the matrix are randomly flashed, eliciting a P300 in the EEG when the user perceives an unexpected flashing on the desired command [3, 11]. Therefore, a P300 is generated when the row or the column that contains the target command are flashed. The system processes the EEG signal of each stimulus, determining if a P300 potential is present. Hence, the target command can be predicted in real time by intersecting the row and the column that contain P300 potentials [11]. In this study, each stimulus lasted for 62.5 ms, followed by a pause of $\sim \mathcal{U}(125,250)$ ms. Due to the low signal-to-noise ratio of the P300 responses, several repetitions (i.e. sequences) of the stimuli are required in order to detect a reliable P300 potential [8].

The processing of the P300 potentials is fairly simple because it is intended to work in real time. Once a trial (i.e. character) is finished, relevant features of the signal are extracted. Due to the high sampling rate of the recordings (256 Hz) in comparison with the low frequency of the P300 responses, a dimensionality reduction step is beneficial for the classification [45]. Therefore, a down-sampling procedure is applied to the EEG signals in a window of 800 ms after the stimuli onsets [24, 31, 45]. In this study, signals were decimated to 20 Hz, resulting in a total of 16 features (20 Hz × 0.8 s) for each channel. Features of each channel were then

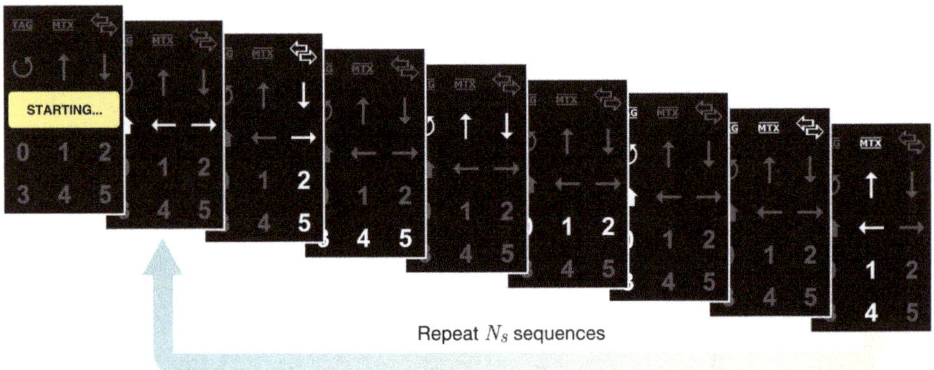

Figure 12.3. Main flow of a sequence of flashings in the row–col paradigm (RCP). Since the matrix size is 5 × 3, a total of eight flashings are required to highlight each row and column. This procedure is repeated N_s times in order to increase the reliability of the P300 potential detection.

concatenated, composing an observation (128 features). Note that there are as many observations as stimuli. The feature matrix is the input of the classification stage, which aims to determine whether a P300 is present in each observation. Step-wise linear discriminant analysis (SWLDA) was employed as a feature selection and classification method [31, 35–37, 45, 46]. SWLDA selects the most relevant features that can discriminate between two classes, using a hyperplane that minimizes the within-class covariance and maximizes the between-class covariance [47]. The selection of the most relevant features is calculated in the calibration session through a step-wise procedure. SWLDA begins with an empty model and adds a new feature when its inclusion is beneficial for the discrimination (i.e. forward step, add if p-value $< p_{in}$). Then, SWLDA removes features that increment the discriminative ability if they are not included in the model (i.e. backward step, remove if p-value $> p_{out}$) [47]. In this study, these forward and backward steps are repeated until the model selects a maximum of 60 features [31, 35, 45, 46, 48]. Selection and elimination criteria were set at $p_{\text{in}} = 0.10$ and $p_{\text{out}} = 0.15$ [45, 46, 48–50]. Before classifying the observations as class 1 (i.e. presence of P300) or class 0 (i.e. absence of P300), classifier weights $\boldsymbol{w}$ must be optimized in a calibration phase. These weights are multiplied to the observation features in order to project them to a space that maximizes the separation between classes [47]. Weights are computed as follows:

$$\boldsymbol{w} \propto \left(\sum\nolimits_0 + \sum\nolimits_1\right)^{-1} (\boldsymbol{\mu}_1 - \boldsymbol{\mu}_0), \tag{12.1}$$

where $\sum_i$ and $\boldsymbol{\mu}_i$ are the covariance matrix and the mean of the class i, where $i \in \{0, 1\}$ [47]. SWLDA output scores can be considered as the log-likelihood of belonging to class 1, under the assumption that noise presents a normal distribution with equal covariances in both classes [51]. In online sessions, the output score for the jth observation is computed as follows:

$$l_j = \|\langle \boldsymbol{w}, \boldsymbol{x}_j \rangle - \langle \boldsymbol{w}, \boldsymbol{\mu}_1 \rangle\|, \tag{12.2}$$

where l_j is the log-likelihood of the observation $\boldsymbol{x}_j$ of containing a P300 potential. In order to predict the selected item, the $\boldsymbol{l}$ vector should be shaped into a $N_r \times N_c$ matrix that indicates the probability of selecting each command. Note that N_r and N_c are the number of rows and columns of the current RCP matrix, respectively. For each cell n, the average of the log-likelihood scores of all the observations that belong to the same row and column is then computed:

$$\lambda_n = \frac{1}{2N_s} \sum_{n=1}^{N_r+N_c} l_{n\in\{\text{row}\bigcup\text{col}\}}, \tag{12.3}$$

where N_s indicates the number of sequences. Finally, the predicted command will be the one that reaches the maximum probability $p = \max(\boldsymbol{\lambda})$.

12.4.3 Asynchrony management

An asynchronous management stage is essential to assure an unsupervised and comprehensive control of the BCI web browser. As aforementioned in section 12.4.2, RCP matrices are synchronous processes that will deliver predicted commands even when the user is not paying attention to the visual stimuli [28]. Therefore, to reach a comprehensive control of the system, the signal processing stage must discern if the user is attending or ignoring the stimuli, usually referred to as control or non-control states, respectively. Indeed, asynchrony is especially useful in this study because sometimes the user will want to read a webpage or watch a video, for example. Since P300 responses will be only present in control state signals, we hypothesize that SWLDA output scores in control signals are higher than in non-control state. In this study, a threshold τ is used to discern between both states [35–37].

The value of τ is calculated in a calibration session, once enough control and non-control state trials are registered. The final probabilities of each trial are concatenated in two different vectors: $\boldsymbol{p}_c$, which contains the probabilities of control trials; and $\boldsymbol{p}_n$, which contains the probabilities of the non-control trials. Both vectors are fed into a receiver operating characteristic (ROC) curve, plotting the true positive rate (TPR) versus the false positive rate (FPR) of a set of possible threshold values (see figure 12.4). The value of τ is chosen offline as the threshold that maximizes the tuple {TPR, FPR}. In other words, τ is the threshold providing the point that minimizes the Euclidean distance to (0,1).

In online sessions, τ is used to determine whether a trial belongs to the control or non-control state. When a new trial is computed, the state is determined as follows:

$$\text{state} = \begin{cases} \text{control}, & \text{if } p > \tau \\ \text{non-control}, & \text{if } p \leqslant \tau \end{cases}. \tag{12.4}$$

When a trial is classified as a control state selection, the command is delivered to the application stage; otherwise, the system considers it as a warning and asks the user for selecting it again.

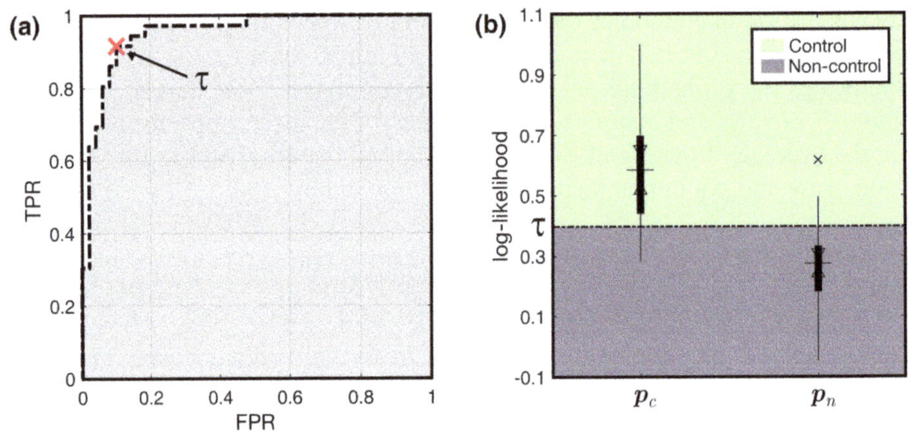

Figure 12.4. Threshold-based asynchronous approach. (a) The ROC curve displays the true positive rate (TPR) versus the false positive rate (FPR) of all possible values of a threshold that discerns between both classes. Data of class 0 and 1 are the log-likelihood scores of the selected trials in control (i.e. p_c) and non-control (i.e. p_n) signals, respectively. The optimal threshold τ is marked with a cross, previously computed as the value that minimizes the distance to the point (0,1). (b) Boxplots that depict the distributions of the normalized log-likelihood scores for both classes. The optimal threshold is indicated as a black dash–dot line. Note that online scores that fall in the green area would be considered as control trials, whereas those in the blue area would be considered as non-control trials.

12.4.4 The web browser application

The last stage receives the selected commands and interprets them in real time, providing visual feedback to the user. The application was developed in JavaScript as an extension of the Google Chrome web browser. Google Chrome was selected as the target browser because it allows developers to install custom extensions that can modify and enhance its functionalities. As can be seen in figure 12.5, the web browser is displayed on the left side of the screen, while the RCP matrix is displayed on the right side.

Due to the high number of commands required to achieve a comprehensive navigation in a modern web browser, two different RCP matrices are used: navigation and keyboard (see figure 12.5). The former is a 5×3 RCP matrix intended to facilitate the navigation through the websites. Its small size provides users a quick way to select commands, since a sequence is composed of only eight flashes. The matrix includes navigation commands, such as up/down scrolls, home page, reload, and back buttons, among others. By contrast, the keyboard matrix is a 9×5 matrix that contains all the alphanumeric characters and a variety of commonly used symbols. The matrix is intended to fill out forms, write e-mails or search. Owing to its size, the selection of a command takes more time than in navigation matrix, requiring a total of 14 flashes per sequence. Note that both matrices include an 'MTX' command that allows users to voluntarily toggle between them when necessary.

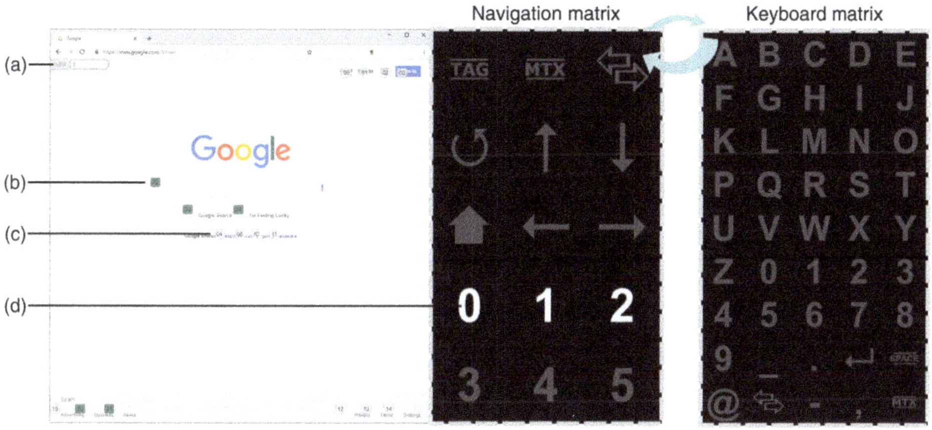

Figure 12.5. Graphical user interface of the BCI web browser application. The currently selected RCP matrix is displayed on the right side of the screen, while the home Google website is shown on the left side. Users can freely toggle between the navigation (left) and keyboard (right) matrices by selecting the command 'MTX'. As shown in the (a) buffer, the user has previously selected the command '2'. Therefore, (b) potential selections are highlighted in green, whereas (c) normal tags remains in grey. In this screenshot, the (d) third row of the navigation matrix is being flashed.

Once a website is loaded, the application computes the number of nodes of the current webpage. A node is considered any clickable item on the web, such as links, images, buttons or forms, among others. When the user selects the command 'TAG', these nodes are identified with a unique numeric code and a custom tag is placed close to them. The numeric tag is composed using numbers from 0 to 5. Note that the length of the codes is the minimum one that allows all nodes to be tagged. As shown in figure 12.5, numbers 0–5 are included in the navigation matrix in order to increase the speed of the BCI web browser. Therefore, users just need to spell the tag to simulate a click on the node. With the objective of avoiding extra selections to confirm a link selection, the system automatically executes the link provided the user has previously included a valid tag. Several feedback aids are also included to favor the ease of use of the application. On the one hand, when tagging is enabled, the application initializes a buffer in the top left corner that displays the previous selections. In the case of a selection error, users can delete previous selections with the navigation matrix. On the other hand, potential selections (i.e. nodes whose tags begin with the previously introduced numbers) are also highlighted in green, as can be noticed in figure 12.5.

12.4.5 Assessment

The developed P300-based BCI web browser was evaluated with a total of 5 CS and 16 MS. Each participant carried out a total of four different sessions: two calibration sessions (CAL1, CAL2) and two evaluation (EVA1, EVA2) sessions, which are described below. A schematic view of the assessment process is depicted in figure 12.6.

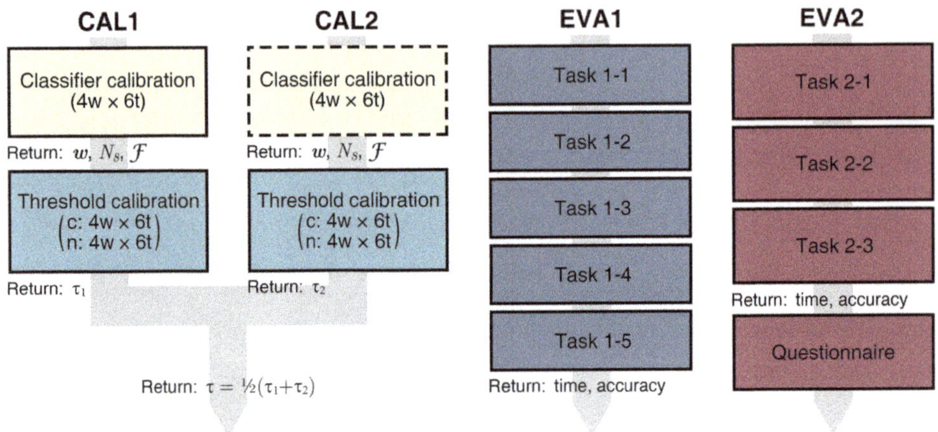

Figure 12.6. Scheme of the assessment procedure, composed of four different sessions: two calibration sessions (CAL1, CAL2) and two evaluation sessions (EVA1, EVA2). CAL1 began with a classifier calibration, intended to compute optimal weights w, number of sequences N_s and the feature set $\mathcal{F}$ of each user. Then, a threshold calibration was performed. In CAL2, classifier was calibrated again for users that did not reach a minimal accuracy of 70% in CAL1. CAL2 ended with other threshold calibration, aimed to increase the robustness of the final value τ. EVA1 was composed by five different tasks, in which only the fifth one required an asynchronous control. EVA2, by contrast, was composed by three different tasks that involved an asynchronous control using τ. Finally, a qualitative questionnaire was handed to the participants in order to collect their opinions and suggestions.

1) *Calibration sessions:* Calibration sessions were intended to compute the customized number of sequences, the classifier weights, the selected features and the asynchrony threshold for each participant. The classifier weights were firstly calibrated in the beginning of CAL1, when users were asked to spell 4 words of 6 trials. In order to help participants to sustain their attention to the task, they were recommended to count how many times the target character was highlighted. Since the initial number of sequences was set at 15, they should perceive 30 flashes in a single trial. The keyboard matrix was used due to the higher number of commands that contains. Then, SWLDA was applied in order to determine the feature set, the classifier weights and the number of sequences that should have each user reaching a proper performance (refer to section 12.4.2). These optimal parameters were used thereafter. In the end of CAL1, the first part of the threshold calibration was performed. Users were asked to spell 8 words of 6 trials with the navigation matrix. Half of them were intended to record the control state, paying attention to the stimuli; whereas the rest were intended to record the non-control state, asking users to ignorie the stimuli. In order to not pay attention to the visual stimuli, users were ordered to read a website. CAL2 was only composed by another threshold calibration step. This is required due to the high inter-session variability of the P300 amplitude and latency depending on cap position shifts, user attention, attitude or drowsiness, among other reasons [26]. The final threshold τ value was calculated as the average of the thresholds of CAL1 and CAL2, which were computed following the procedure described in the section 12.4.3.

For users that did not achieve a minimum training accuracy of 70% in CAL1, a new classifier calibration procedure was trained in CAL2. Users that did not reach 70% after both sessions were discarded from the subsequent assessment. Note that an accuracy of 70% is usually considered as the minimum rate for experiment of a satisfactory control of a BCI system [24, 48].

2) *Evaluation sessions:* Evaluation sessions were intended to assess the usefulness and efficacy of the developed P300-based BCI web browser. However, the threshold was not applied in EVA1 in order to assess if its application entails an improvement to the general performance. EVA1 was made up of five different tasks: the first four were intended to assess the control state selections, whereas the last one was intended to evaluate the non-control state performance. EVA1 tasks are described below:

   Task 1-1. Link selection. Users had to scroll up and down a Wikipedia page and select a link (6 items).

   Task 1-2. Google searching. Users had to select the Google form, spell 'BCI' and select 'ENTER' to make the search (8 items).

   Task 1-3. *Tweet* publishing. Users had to select the Twitter form, spell a *tweet* of 2 characters and send it (6 items).

   Task 1-4. E-mail writing. Users had to read an inbox e-mail in Gmail and reply to it by introducing a single number (13 items).

   Task 1-5. Passive reading. With the threshold enabled, users had to read a piece of news while ignoring the stimuli (10 items).

   The second evaluation session was intended to assess the performance of the BCI system when asynchrony is enabled. In EVA2, users were asked to complete three slightly different tasks that involve the use of control and non-control states (i.e. alternating website reading and web surfing). EVA2 tasks are described below:

   Task 2-1. Reading and link selection. Users had to scroll a Wikipedia page, read the information and select a link (8 items).

   Task 2-2. *Tweet* publishing. Users had to follow the same procedure as Task 1-3 (6 items).

   Task 2-3. Active reading. Users had to read a piece of news, scrolling down the webpage if needed (4 items).

During the evaluation sessions, both quantitative and qualitative metrics were measured. Average accuracy, number of selections, number of errors, time to finish the tasks and number of false negatives were measured as quantitative metrics. Regarding the qualitative ones, a questionnaire was provided to the users at the end of EVA2. The survey consisted on 20 items that had to be ranked in a 7-point Likert scale, where positive and negative statements were shuffled to avoid acquiescence bias [52]. The questionnaire was intended to collect the subjective opinions of the participants about the browser interface, the speed, the ease of use and the duration of the sessions, as well as users' expectations, motivation and previous experience with BCIs. An open-ended question was added at the end in order to allow users to write personal suggestions for further improvements.

Table 12.3. Results of both calibration sessions.

	Subject	CAL1		CAL2		Average accuracy	Number of sequences	Discarded?
		Accuracy	Wrong selections	Accuracy	Wrong selections			
CS	H01	100.0%	0	100.0%	0	100.0%	7	No
	H02	100.0%	0	91.67%	2	95.84%	11	No
	H03	100.0%	0	100.0%	0	100.0%	6	No
	H04	100.0%	0	91.67%	2	95.84%	10	No
	H05	100.0%	0	91.67%	2	95.84%	9	No
	Mean	**100.0%**	**0**	**95.00%**	**1.2**	**97.50%**	**8.60**	—
	SD	0.00%	0	4.56%	1.1	2.28%	2.07	—
MS	P01	87.50%	3	79.17%	5	83.34%	10	No
	P02	91.67%	2	87.50%	3	89.59%	6	No
	P03	41.67%	14	75.00%	6	58.34%	15	No
	P04	79.17%	5	95.83%	1	87.50%	13	No
	P05	<70%	—	<70%	—	—	—	Yes
	P06	83.33%	4	66.67%	8	75.00%	15	No
	P07	83.33%	4	91.67%	2	87.50%	7	No
	P08	83.33%	4	70.83%	7	77.08%	6	No
	P09	75.00%	6	95.83%	1	85.42%	10	No
	P10	91.67%	2	75.00%	6	83.34%	13	No
	P11	<70%	—	<70%	—	—	—	Yes
	P12	66.67%	8	70.83%	7	68.75%	9	No
	P13	83.33%	4	66.67%	8	75.00%	8	No
	P14	87.50%	3	87.50%	3	87.50%	10	No
	P15	91.67%	2	75.00%	6	83.34%	6	No
	P16	<70%	—	<70%	—	—	—	Yes
	Mean	**80.45%**	**5.14**	**79.81%**	**4.85**	**80.13%**	**9.85**	—
	SD	13.65%	3.57	10.60%	2.54	12.13%	3.29	—

CS: control subjects, MS: multiple sclerosis patients. Note that each session was composed of a total of 24 selections. Mean and standard deviation were computed regardless of the discarded users.

12.5 Results

Results of the calibrations sessions CAL1 and CAL2 are shown in table 12.3. Training accuracies and wrong selections of both sessions are detailed. Optimal number of sequences per user are detailed as well. As can be noticed, three MS patients (P05, P11 and P16) could not obtain a minimum training accuracy of 70% at the end of CAL2 and thus, they were removed from the assessment. As expected, CS obtained higher training accuracies and a lower number of sequences (97.5% w/ 8.60 seq.) than MS patients (80.13% w/ 9.85 seq.).

Table 12.4. Results of the first evaluation session.

	Subject	Link selection		Google searching		*Tweet* publishing		E-mail writing		Passive reading		Average accuracy[1]
		Time	Acc.	Time	Acc.	Time	Acc.	Time	Acc.	Time	Acc.	
CS	H01	2:16	100.0%	3:40	100.0%	2:14	100.0%	3:39	100.0%	3:39	100.0%	100.0%
	H02	2:51	00.00%	5:56	75.00%	3:16	100.0%	9:06	75.00%	5:00	100.0%	82.50%
	H03	2:00	100.0%	3:16	100.0%	2:00	100.0%	4:20	100.0%	3:20	100.0%	100.0%
	H04	2:50	100.0%	4:45	100.0%	2:50	100.0%	6:06	92.31%	4:41	90.00%	96.97%
	H05	2:50	100.0%	4:44	100.0%	2:50	83.33%	8:18	87.50%	4:46	90.00%	91.67%
	Mean	**2:33**	**100.0%**	**4:28**	**95.00%**	**2:38**	**96.67%**	**6:18**	**90.96%**	**4:17**	**96.00%**	**94.23%**
	SD	0:24	0.00%	1:03	11.18%	0:31	7.45%	2:13	10.39%	0:45	5.48%	7.39%
MS	P01	3:35	100.0%	6:05	100.0%	5:20	77.78%	15:04	66.67%	5:30	90.00%	79.54%
	P02	2:22	100.0%	4:02	100.0%	4:24	100.0%	5:17	100.0%	3:18	100.0%	100.0%
	P03	N.c.	25.00%	6:42	85.71%	N.c.	57.14%	N.c.	—	8:15	100.0%	61.11%
	P04	2:48	100.0%	4:45	100.0%	2:49	100.0%	6:24	92.86%	7:09	87.50%	96.97%
	P06	4:20	87.50%	8:05	72.73%	4:49	77.78%	8:54	75.00%	8:15	87.50%	77.27%
	P07	4:45	72.73%	N.c.	40.00%	3:37	83.33%	N.c.	50.00%	3:51	60.00%	63.33%
	P08	3:12	100.0%	6:20	100.0%	4:50	88.89%	6:58	100.0%	3:18	90.00%	97.20%
	P09	7:35	100.0%	N.c.	70.00%	3:20	100.0%	N.c.	62.50%	5:30	50.00%	82.35%
	P10	3:41	100.0%	N.c.	66.67%	5:01	75.00%	N.c.	62.50%	7:09	100.0%	76.00%
	P12	N.c.	66.67%	8:00	72.73%	7:02	63.64%	N.c.	53.33%	4:57	90.00%	62.79%
	P13	N.c.	71.43%	4:26	88.89%	2:13	100.0%	7:12	80.00%	2:45	90.00%	83.78%
	P14	3:48	75.00%	N.c.	75.00%	3:08	57.14%	N.c.	46.15%	5:30	80.00%	62.50%
	P15	N.c.	42.86%	5:31	70.00%	3:57	75.00%	N.c.	64.29%	3:18	90.00%	64.10%
	Mean	**4:01**	**80.09%**	**6:00**	**80.13%**	**4:13**	**81.21%**	**8:18**	**71.11%**	**5:17**	**85.77%**	**77.46%**
	SD	1:31	24.48%	1:28	17.84%	1:19	15.93%	3:31	18.67%	1:56	14.94%	14.24%

CS: control subjects, MS: multiple sclerosis patients, Acc.: accuracy, N.c.: not completed. MS patients M05, M11 and M16 were removed from the assessment because they did not achieve a minimum accuracy of 70% in the calibration sessions.

[1] Averaged accuracy includes only the tasks in which threshold was enabled (i.e. it does not include the passive reading task).

Assessment results of sessions EVA1 and EVA2 are detailed in tables 12.4 and 12.5, respectively. Task durations and accuracies are detailed for each subject. In the EVA2 results, the false negative rate (FNR) is detailed in order to indicate the threshold performance. FNR is defined as the ratio of false negatives (i.e., control trials labeled as non-controls) to the total number of selections. In general, CS reached higher performances than MS in both sessions. EVA1 results show that CS and MS reached average accuracies of 94.23% and 77.46%, respectively. These results were improved in EVA2, especially for MS patients, reaching average accuracies of 95.75% and 84.14%.

Finally, questionnaire results are shown in table 12.6. Participants were quite satisfied with the BCI web browser. All positive statements were evaluated above the mean value and almost all negative statements below it. The exceptions were questions 3 and 13. The former reflected the speed of the browser. Some MS indicated that it took too long to surf the Internet. For the latter, both CS and MS participants declared to be slightly happy that assessment sessions were over. Regarding the last open-ended question, MS patients suggested improving the selection speed, adding a tabulation command, planning shorter sessions, make flashing less annoying and trying to reduce the number of sequences. CS suggested that extra symbols could be added in other RCP matrix and reported that they sometimes focused unintentionally their sight on adjacent cells.

12.6 Discussion

As shown in table 12.3, three MS patients (P05, P11 and P16) were not able to reach a minimal accuracy of 70% in the calibration sessions and thus, they were removed from the subsequent assessment of the P300-based BCI web browser. This issue may lie in the shape of their P300 evoked potentials, whose amplitude may be too attenuated or their latency may show a high variability among trials. These accuracies were expected in the case of P05 owing to his lack of sustained attention capabilities. However, the clinical characteristics of P11 or P16 do not provide an apparent reason for this poor calibration performance.

Regarding table 12.4 results of EVA1, CS reached an average accuracy of 94.23%, while MS reached 77.46%. Although all CS were able to finish all the tasks, not all MS patients could finish them. Despite this issue, four MS patients reached average accuracies over 80%. Indeed, M02 stands out for achieving a perfect control of the browser (100%) in all tasks. In the case of CS, all of them obtained average accuracies greater than 80%, and H02 and H03 reached an accuracy of 100%. Sorted by decreasing accuracy, CS reached average accuracies of 100% in Task 1-1, 96.67% in Task 1-3, 96.00% in Task 1-5, 95.00% in Task 1-2 and 90.96% in Task 1-4. Considering MS patients, they obtained 85.77% in Task 1-5, 81.21% in Task 1-3, 80.13% in Task 1-2, 80.09% in Task 1-1 and 71.11% in Task 1-4. Clearly, Task 1-4 proved to be the most difficult one for CS and MS, likely due to the large number of selections involving the use of both RCP matrices. It is noteworthy that Task 1-5, the only one in EVA1 that employed the asynchronous threshold, resulted as the easiest task for MS patients. This means that the asynchrony management was beneficial

Table 12.5. Results of the second evaluation session.

	Subject	Reading & Link			*Tweet* publishing			Active reading			Average accuracy[1]
		Time	FNR	Acc.	Time	FNR	Acc.	Time	FNR	Acc.	
CS	H01	2:58	0.00	100.0%	2:17	0.00	83.33%	1:29	0.00	100.0%	94.44%
	H02	7:02	0.23	92.31%	5:20	0.10	100.0%	2:44	0.00	60.00%	89.29%
	H03	2:40	0.00	100.0%	2:04	0.00	100.0%	1:20	0.00	100.0%	100.0%
	H04	4:32	0.00	100.0%	4:36	0.25	87.50%	2:20	0.00	100.0%	95.00%
	H05	4:18	0.11	100.0%	2:48	0.00	100.0%	1:55	0.00	100.0%	100.0%
	Mean	**4:18**	**0.07**	**98.46%**	**3:25**	**0.07**	**94.17%**	**1:58**	**0.00**	**92.00%**	**95.75%**
	SD	1:44	0.10	3.44%	1:28	0.11	8.12%	0:35	0.00	17.89%	4.48%
MS	P01	6:05	0.30	92.31%	N.c.	0.00	44.44%	1:45	0.00	100.0%	76.92%
	P02	4:02	0.25	91.67%	2:31	0.13	85.71%	2:48	0.00	100.0%	92.00%
	P03	N.c.	0.13	100.0%	N.c.	0.13	62.50%	2:39	0.00	100.0%	85.00%
	P04	3:50	0.00	100.0%	2:48	0.00	100.0%	1:53	0.00	100.0%	100.0%
	P06	5:42	0.00	77.78%	3:45	0.00	85.71%	4:30	0.00	85.71%	82.61%
	P07	N.c.	0.40	100.0%	3:21	0.22	88.89%	1:29	0.00	100.0%	95.65%
	P08	3:22	0.00	70.00%	3:42	0.09	81.82%	2:08	0.00	75.00%	76.00%
	P09	N.c.	0.17	83.33%	N.c.	0.36	92.86%	N.c.	0.00	75.00%	86.67%
	P10	N.c.	0.08	63.64%	N.c.	0.14	71.43%	N.c.	0.00	75.00%	68.18%
	P12	N.c.	0.17	33.33%	N.c.	0.00	75.00%	N.c.	0.33	83.33%	72.00%
	P13	5:24	0.33	91.67%	5:24	0.20	100.0%	1:54	0.00	100.0%	96.30%
	P14	N.c.	0.18	72.73%	4:37	0.00	100.0%	1:56	0.00	100.0%	87.50%
	P15	N.c.	0.07	85.71%	N.c.	0.56	66.67%	N.c.	0.00	75.00%	75.00%
	Mean	**4:44**	**0.16**	**81.71%**	**3:44**	**0.14**	**81.16%**	**2:20**	**0.03**	**83.93%**	**84.14%**
	SD	1:08	0.13	18.78%	1:00	0.17	16.69%	0:55	0.09	11.77%	10.08%

CS: control subjects, MS: multiple sclerosis patients, FNR: false negative rate, Acc.: accuracy, N.c.: not completed. MS patients M05, M11 and M16 were removed from the assessment because they did not achieved a minimum accuracy of 70% in the calibration sessions.

[1] Averaged accuracy includes only the tasks in which threshold was enabled (i.e. it does not include the passive reading task).

Table 12.6. Results of the questionnaire.

#	Statement	CS		MS	
		Mean	SD	Mean	SD
1	I am not used to surfing the Internet	1.2	0.4	3.2	2.3
2	I have found it interesting to use the BCI web browser	6.4	0.5	6.2	0.9
3	In my opinion, it takes much too long to surf the Internet with the BCI browser	4.0	1.0	4.8	0.9
4	My expectations for the browser were completely met	6.4	0.5	5.7	1.2
5	I was bored during the assessment sessions	2.8	1.3	2.7	2.0
6	I can imagine myself using this browser in my daily life	3.4	1.1	4.6	1.7
7	I became impatient during the assessment sessions	2.2	0.8	2.8	1.8
8	I found the assessment sessions entertaining	5.2	0.4	5.4	1.2
9	It was stressful to concentrate when it was required	2.0	1.0	2.9	1.7
10	I would gladly carry out more testing sessions with the BCI browser	6.6	0.5	5.6	1.2
11	The assessment sessions made me feel tired	2.8	1.8	3.0	1.9
12	User interface is intuitive and easy to understand	5.4	2.1	5.9	1.3
13	I am happy that the assessment sessions are over	4.6	0.9	4.2	1.9
14	I found it easy to select keyboard matrix commands	4.6	1.7	5.3	1.3
15	I found it difficult to select navigation matrix commands	2.4	1.1	2.5	1.3
16	I like computers and information technologies	6.0	1.0	4.9	2.4
17	Flickering stimuli are annoying	1.8	0.8	3.7	2.1
18	I would love to participate in other similar studies	6.0	1.0	5.2	1.5
19	The duration of the assessment sessions was too long	3.0	1.0	2.4	1.4

CS: control subjects, MS: multiple sclerosis patients. Each statement was ranked in a 7-point Likert scale where 0 means 'strong disagreement', 4 means 'neutral' and 7 means 'strong agreement'.

for MS patients in EVA1, suggesting that the use of a threshold could improve the general performance.

In relation to table 12.5 results of EVA2, CS reached an average accuracy of 95.75%, while MS reached 84.14%. As in EVA1, there were several MS patients that could not finish the tasks. A total of eight MS patients reached average accuracies over 80%, and M04 reached a perfect control of the browser (100%) in all tasks. Regarding CS, all of them obtained performances over 80%, and two of them, H03 and H05, reached an accuracy of 100%. Sorted by decreasing accuracy, CS obtained average accuracies of 98.46% in Task 2-1, 94.17% in Task 2-2 and 92.00% in Task 2-3. Concerning MS, they obtained 83.93% in Task 2-3, 81.71% in Task 2-1 and 81.16% in Task 2-3. The results of MS in Task 2-3, together with the low value of FNR for that task (0.03), reinforce the fact that the inclusion of the asynchronous threshold could have been beneficial for MS patients. Precisely, threshold only causes an average of 4.61% ± 8.71% and 10.87% ± 14.33% of false negative errors to the total number of performed selections in CS and MS participants, respectively.

In comparison with EVA1 (CS: 94.23%, MS: 77.46%), average accuracies of EVA2 (CS: 95.75%, MS: 84.14%) are slightly higher. Taking into account that threshold was only enabled in EVA2, results show an apparent improvement in performance when asynchrony is provided. However, this improvement is not significant for CS users (Wilcoxon signed-rank test, p-value = 0.63) and the threshold has avoided less uncertain selections for CS than for MS subjects. This fact suggests that the threshold does not provide an improvement in terms of accuracy for subjects with full cognitive and physical capabilities, although it may provide a less demanding experience and a higher control of the BCI system. For MS subjects, even though the increase in accuracy between both sessions is also not significant (Wilcoxon signed-rank test, p-value = 0.11), tasks that involved a demanding use of the non-control state turned out to be easier for them. Despite the advantages of the asynchronous threshold, a badly optimized τ value could lead to an increase of the FNR and the duration of the tasks. This issue occurred in the case of H02, who reached an accuracy of 100% in Task 1-3 and Task 2-2 (both tasks were intended to publish a *tweet*). The duration of Task 2-2 for H02 was increased in comparison with Task 1-3, because up to 10% of his selections were false negatives. This issue is due to the inability of the threshold to follow nonstationary changes of the EEG across different sessions, generating a trade-off between navigation speed and accuracy. These changes are emphasized as more sessions are carried out without updating classifier's weights $\mathbf{w}$, and actually constitute one of the greatest limitations of practical BCI systems [53]. Besides, τ values must be re-calculated if $\mathbf{w}$ is updated, since the threshold relies on the log-likelihood scores that are returned by SWLDA. Despite this issue, results still reinforce the fact that the BCI browser performance is improved when threshold is enabled, especially for MS patients. This way, end users can successfully avoid selection errors when the intensity of their P300 potentials is not enough to be considered as strong deliberate selections.

As the qualitative results of table 12.6 show, participants were quite satisfied with the developed BCI web browser. All positive statements were ranked above the neutral value (i.e. 4), and all negative statements were ranked below it with the exception of questions 3 and 13. The former was intended to assess the navigation speed, where CS returned a neutral response (4.0 ± 1.0) and MS slightly agreed that it takes much too long to surf the Internet (4.8 ± 0.9). Unfortunately, browser speed is directly related with the optimal number of sequences of each user, which is calculated in calibration sessions and depends on the training accuracy of the SWLDA classifier. Therefore, navigation speed could be increased by improving the classifier robustness, either getting more training samples (increasing the duration of CAL1) or using more complex signal processing algorithms. It is worth mentioning that CS ranked the statement with a neutral value, probably because their number of sequences was lower (8.60 ± 2.07) than for MS (9.85 ± 3.29). The thirteenth question reflects that participants were slightly happy that the assessment sessions were over (CS: 4.6 ± 0.9, MS: 4.2 ± 1.9). This result reveals that their participation implied an effort, a fact that should be borne in mind when designing the contents and duration of the assessment sessions. At the same time, all participants declared that they would gladly carry out more sessions with the browser (CS: 6.6 ± 0.5, MS: 5.6 ± 1.2) and that they would love to participate in further studies (CS: 6.0 ± 1.0, MS: 5.2 ± 1.5). Moreover, the top-rated aspect was the user interface, due to its user-friendliness and simplicity.

CS users also pointed out that sometimes they unintentionally focused their sight on adjacent cells. This issue is known as the adjacency-distraction (AD) problem, and causes adjacent non-target flashes to distract users and make selection errors. These errors are usually found in the same row or column as the target command. In our assessment, all the errors of CS were caused by this issue (100% out of 14 errors). For MS patients, the AD problem caused 85.57% of their errors (out of 141). Since the probabilities of randomly select adjacent cells or cells that belong to the target's row or column are 44.66%–66.66% in navigation matrix and 28.88%–35.55% in keyboard matrix, it is clear that the majority of errors are due to the AD problem. Further endeavors could be focused on implementing the checkerboard paradigm, another version of the RCP that solves the AD problem and the double-flash problem at the same time [54].

A comparison among related studies is shown in table 12.7. As shown, initial BCI web browsers employed endogenous control signals that forced users to make dichotomous decisions to select web links [7, 17, 18, 29]. These approaches not only suffered from a lack of speed in selecting a command, but also required users to make an intense training for learning how to regulate the signals themselves [7, 17, 18, 29]. The selection slowness was overcome by means of using P300 evoked potentials as control signals [24, 31, 42]. RCP matrices allowed researchers to provide users with a wide variety of commands, making possible strategies such as node tagging [24] or virtual cursor movements [31, 42]. The latter is more rigid, allowing users to move a discrete number of pixels that must be fixed prior to the assessment [31]. Moreover, intense training is still present in Yu *et al*, since users should learn to self-regulate the SMR signals [42]. Besides the fact that P300 potentials and node tagging makes our proposal faster and more self-sufficient than

Table 12.7. Comparison with previous studies.

Author	Year	Control signal	Type of signal	Functionalities		Assessment		
				Link selection	Asynchrony	Subjects		Avg. accuracy
Mankoff *et al* [7]	2002	N.d.	Endogenous	Dichotomous tree	None	—	—	—
Tomori and Moore [29]	2003	N.d.	Endogenous	Dichotomous tree	None	—	—	—
Karim *et al* [17]	2006	SCP	Endogenous	Dichotomous tree	None	1	ALS	80.00%
Bensch *et al* [18]	2007	SCP/SMR	Endogenous	Dichotomous tree	None	—	—	—
Mugler *et al* [24]	2010	P300	Exogenous	Node tagging	Read command	3	ALS	72.00%
						10	CS	93.40%
Sirvent Blasco *et al* [31]	2012	P300	Exogenous	Virtual cursor	Read command	4	CS	93.00%
Yu *et al* [42]	2012	P300/SMR	Both	Virtual cursor	Threshold	7	CS	93.21%
Present study	2019	P300	Exogenous	Node tagging	Threshold	16	MS	84.14%
						5	CS	95.75%

N.d.: not defined, SCP: slow cortical potentials, SMR: sensory-motor rhythms, ALS: amyotrophic lateral sclerosis patients, MS: multiple sclerosis patients, CS: control subjects.

other previous approaches [7, 17, 18, 29, 31, 42], the main advantage lies in the asynchronous management. In our study, users can experiment a free surfing navigation without undesirable selections, even if they are not paying attention to the visual stimuli. The threshold-based approach therefore avoids the use of constant supervision [7, 17, 18, 29] or the inclusion of a 'read mode' command [24, 31]. As a result, users can read a website or watch a video without pausing the application. This strategy makes the control of the system smoother and less demanding, which is especially desirable for end users that suffer from physical limitations.

Table 12.7 also reflects one of the greatest drawbacks of the BCI literature, which is the lack of evaluation with end users. Indeed, Mankoff *et al*, Tomori and Moore and Bensch *et al* did not test their approaches with any subject [7, 18, 29]; while Sirvent Blasco *et al* and Yu *et al* only tested their BCI web browsers with healthy subjects [31, 42]. Since CS accuracies have been observed to be higher than those obtained by motor-disabled subjects [24], care must be taken when generalizing those results for a population of end users. Moreover, there has been observed a great inter-session variability in the performance of MS patients. In our evaluation, MS patients achieved an average accuracy of 84.14%, which is higher than those reported in previous studies with ALS patients [17, 24]. Indeed, significant differences have been found between our work and Mugler *et al* (Mann–Whitney U Test, p-value: 0.0193) [24]. Note that Karim *et al* only tested the system with 1 ALS patient, and thus the statistical analysis cannot be performed [17]. It is also worth mentioning that our study has been tested with a larger population of end users (16). Similarly, CS users reached a higher average accuracy (95.75%) than those reported by Mugler *et al* (93.40%), Sirvent Blasco *et al* (93.00%) or Yu *et al* (93.21%) [24, 31, 42], although this increase is not significant (Mann–Whitney U Test, p-value>0.05).

According to the experimental outcomes, it has been demonstrated that our P300-based BCI web browser allows disabled users to experiment a comprehensive navigation through the Internet. Nevertheless, several limitations can be pointed point. The asynchronous mode of the system is handled by a threshold-based technique, whose value depends on the classifier scores. Therefore, the threshold is no longer useful if the SWLDA classifier is updated, for instance, due to inter-session variability issues. In the end, this fact entails additional time consuming tasks to update the threshold when classifier weights change. Further endeavors could be aimed at developing filter asynchrony metrics that work independently of the classifier [28, 38–40]. Notwithstanding our assessment with end users, all of them were MS patients. The cognitive disability that commonly is present on MS is rarely presented in ALS patients, since their neurological damage is more focused in motor neurons. According to this rationale, it is suggested to test the developed BCI web browser with a population of ALS patients as a future research line. As pointed out by several participants, our browser does not allow users to alternate between lower case and capital letters, which is especially useful in user/password forms. A further improvement must be aimed at overcoming this limitation by adding an extra command with the aforementioned functionality.

12.7 Conclusion

The present chapter has introduced BCI systems as novel tools to support the communication of MS patients. In addition, an asynchronous P300-based BCI web browser to surf the Internet has been designed, developed and tested with CS and MS users. The system monitors the EEG signals of the users and processes P300 potentials to translate their intentions into application commands. Two different RCP matrices control the visual stimulation: the navigation matrix, intended to provide a fast navigation through websites; and the keyboard matrix, intended to fill out forms or write e-mails. Moreover, a threshold-based asynchronous metric has been implemented in order to avoid selections when users want to read a website. Selected commands are sent to the web browser, which provides visual feedback in real time. The BCI web browser has been tested with 5 CS and 16 MS patients, reaching average accuracies of 95.75% and 84.14%, respectively. Results also show that the reached accuracies are significantly higher those that obtained by previous approaches. All participants reported to be satisfied with the browser, which was easy to understand and use. To conclude, our P300-based BCI system has proved to be a suitable solution to provide a comprehensive navigation for disabled users, improving their personal autonomy and quality of life.

References

[1] Wolpaw J R and Wolpaw E W 2012 *Brain–Computer Interfaces: Principles and Practice* (New York: OUP)

[2] Wolpaw J R, Birbaumer N, Heetderks W J, McFarland D J, Peckham P H, Schalk G, Donchin E, Quatrano L A, Robinson C J and Vaughan T M 2000 Brain–computer interface technology: a review of the first international meeting *IEEE Trans. Rehabil. Eng.* **8** 164–73

[3] Wolpaw J R, Birbaumer N, McFarland D J, Pfurtscheller G and Vaughan T M 2002 Brain–computer interfaces for communication and control *Clin. Neurophysiol.* **113** 767–91

[4] World Health Organization 2008 Atlas: multiple sclerosis resources in the world *Vasa.* [Online]. Available: http://medcontent.metapress.com/index/A65RM03P4874243N.pdf

[5] Compston A and Coles A 2008 Multiple sclerosis *Lancet* **372** 1502–17

[6] Kemp S 2018 Digital in 2018 *Tech. Rep.* [Online]. Available: https://www.slideshare.net/wearesocial/digital-in-2018-in-southeast-asia-part-2-southeast-86866464; https://www.slideshare.net/wearesocial/digital-in-2018-in-southeast-asia-part-1-northwest-86866386; https://www.slideshare.net/wearesocial/digital-in-201

[7] Mankoff J, Dey A, Batra U and Moore M 2002 Web accessibility for low bandwidth input *Proc. Fifth Int. ACM Conf. on Assistive Technologies* **vol 9** pp 17–24 [Online]. Available: http://dl.acm.org/citation.cfm?id=638255

[8] Nicolas-Alonso L F and Gomez-Gil J 2012 Brain computer interfaces, a review *Sensors* **12** 1211–79

[9] Pastor M A, Artieda J, Arbizu J, Valencia M and Masdeu J C 2003 Human cerebral activation during steady-state visual-evoked responses *J. Neurosci.* **23** 11621–7

[10] Volosyak I, Cecotti H and Gräser A 2009 Optimal visual stimuli on LCD screens for SSVEP based brain–computer interfaces *2009 4th Int. IEEE/EMBS Conf. on Neural Engineering, NER '09* pp 447–50

[11] Farwell L A and Donchin E 1988 Talking off the top of your head: toward a mental prosthesis utilizing event-related brain potentials *Electroencephalogr. Clin. Neurophysiol.* **70** 510–23

[12] Vilic A 2013 *The AVI SSVEP Dataset* pp 1–6 [Online]. Available: http://www.setzner.com/avi-ssvep-dataset/

[13] Martínez-Cagigal V, Santamaría-Vázquez E, Gomez-Pilar J and Hornero R 2019 Towards an accessible use of smartphone-based social networks through brain–computer interfaces *Expert Syst. Appl.* **120** 155–66

[14] Real R, Erlbeck H, Herweg A, Sollfrank T, Kübler A and Kleih S C 2004 *Slow Cortical Potential Training in Stroke* p 1 [Online]. Available: http://bnci-horizon-2020.eu/database/data-sets

[15] Pfurtscheller G and Schlögl A 2003 *Competition II - Dataset III (Motor Imagery)* pp 1–2 2003. [Online]. Available: http://www.bbci.de/competition/ii/

[16] Hinterberger T, Schmidt S, Neumann N, Mellinger J, Blankertz B, Curio G and Birbaumer N 2004 Brain-computer communication and slow cortical potentials *IEEE Trans. Biomed. Eng.* **51** 1011–8

[17] Karim A A, Hinterberger T, Richter J, Mellinger J, Neumann N, Flor H, Kubler A and Birbaumer N 2006 Neural internet: web surfing with brain potentials for the completely paralyzed *Neurorehabil. Neural Repair* **20** 508–15

[18] Bensch M, Karim A A, Mellinger J, Hinterberger T, Tangermann M, Bogdan M, Rosenstiel W and Birbaumer N 2007 Nessi: An EEG-controlled web browser for severely paralyzed patients *Comput. Intell. Neurosci.* **2007** 71863

[19] Reilly B 2013 *Mu Rhythm* (New York: Springer) pp 1940–41

[20] Pfurtscheller G and Lopes da Silva F H 1999 Event-related EEG/MEG synchronization and desynchronization: basic principles *Clin. Neurophysiol.* **110** 1842–57

[21] Neuper C, Scherer R, Reiner M and Pfurtscheller G 2005 Imagery of motor actions: Differential effects of kinesthetic and visual-motor mode of imagery in single-trial EEG *Cogn. Brain Res.* **25** 668–77

[22] Wierzgała P, Zapała D, Wojcik G M and Masiak J 2018 Most popular signal processing methods in motor-imagery BCI: a review and meta-analysis *Front. Neuroinform.* **12** 1–10

[23] Kübler A, Holz E and Kaufmann T 2013 Bringing BCI controlled devices to end-users: a user centred approach and evaluation *Converging Clinical and Engineering Research on Neurorehabilitation* (Berlin: Springer) pp 1271–4

[24] Mugler E M, Ruf C A, Halder S, Bensch M and Kübler A 2010 Design and implementation of a P300-based brain–computer interface for controlling an internet browser *IEEE Trans. Neural Syst. Rehabil. Eng.* **18** 599–609

[25] McCane L M, Sellers E W, Mcfarland D J, Mak J N, Carmack C S, Zeitlin D, Wolpaw J R and Vaughan T M 2014 Brain–computer interface (BCI) evaluation in people with amyotrophic lateral sclerosis *Amyotroph. Lateral Scler. Frontotemporal Degener.* **15** 207–15

[26] Picton T W 1992 The P300 wave of the human event-related potential *J. Clin. Neurophysiol.* **9** 456–79

[27] Nicolas-Alonso L F, Corralejo R, Gomez-Pilar J, Álvarez D and Hornero R 2015 Adaptive semi-supervised classification to reduce intersession non-stationarity in multiclass motor imagery-based brain-computer interfaces *Neurocomputing* **159** 186–96

[28] Pinegger A, Faller J, Halder S, Wriessnegger S C and Müller-Putz G R 2015 Control or non-control state: that is the question! An asynchronous visual P300-based BCI approach *J. Neural Eng.* **12** 14001
[29] Tomori O and Moore M 2003 The neurally controllable internet browser (BrainBrowser) *CHI '03 extended abstracts on Human factors in computing systems - CHI '03* p 796
[30] Moore M M 2003 Real-world applications for brain–computer interface technology *IEEE Trans. Neural Syst. Rehabil. Eng.* **11** 162–5
[31] Sirvent Blasco J, Iáñez E, Úbeda A and Azorín J 2012 Visual evoked potential-based brainmachine interface applications to assist disabled people *Expert Syst. Appl.* **39** 7908–18
[32] Zhang H, Guan C and Wang C 2008 Asynchronous P300-based brain–computer interfaces: a computational approach with statistical models *IEEE Trans. Biomed. Eng.* **55** 1754–63
[33] Li Y, Pan J, Wang F and Yu Z 2013 A hybrid BCI system combining P300 and SSVEP and its application to wheelchair control *IEEE Trans. Biomed. Eng.* **60** 3156–66
[34] He S, Zhang R, Wang Q, Chen Y, Yang T, Feng Z, Zhang Y, Shao M and Li Y 2017 A P300-based threshold-free brain switch and its application in wheelchair control *IEEE Trans. Neural Syst. Rehabil. Eng.* **25** 715–25
[35] Aloise F, Schettini F, Aricò P, Leotta F, Salinari S, Mattia D, Babiloni F and Cincotti F 2011 P300-based brain-computer interface for environmental control: an asynchronous approach *J. Neural Eng.* **8** 025025
[36] Breitwieser C, Pokorny C and Müller-Putz G R 2016 A hybrid three-class brain–computer interface system utilizing SSSEPs and transient ERPs *J. Neural Eng.* **13** 066015
[37] Tang J, Liu Y, Jiang J, Yu Y, Hu D and Zhou Z 2018 Toward brain-actuated mobile platform *Int. J. Hum.-Comput. Interact.* **35** 846–58
[38] Panicker R C, Puthusserypady S, Pryana A P and Sun Y 2010 Asynchronous P300 BCI: SSVEP-based control state detection *Eur. Signal Process. Conf.* **58** 934–8
[39] Liu Y, Ayaz H, Curtin A, Shewokis P A and Onaral B 2012 Detection of attention shift for asynchronous P300-based BCI *Proc. of the Annual Int. Conf. of the IEEE Engineering in Medicine and Biology Society, EMBS* pp 3850–3
[40] Ma Z and Qiu T 2018 Quasi-periodic fluctuation in Donchin's speller signals and its potential use for asynchronous control *Biomed. Tech.* **63** 105–12
[41] Minguillon J, Lopez-Gordo M A and Pelayo F 2017 Trends in EEG-BCI for daily-life: Requirements for artifact removal *Biomed. Signal Process. Control* **31** 407–18
[42] Yu T, Li Y, Long J and Gu Z 2012 Surfing the internet with a BCI mouse *J. Neural Eng.* **9** 036012
[43] Jasper H H 1958 The ten-twenty electrode system of the international federation *Electroencephalogr. Clin. Neurophysiol.* **10** 371–5
[44] Schalk G, McFarland D J, Hinterberger T, Birbaumer N and Wolpaw J R 2004 BCI2000: A general-purpose brain–computer interface (BCI) system *IEEE Trans. Biomed. Eng.* **51** 1034–43
[45] Krusienski D, Sellers E, McFarland D, Vaughan T and Wolpaw J 2008 Toward enhanced P300 speller performance *J. Neurosci. Methods* **167** 15–21
[46] Krusienski D J, Sellers E W, Cabestaing F, Bayoudh S, McFarland D J, Vaughan T M and Wolpaw J R 2006 A comparison of classification techniques for the P300 Speller *J. Neural Eng.* **3** 299–305
[47] Keinosuke F 1990 *Introduction to Statistical Pattern Recognition* (New York: Academic)

[48] Corralejo R, Nicolás-Alonso L F, Álvarez D and Hornero R 2014 A P300-based brain-computer interface aimed at operating electronic devices at home for severely disabled people *Med. Biol. Eng. Comput.* **52** 861–72

[49] Sellers E W and Donchin E 2006 A P300-based brain–computer interface: initial tests by ALS patients *Clin. Neurophysiol.* **117** 538–48

[50] Sellers E W, Krusienski D J, McFarland D J, Vaughan T M and Wolpaw J R 2006 A P300 event-related potential brain–computer interface (BCI): the effects of matrix size and inter stimulus interval on performance *Biol. Psychol.* **73** 242–52

[51] Narsky I and Porter F C 2013 *Statistical Analysis Techniques in Particle Physics: Fits, Density Estimation and Supervised Learning* (New York: Wiley)

[52] Likert R 1932 A technique for the measurement of attitudes *Arch. Psychol.* **22** 55

[53] Nicolas-Alonso L F, Corralejo R, Gomez-Pilar J, Álvarez D and Hornero R 2015 Adaptive semi-supervised classification to reduce intersession non-stationarity in multiclass motor imagery-based brain–computer interfaces *Neurocomputing* **159** 186–96

[54] Townsend G, LaPallo B K, Boulay C B, Krusienski D J, Frye G E, Hauser C K, Schwartz N E, Vaughan T M, Wolpaw J R and Sellers E W 2010 A novel P300-based brain-computer interface stimulus presentation paradigm: moving beyond rows and columns *Clin. Neurophysiol.* **121** 1109–20

IOP Publishing

Neurological Disorders and Imaging Physics, Volume 2
Engineering and clinical perspectives of multiple sclerosis
Ayman El-Baz and Jasjit S Suri

Chapter 13

Language, speech and voice symptomatology (dysarthria) in multiple sclerosis: electroglottographic and acoustic analysis for assessment

Kostas Konstantopoulos and Dimitrios Karangioules

Multiple sclerosis (MS) is defined as an adult onset incurable and chronic autoimmune neurodegenerative disease of the central nervous system (CNS) of unknown etiology. The disease affects white matter and periventricular areas in the brain, brainstem, cerebellum, spinal cord, and optic nerves.

The general neurological symptomatology of MS involves sensory disturbances, bowel and bladder dysfunction, unilateral loss of vision or double vision, limb weakness, fatigue, ataxia, dysphagia, cognitive deficits, language abnormalities, and dysarthria (speech/voice disturbances). Respiratory and facial paralysis are also involved in 10% of the patients, as well as facial myokymia and trigeminal neuralgia. Body tremor is often noticed, while less often, tremor of speech is observed [1].

Cognitive dysfunctions in MS affect the perception, intelligence, imagination, memory planning, reasoning and lead to difficulties in information processing speed, memory and executive functions including language [2, 3]. There is some literature discussing the relationship of cognition to language in MS [4, 5]. One longitudinal study involving 38 patients, found that from one point of view, depressed mood and anxiety were predictors of cognitive change while from another point of view patients' negative affect was a predictor of a decline in episodic memory in newly learned verbal information [4]. Another study, showed that depression and fatigue were correlated with slowing of information processing, lower verbal fluency, fewer digits recalled from immediate memory, long-term memory, and difficulties in immediate and delayed recall of complex visual information [5].

One meta-analysis study included 57 studies with 2042 participants diagnosed with relapsing–remitting MS and found that general cognitive ability, attention/

executive ability and memory/learning, were significantly more affected than verbal functions/language, and concept formation/reasoning. However, language deficits and verbal functions were found to distinguish patients with MS as compared to healthy controls [6]. A fairly recent systematic review [7] examined language impairments in 1745 MS patients. The study found that language impairments were infrequent but affected verbal fluency, lexical access, and language comprehension. There was also found a correlation between language and executive functions.

Cognitive-linguistic deficits were also strongly related to dysarthria (speech/voice abnormalities). The deterioration of the corresponding functions was global, affecting language, comprehension, while episodic memory and linguistic expression were significantly affected [8].

In contrast to language dysarthria is frequently affected at the early stages of the disease and worsens as the disease advances [1, 9]. Later on, reduced vital capacity, inadequate ventilation and breathing disturbances are the most common symptoms that may affect speech/voice and they are more apparent during disease exacerbations. Generalized respiratory or diaphragmatic muscle weakness, difficulties in breathing, voice coordination and bulbar weakness may also contribute to the severity of dysarthria. Regarding speech, some researchers emphasize that the tongue function is severely more affected than the lips function [10].

Dysarthria is defined as a neurological motor deprivation that is followed by lack of muscle control affecting the subsystems of speech (respiration, voice, resonance, articulation, prosody). According to various researchers, it is produced by impairment of any of the basic motor processes and the outcome consists of slow, weak/asthenic inaccurate and uncoordinated speech muscle movements [1, 11, 12].

The dysarthria type in MS is variable mostly mixed, spastic and/or ataxic reflecting the variability of lesions in the CNS. So, most of the studies that investigate dysarthria in MS involve patients with a mixed type dysarthria. However, other types are also found and include, the flaccid, the hypokinetic and the hyperkinetic dysarthria types. Each dysarthria can appear individually or combined, for example mixed flaccid–spastic, mixed ataxic–hypokinetic, etc [1, 11, 12]. Rarely, one type of sudden dysarthria characteristics, also called paroxysmal dysarthria, occurs in MS.

Neuroanatomically, ataxic dysarthria relates to damage to the cerebellar control circuit [1]. Bilateral lesions have been associated with the most severe dysarthria deficits and unilateral lesions with mild to moderate dysarthria [13, 14]. Spastic dysarthria is due to damage to the direct and indirect pathways of the CNS. Unilateral lesions do not have an important effect on jaw, velopharyngeal, laryngeal and lingual speech movements while the opposite occurs with bilateral lesions. Also, when acute lesions are confirmed, muscle tone is affected and weakness emerges, further evolving to spasticity and increased tone. Since the muscles that are involved in speech movements, are interwoven with fine and discrete movements, they tend to be significantly affected [1].

The prevalence of dysarthria in MS varies between 34%–56% [1, 9, 15–21]. The different percentages in the prevalence of dysarthria may be due to different numbers of participants and/or different stages of the disease.

Instead of dysarthria and articulation alone, there are a number of studies that give emphasis on voice characteristics [9, 17, 18, 22]. Some studies show that the voice abnormalities are more frequent than speech abnormalities. Hartelius [17] employed a large sample of 200 MS participants and found that the most frequent dysarthria symptoms were weak voice (43%), difficulty getting started (34%) and imprecise articulation (33%). Konstantopoulos [18] reported 45.3% of 64 MS patients presented voice and/or articulation difficulties and Yamout [22] reported that vocal fatigue and vocal breaks were the most occurrent symptoms, but it was stated that they may coexist with dysarthria. Finally, one study [9] found many voice symptoms that were in high occurrence including glottal fry (88%), harshness (86%), loudness level (68%), pitch variation (69%), strained/strangled (62%) and pitch level (57%), with the first three being the most prevalent.

Most of the researches show that dysarthria in MS is generally mild to moderate in severity [20, 21, 23], even though there have been some studies that also found a severe type of dysarthria [9]. The dysarthria is mostly common in primary progressive and secondary progressive MS types [9, 22]. It also affects the quality of life in MS patients [20], even though it is not directly related to disease duration. Medication does not seem to improve dysarthria in MS. It is only reported in single case studies and involves only one form of dysarthria, paroxysmal ataxia and dysarthria [24].

The severity of dysarthria signs results in a reduction of the speaker's speech intelligibility, rhythm, and communication proficiency. The combination of ataxic and spastic characteristics in MS dysarthria contribute to the disturbed prosodic functions showing slowness of individual movements and repetition. In turn, the reduction of range and force of the articulation structures and velopharyngeal movements results in the appearance of imprecise consonants, vowel distortions, and hypernasality. As a result, speech rate is compromised resulting in reduced loudness and vowel duration.

Rarely, paroxysmal dysarthria (PD) and paroxysmal dysarthria with ataxia (PDA) has been found in patients with MS [25, 26]. This dysarthria type is characterized by sudden short-timed episodes of dysarthria. PD shows higher prevalence than PDA according to one study [27]. It is also acknowledged that these types coexist with other pathological findings such as trigeminal neuralgia, tonic seizures, ataxia, and paroxysmal akinesia, that indicate an underlying neurological pathology [25, 27]. However, one study [28] reported that there are disagreements in the scientific community about the existence of PDA and/or PD symptomatology exclusively in MS and not in other neurological diseases.

In order to help the reader to understand the relation between perceptual dysarthria signs and objective quantitative assessment, a discussion of the theoretical aspects of objective quantitative assessment of voice (electroglottography) and speech (acoustic analysis) will be mentioned first, and a discussion about perceptual symptomatology/objective quantitative assessment with follow.

13.1 Objective instrumental measurements of voice (electroglottography)

Standardization of voice quality assessment includes assessments such as the subjective self-evaluation of voice, the perceptual ratings of voice and the objective/instrumental measures [29]. In standard clinical practice, self-assessment (completed by the patient) and perceptual assessment (completed by the examiner) are most common but they have the disadvantage of low inter-rater agreement.

In general, instrumental measures have the advantage of providing more objectivity in the quantification to the measurement and often include methods such as electroglottography, videostroboscopy, acoustic analysis, aerodynamics and speed single-line scanning (video-kymography) [30]. In MS, electroglottography and acoustic analysis are mostly used for voice/speech analysis and so our discussion will be limited to these two methods. Rarely, physiological methods and measures such as tongue transducers were used to search range, force, and rapid alternating movements (diadochokinesis) of lip and tongue function [10]. The results of this study showed the importance of the assessment of the tongue by finding correlations of its movement with the severity of neurological deficit and years of disease progression. Since 2003, the results of this study however, were not replicated.

13.2 Electroglottography definition and description

Electroglottography (EGG) or electrolaryngography [31] is a noninvasive electrical method invented by Fabre [32] to measure rate and regularity of vocal fold vibration during voicing. The aim of electroglottography is to monitor vocal fold closure and to record changes of vocal fold vibration during voiced sounds. More specifically, the electroglottographic signal is the product of conductance (ease with where electric current flows through a substance, in our case human tissue) or impedance (opposition that an electric circuit offers to electric current) by using two isolated ring electrodes at the level of thyroid alae and passing a current of 0.3–0.5 MHz between them during the production of voiced sounds. Air is considered a poor conductor of electricity (vocal folds open) while tissue is a moderately good conductor of electricity (vocal folds closed and vibrate). When the vocal folds are closed, the impedance of the electrical current flow across the neck is reduced while the opposite occurs when the vocal folds are open. This phenomenon causes a detectable signal change at the receiving electrode which can be converted into a waveform representing variations in impedance. So, during the glottal cycle (opening and closing of the vocal folds) the electrical impedance in the larynx is increased when the glottis is open (air between the vocal folds) and decreased when the glottis gradually closes. Figure 13.1 shows a generic diagram of a typical electroglottographic setting for recording.

In electroglottography, there is production of two waveform signals during the stages of a vocal fold cycle. In Fourcin's electroglottography these are defined as the Gx signal and Lx signal (see figure 13.1). The Lx signal shows the glottal behavior that is taking place while the Gx signal shows additional changes in impedance

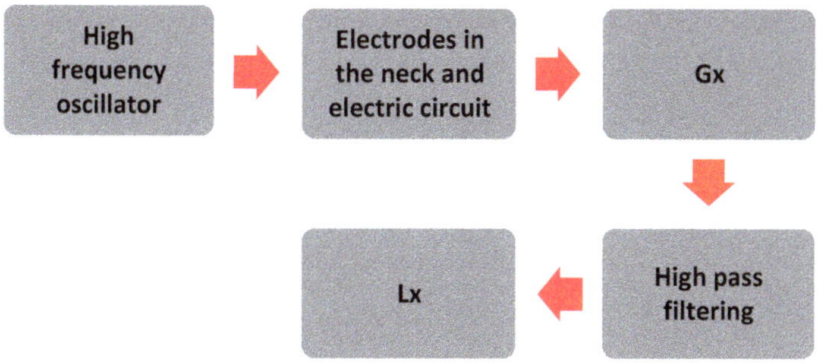

Figure 13.1. Block diagram of a typical electroglottograph.

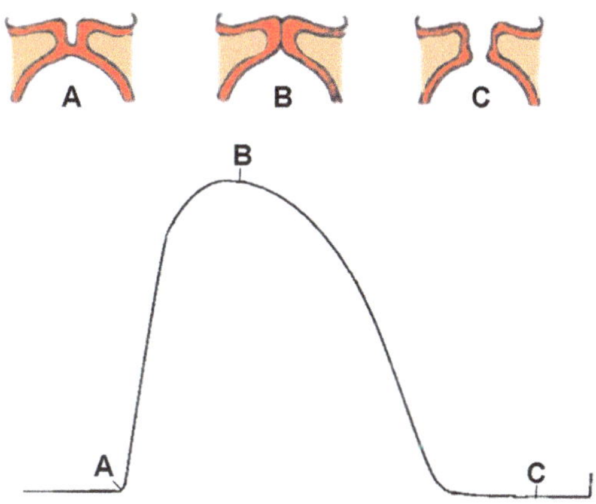

Figure 13.2. Closing and opening phases of the vocal folds in a cycle.

before and after phonation such as changes due to tissue characteristics or swallowing during voicing. Filtering of unwanted movements in the vocal tract is useful to produce the Lx signal from the Gx signal in order to show impedance variations during voicing. The end product (Lx signal) has peaks when there is contact of the vocal folds (minimal impedance) and troughs when there is no contact of vocal folds (maximal impedance). More specifically, the start of each steep rise in the Lx output is associated with the onset of vocal fold closure, the peak of each cycle is associated with maximal closure (horizontal and vertical) and the trough is associated with vocal fold separation [33]. Figure 13.2 shows the electroglottographic view of a typical cycle and three corresponding positions of the vocal folds. In this figure, letter A corresponds to the beginning of the closing phase of the vocal folds, letter B corresponds to the maximum closure of the vocal folds and letter C corresponds to the full opening phase of the vocal folds.

Fourcin [34] reports that uniform Lx peaks are associated with uniform acoustic output, a sharp Lx contact (point A) is associated with good acoustic excitation and a long closure duration is associated with undamped formants (they will be explained in the section about acoustic analysis). Even though some authors have doubts about the exact agreement between vocal fold contact and the Lx waveform [35], others report that the EGG signal helps in the accurate analysis of voice by giving emphasis on the vocal fold contact and so improves accuracy in acoustic measurements where other methods are less efficient [36].

Commercially, there are many software programs of electroglottography but in this discussion we will give emphasis to the definitions in the electroglottographic variables given by Abberton [33] in order to help the reader to understand the results of the studies that measured voice in MS.

Most of the measures that can be derived from electroglottography will be discussed in the findings of voice in MS below but generally include measures derived from the vibration of the vocal folds such as mean fundamental frequency, fundamental frequency range, durations of continuous laryngeal activity corresponding to voiced portions and speech, measures of vocal fold closed and open phases in each vibratory cycle, etc.

13.3 Acoustic analysis of speech

According to the acoustic theory of speech production [37], the speech sounds are produced with different modifications of the vocal tract. So, fricatives are produced with a constricted vocal tract, nasals are produced with an open nasal cavity while vowels are produced with an open vocal tract. In this way, the vocal tract functions as a resonator or as a filter that enhances specific frequencies from the acoustic energy (the product of the vibrating vocal folds). Having in mind that sounds, words and sentences are produced with different shapes of the vocal tract, different resonant frequencies (spectral peaks) are produced.

In acoustic theory (source–filter theory of vowel production), the output may be explained by the equation [38]:

$P(f) = U(f)\ T(f)\ R(f)$ where

$P(f)$ = speech sound pressure when the sound comes out of the mouth

f = frequency

U = Volume velocity (voice source of the vocal folds)

T = Transfer function (resonances)

R = Radiation characteristic (changes when speech comes out of the oral cavity)

According to Fant [37] lower resonant frequencies are produced by a longer vocal tract and higher resonant frequencies are produced by a shorter vocal tract. So, the length of the vocal tract and its cross-sectional area are important factors to determine each sound.

A spectrum is a graph that shows the distribution of energy and more specifically the frequency in the horizontal axis (measured in Hz) and amplitude in vertical axis (measured in dB). The spectrum is shaped by the resonances (formants) of the vocal tract. A formant of a sound is related to the shape of the vocal tract at a specific time and it produces the characteristic quality of this sound. In the spectrum, there are peaks that represent harmonics (multiples) of the fundamental frequency in the vibrating vocal folds. Harmonics are tones whole-number multiples of fundamental frequency. In each speech sound, there are 3–4 formants with numerical values (in

Hz) that can distinguish one sound from another but more especially the vowels. Each formant has a center frequency and a bandwidth (rate of damping in energy).

The acoustic analysis of speech calculates the formants of sounds that modify the energy produced by the vocal folds. The frequency of the first formant varies inversely with the height of tongue during the production of a vowel. So, a higher first formant frequency is produced with a lower tongue position. Along the same lines, the frequency of the second formant is related to tongue advancement and so, as the position of the tongue advances in the oral cavity the frequency of the second formant is increased. Finally, a longer vocal tract in length (as when the lips are rounded) produces lower formant frequencies. Each vowel, it is characterized by the patterns of its formants, the peaks, its duration, and its fundamental frequency. Produced speech frequencies are below 8000 Hz while our ears may detect frequencies from 16–20 000 Hz. Even though the vowels can easily be characterized, the consonants have inherent difficulties in description based on differences in their characteristics of production such as noise, obstruction of the vocal tract, nasal quality (such in /m/ and /n/), etc.

The perturbation theory predicts formant frequencies based on the constrictions of the vocal tract when different sounds are produced. As a general rule, a constriction in an area close to larynx increases the three formant frequencies while a constriction in the lips decreases the three formant frequencies, etc. As was mentioned before, the decrease of all formant frequencies can also be accomplished by the lengthening of the vocal tract and this is the result of lip protrusion, and a decreased movement of the larynx.

The acoustic analysis of speech can also be attained in a graph showing energy change over time, called a spectrogram. The spectrogram is depicted in a graph in which time is on the horizontal axis, frequency is on the vertical axis and intensity varies by the colour (black) of the graph. The spectrogram is an efficient way to depict speech because speech is produced rapidly and the spectrogram has the adequate sensitivity for such measurement [38]. Figure 13.3(a) shows one spectrogram of a pair-matched healthy control participant (age, gender, education) to an MS patient (figure 13.3(b)). In both figures, there is a quick repetition of three syllables of /pa/ (in speech assessment this task is called diadochokinesis). The acoustic analysis of the healthy participant shows the duration of the sound /p/in the first /pa/ syllable (6 ms), the duration of the vowel /a/ in the first /pa/ syllable (124 ms), the silence between the first /pa/ syllable and the second /pa/ syllable (83 ms), and so on.

Figure 13.3(b) shows the same /pa/ production of an MS patient exhibiting severe dysarthria. Notice the production of the first sound /p/ (9 ms) and the lack of production of the sound /p/ in all other /pa/ syllables. Also, there is an increase in the duration in all vowels as compared to the healthy control participant (first /a/ = 200 ms, second /a/ = 292 ms, and third /a/ = 311 ms). Finally, the silence between the first /pa/ and the second /pa/ was increased as compared to the healthy control participant (198 ms). Note, that severe dysarthria in figure 3b results in vowel production with a continuous energy repetition and no silence (lack of consonant in the 2nd and 3rd /a/ production).

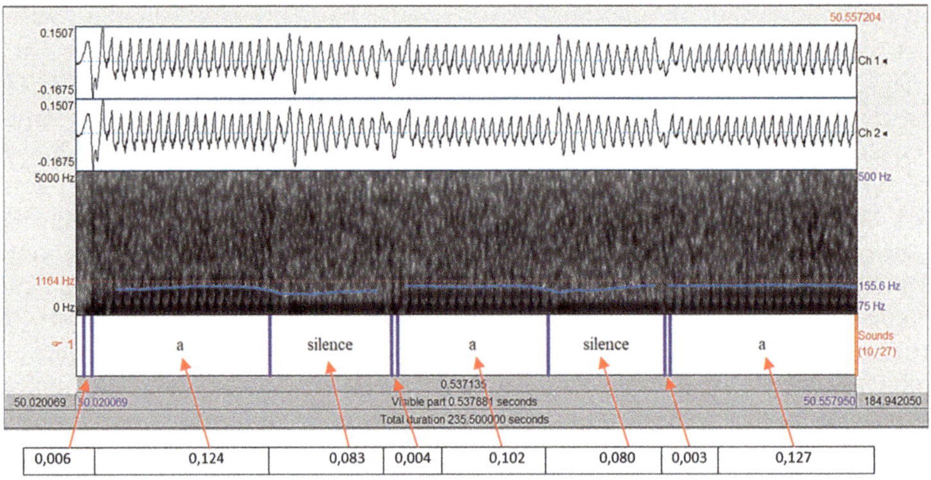

(a)

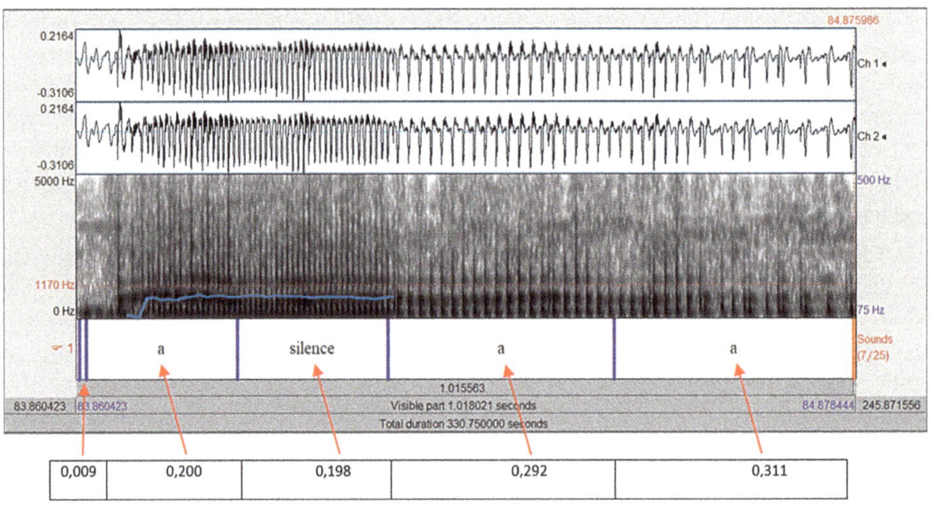

(b)

Figure 13.3. (a) Rapid production of diadochokinesis of the sound /pa/ in a healthy participant. (b) Rapid production of diadochokinesis of the sound /pa/ in a MS patient with severe dysarthria.

The comparison between acoustic analysis and EGG shows that the first gives emphasis to the acoustic characteristics of the whole vocal tract as opposed to electroglottography which gives emphasis on the product of vocal folds while vibrating. In both methods, there are variables that overlap, but acoustic analysis and electroglottography have different ways to extract these variables.

Technically, the acoustic analysis is using a high-quality recording of a voice sample through a microphone, a digitization technique (analog to digital process) and a software analysis of the signal. A variation in an electrical voltage from speech will be received by the microphone that is sensitive to voltage changes in the air pressure. The amount of movement is related to the amplitude of a sound and so, a large speech movement is perceived as a loud sound and a short speech movement is perceived as a soft sound. Filtering, either inverse filtering or commonly linear predictive coding (LPC) is also used for the provision of a clear acoustic signal.

A number of acoustic variables extracted by the acoustic signal involve durations, the short-term fundamental frequency perturbation, the short-term amplitude perturbation, the harmonics to noise ratio, the long-term frequency and amplitude modulation, the formant frequencies, etc. Most of them will be discussed under the electroglottographic results in MS and so no further discussion will be given here.

The calculation of duration, amplitude and fundamental frequency of a speech sample that is depicted as a sound pressure waveform (spectrum or spectrogram) takes place by selecting the part of the sample we prefer to analyze. The basic concept of Fourier, a French mathematician, is that periodic waveforms can be analyzed as sinusoidal components. This concept may be applied to speech because the resonant frequencies of the vocal tract are periodic waveforms. As another method of analysis, Fast Fourier Transform (FFT) can also be used for speech analysis due to the quasiperiodic nature of speech. Its product is a spectrum having components such as harmonics. Also, the LPC is based on the assumption that any speech sample is a linear function of those that precede it. LPC analysis is based on formant frequencies and resonances rather than harmonics of the fundamental (Fourier analysis).

The product of acoustic analysis in voice assessment is fundamental frequency or frequency of the vibrating vocal folds, and it takes place after a software application from the recorded sample received by the microphone through the mouth of the speaker. However, period by period analysis of fundamental frequency in electroglottography is preferable rather than acoustic analysis because it systematically records voice cycle by cycle.

Regarding the tasks for assessment, in either electroglottography or acoustic analysis, the objective assessment of speech/voice requires a high quality digital recording taking place in a sound-proofed or a quiet room, a 10 cm mouth-to-microphone distance and tasks such as sustained vowel production (maximum prolongation of a sound), reading or monologue and diadochokinesis. The logic behind the sustained vowel production (usually the /a/ sound and less often the /i/ sound) is that there is no influence of articulation and other phenomena that are produced in the vocal tract during phonation. Additionally, reading is preferred over monologue because it provides a standard passage for comparison among patients.

13.4 Variables of electroglottographic analysis during sustained phonation

In sustained phonation, either electroglottography or acoustic analysis can be used to measure variables such as fundamental frequency, jitter, shimmer, and signal-to-noise ratio (SNR).

The frequency of a sound wave is defined as the number of regular fluctuations which occur in a given period of time. So, a waveform that is repeated every 0.02 s has a frequency of 200 Hz. In voice, frequency is the rate at which a voicing source vibrates creating vocal fold vibration repetition and it correlates perceptually with pitch. It is measured in Hz (number of cycles per second). The fundamental frequency (Fx in Fourcin's electroglottograph) can be defined as the lowest frequency of a periodic waveform. Fx in EGG is considered as a more reliable measure than acoustics because it measures fundamental frequency directly from the voice source, the vibrating vocal folds [36].

In sustained phonation, variables such as the average fundamental frequency and the jitter are calculated from the Lx waveform on a cycle-by-cycle basis as a contrast to the acoustic signal in which they are derived from the end product in the mouth. The average fundamental frequency of the vibrating vocal folds is defined as the addition of a number of cycles (1 divided by the time to complete one vibratory cycle) and divided by the number of cycles. Jitter is the perturbation of the waveform frequency and percent jitter is defined as the average temporal perturbation divided by the average vocal fold cycle duration and multiplied by 100 (percent change in cycle duration between cycles). In other words, jitter is the percentage of change in cycle duration between cycles. It is referred as a measure of vocal stability and in normal voice is less than 1% of frequency variability. Elevated jitter corresponds to hoarse, harsh or rough voice quality.

Shimmer is alternative to jitter in amplitude, it is defined as the amplitude perturbation of changes and it is measured on the peak amplitude of the waveform. Elevated shimmer corresponds to abnormal voice quality such as hoarseness, and shimmer like jitter is regarded as a measure of vocal stability. Shimmer is measured in decibels (dB).

Another variable to measure voice quality in sustained phonation is called contact quotient (Qx in electroglottography). It is defined as the mean percentage of time the vocal folds are closed, with a closure width 70% down from positive peak (maximum closure) and it is divided by the mean total closure time. There is a relationship between closed quotient and voice quality and so, less vocal fold contact during the vocal cycle corresponds to a breathier voice. Qx is expressed as a percentage and a 50% value indicates vocal fold in contact for half the time period of the cycle. The MDVP program (Laryngograph Ltd) measures contact during the cycle if it is at the upper 70% or above of the peak amplitude, covering all stages of the cycle where there is some vocal fold contact.

13.5 Variables of electroglottographic analysis during connected speech

Connected speech analysis (reading a standard passage and/or monologue) has the advantage of more representation of normal conversation instead of sustained phonation. The speech studio software (Laryngograph Ltd) provides quantitative analysis of connected speech including frequency, amplitude, contact quotient and different combinations of these measures. The frequency is illustrated in a histogram with variables such as DFx1 mean (distribution of frequencies 1), DFx2 mean (distribution of frequencies 2), CFx, DQx1 mean (distribution of closed phases of vocal folds 1), DQx2 mean (distribution of closed phases of vocal folds 2), or combined measures such the QxFx mean measure.

According to the specific software program, Dx is the general distribution of fundamental frequencies during voiced speech on a probability histogram and it gives a measure of vocal fold closure regularity. Dx is plotted on a logarithmic scale corresponding to perceived pitch. Its frequency axis is divided into 128 logarithmically equal spaced 'bins' having an overall range from 30.52–1000 Hz. Each bin is a few Hz in width [33] and it is presented in two orders (first order and second order).

The first order (DFx1 mean) gives the raw data while the second order (DFx2 mean) includes pairs of laryngeal periods that occurred twice in the same statistical 'bin'. Both orders represent vocal fold regularity [33, 34, 39] and are explained in the next paragraphs.

More specifically, DFx1 mean (first order distribution) is defined as the probability larynx frequency distribution (frequency regularity) of each vocal fold cycle during voice speech. It is measured in Hz. The software program splits the frequency range into consecutive intervals and divides the number of vocal fold cycles into 3% steps falling in each interval by the total number of vocal fold cycles in the speech sample [40]. It is plotted horizontally on a logarithmic scale and vertically on the probability of occurrence of a particular frequency. It takes into account all periods of the vibrating vocal folds (Tx).

DFx2 mean is defined as the distribution of **successive pairs** of vocal fold cycles in a 3% frequency bin and it represents regular periodic vocal fold cycles over at least two cycles. Theoretically, the second order distribution is preferable to the first order because it does not include data irrelevant to voicing such as swallowing or excessive gross laryngeal movement during recording.

CFx is an indicator of pitch irregularity. It is actually a scatterplot of each fundamental frequency against the one following and it is comparable to first order Dx plot. In this measure the frequency of each vocal fold cycle is plotted against the frequency of the next cycle. In normal voice this is depicted as a diagonal plot. So, when irregularity increases there is an increase in the amount of scatter of frequencies. CFx is depicted as a scattergram (representation of points referencing two variables and showing their relationship, stronger where the points are clustered closest together) that plots successive Fx period by period and looks at the differences in the frequencies of successive periods. It is a reflection of vocal regularity expressed as a percentage (similar to jitter in sustained phonation).

Qx is defined as the mean percentage of time the vocal folds are closed (measured 70% down from the waveform peak) to the total period and it is related to the quality of excitation of the vocal tract as the vocal folds vibrate [39, 41, 42]. It is derived from the electroglottographic waveform (Lx) by determining the period of time between closing and opening of the vocal folds. Like frequency it may be represented in two orders, first order and second order (DQx1 mean and DQx2 mean). DQx1 mean is a probability distribution for the closed phases of each vocal fold cycle. The peak of plot is the most commonly occurring value (modal voice).

DQx2 mean is an indicator of irregularity, and it includes the adjacent vocal cycles. A breathy voice corresponds to decreases in Qx value and a suppressed voice with values above normal. A better closed phase includes similar DQx1 and DQx2 mean measures.

13.6 Findings of perceptual, acoustic and electroglottographic variables in MS

In MS, the literature states variable dysarthria symptomatology including voice quality, articulation/speech rate, and prosody [1, 19–23, 43] and more specifically:

- Vocal tension control (tension in the muscles that affect the production of voice).
- Hoarseness (voice sounds strained and raspy).
- Breathy voice (more air than normal flows causing a murmured sounding voice).
- Vocal tremor (tremulous unsteady voice).
- Reduced maximum phonation (maximum time someone can sustain a vowel during exhalation).
- Vocal fatigue (fatigued voice).
- Voice breakdowns (voice stops).
- Episodes of sudden articulation breakdowns (sudden articulatory stops or deterioration).
- Slower speech rate.
- Scanning speech (increased stress on unstressed syllables).
- Vowel distortion.
- Difficulty in pitch control.
- Deficits in prosody (intonation, stress, tempo, rhythm, pause).
- Monotony of speech (no variety of voice pitch).
- Hypernasality (using mostly the nasal area as a resonator).
- Impaired respiratory functions.

In the last decade, there have been a number of acoustic and electroglottographic studies in MS aimed at finding markers of the disease based on speech/voice. Most of the studies use either acoustic methods or electroglottographic methods or both for the quantification of speech/voice characteristics (dysarthria) in MS. There are inherent characteristic difficulties with this search involving the variable nature of symptomatology and lesion topography in this disease, the different forms of the disease and the mild-moderate form of dysarthria [44, 45].

Many studies compare the dysarthria in MS with the dysarthria of Parkinson's disease (PD) to show differences in speech rate, such as slow rate (MS) as compared to faster speech rate (PD) [46]. The specific results of these studies will be discussed below, under voice quality, articulation/speech rate, and prosody.

13.7 Voice quality

In MS, the perceptual assessment of voice quality showed **asthenic weak voice** [47, 48], **phonatory instability** [9, 22, 49, 50] and **breathiness** [48, 51].

The electroglottographic results proved that correlates to **asthenic voice** were the mean closed quotient in five patients with dysphonia [52] and DQx1 mean in monologue, CQx mean in monologue, DFx1 90% range in monologue, DQx1 90% range in reading, and DQx1 90% range in monologue in 64 patients with MS as compared to 64 pair-matched controls [53].

Other electroglottographic studies found that correlates to **phonatory instability** and/or **breathiness** were the vocal jitter and the standard deviation of the average fundamental frequency (sustained phonation) as well as the mean fundamental frequency of the vibrating vocal folds (reading) [18]. Dogan [48] found that jitter and shimmer were higher in the MS patients while the maximum phonation time was lower. However, the mean fundamental frequency was found not to differ in the two groups. Feijo [54] used acoustic methods and found that fundamental frequency was higher in the MS patients, while the standard deviation of fundamental frequency was higher in females with MS and jitter was higher in males with MS. Hartelius [55] analyzed the sustained phonation of 20 MS patients using acoustic methods with the FFT and found that the frequency-based analysis of spectral components distinguished the patients from the controls. Very slow fluctuation of 1–2 Hz (wow), vocal tremor (8 Hz) and flutter (17–18 Hz), distinguished the MS patients from the controls.

13.8 Articulation and speech rate

Tjaden searched the effect of different reading conditions and rate in a number of acoustic studies [23, 56–58]. One study [23] compared two groups of dysarthric patients (MS and Parkinson's disease) and one group of healthy controls. The dysarthric patients in both diseases exhibited more difficulty in adjusting their speaking rate (slow and fast conditions) while reading a passage, and this difficulty was proposed to function as a clinical marker of mild to moderate dysarthria. The strategy of a slow rate was accompanied with lengthened average pause durations in the reading passage. However, no statistical differences between the clinical groups were found.

The same authors did not find differences among the clinical groups of MS versus PD patients in acoustic measures of articulation rate, pause characteristics, vocal intensity and segmental articulation when the patients read a passage in three conditions (slow, loud and habitual) [56]. In a similar study [57] there were found differences in articulatory rate between MS and the parkinsonian group. Higher reading rate, lower intensity, and greater duration in some vowels were found in the MS group. Tjaden [58] compared patients with MS versus PD while reading sentences in habitual, clear and loud conditions to find spectral coefficients in the consonants /s/, /ʃ/, /t/, and /k/ at initial and medial positions in words. The results showed that the word-initial position of the consonants during loud reading differed from the other two conditions and the authors proposed this finding to improve intelligibility during speech therapy techniques.

At the syllabic level, the form of dysarthria that is produced by lesions in the cerebellum (ataxic dysarthria as one type of dysarthria in MS) was measured acoustically in patients with MS as compared to healthy controls [59]. Perceptually, the speech in these patients exhibited decreased variation for loudness, decreased phrase length, slow rate, difficulty in maintaining the appropriate loudness, stress, respiration and showed prolongation in phonemes as well as imprecise consonants. The acoustic findings supported the perceptual impressions. The MS patients exhibited increased syllable durations and isochrony (equalized syllables in stress) as well as increased durations for the intervals between stress.

Specific acoustic measures such as the second formant across sentences were used to compare the speech of MS patients versus the speech of healthy controls as they were reading a standard passage [60]. The results showed that the extremely rapid changes in the secod formant in specific sentences and specific phonetic combinations were important to describe the mild-moderate dysarthria in the MS.

13.9 Prosody

The slowness of tongue movements may result in a lower speech rate (measured in syllables or words per minute). Indeed, perceptual studies showed that the speech rate was slower in MS patients as compared to healthy controls [49, 50]. One study reported correlations of speech rate to scores in neuropsychological tests [61]. The authors found that multisyllabic combinations (as a correlate of speech rate) were slower in MS patients, and it was related to the performance in tests measuring cognition such as the verbal fluency test (COWAT), the Paced Auditory Serial Addition Test (PASAT), the Animal Naming test, and the Symbol Digits Modality Test (SDMT).

Acoustic studies proved the results of the perceptual studies [9, 50, 51, 59, 60]. The speech rate was found to be slower due to increased number of pauses in connective speech of the patients with MS.

13.10 Summary of findings and conclusions

In summary, the electroglottographic/acoustic results showed that MS patients exhibit decreases in mean closed quotient, average fundamental frequency in sustained phonation, mean fundamental frequency in reading, maximum sustained phonation while prolongating a vowel and speech rate. Also, there were found to be increases in variables such as jitter and shimmer showing instability in the short-term variability of voice. Finally, the patients exhibited difficulty in adjusting their speech rate and showed extremely rapid changes in the second formant in multisyllabic repetition of words. So, the objective instrumental techniques such as EGG/acoustic analysis are able to prove the perceptual findings with accuracy and probably to compare the speech before and after speech therapy.

Further research is needed to relate these findings to the specific subtype of MS by using larger patient samples. Speech/voice is important to show changes from mild to moderate or severe disease states. Along the same lines, a recent review of dysarthria characteristics in MS proposed that speech assessment methods are very important to monitor change in disease progression [62].

References

[1] Duffy J R 2013 *Motor Speech Disorders: Substrates, Differential Diagnosis, and Management* (St. Louis, MO: Elsevier)

[2] Chiaravalloti N D and Deluca J 2008 Cognitive impairment in multiple sclerosis *Lancet Neurol.* **7** 1139–51

[3] Winkelmann A, Engel C, Apel A and Zettl U K 2007 Cognitive impairment in multiple sclerosis *J. Neurol.* **254** 35–42

[4] Christodoulou C *et al* 2009 Negative affect predicts subsequent cognitive change in multiple sclerosis *J. Int. Neuropsychol. Soc.* **15** 53–61

[5] Diamond B, Johnson S, Kaufman M and Graves L 2008 Relationships between information processing, depression, fatigue and cognition in multiple sclerosis *Arch. Clin. Neuropsychol.* **23** 189–99

[6] Prakash R S, Snook E M, Lewis J M, Motl R W and Kramer A F 2008 Cognitive impairments in relapsing–remitting multiple sclerosis: a meta-analysis *Mult. Scler.* **14** 1250–61

[7] Renauld S, Mohamed-Saïd L and Macoir J 2016 Language disorders in multiple sclerosis: A systematic review *Mult. Scler. Relat. Disord.* **10** 103–11

[8] Mackenzie C and Green J 2009 Cognitive–linguistic deficit and speech intelligibility in chronic progressive multiple sclerosis *Int. J. Lang. Commun. Disord.* **44** 401–20

[9] Hartelius L, Runmarker B and Andersen O 2000 Prevalence and characteristics of dysarthria in a multiple-sclerosis incidence cohort: relation to neurological data *Folia Phoniatr. Logop.* **52** 160–77

[10] Hartelius L and Lillvik M 2003 Lip and tongue function differently affected in individuals with multiple sclerosis *Folia Phoniatr. Logop.* **55** 1–9

[11] Anderson N B and Shames G H 2014 *Human Communication Disorders: An Introduction* (Harlow: Pearson)

[12] Yorkston K M 1999 *Management of Motor Speech Disorders in Children and Adults* (Austin, TX: Pro-Ed)

[13] Ackermann H, Vogel M, Petersen D and Poremba M 1992 Speech deficits in ischaemic cerebellar lesions *J. Neurol.* **239** 223–7

[14] Kent R D, Duffy J R, Slama A, Kent J F and Clift A 2001 Clinicoanatomic studies in dysarthria: Review, critique, and directions for research *J. Speech Lang. Hear. Res.* **44** 535–51

[15] Danesh-Sani S A *et al* 2013 Clinical assessment of orofacial manifestations in 500 patients with multiple sclerosis *J. Oral Maxillof. Surg.* **71** 290–4

[16] Feenaughty L, Tjaden K, Benedict R H and Weinstock-Guttman B 2013 Speech and pause characteristics in multiple sclerosis: A preliminary study of speakers with high and low neuropsychological test performance *Clin. Linguist. Phon.* **27** 134–51

[17] Hartelius L and Svensson P 1994 Speech and swallowing symptoms associated with Parkinson's disease and multiple sclerosis: a survey *Folia Phoniatr. Logop.* **46** 9–17

[18] Konstantopoulos K, Vikelis M, Seikel J A and Mitsikostas D 2010 The existence of phonatory instability in multiple sclerosis: An acoustic and electroglottographic study *Neurol. Sci.* **31** 259–68

[19] Nordio S *et al* 2018 Expiratory and phonation times as measures of disease severity in patients with Multiple Sclerosis. A case-control study *Mult. Scler. Relat. Disord.* **23** 27–32

[20] Piacentini V *et al* 2014 Relationship between quality of life and dysarthria in patients with multiple sclerosis *Arch. Phys. Med. Rehabil.* **95** 2047–54

[21] Rusz J *et al* 2018 Characteristics of motor speech phenotypes in multiple sclerosis *Mult. Scler. Relat. Disord.* **19** 62–9

[22] Yamout B *et al* 2009 Vocal symptoms and acoustic changes in relation to the expanded disability status scale, duration and stage of disease in patients with multiple sclerosis *Eur. Arch. Oto-Rhino-Laryngol.* **266** 1759–65

[23] Tjaden K and Wilding G 2011 Speech and pause characteristics associated with voluntary rate reduction in Parkinson's disease and Multiple Sclerosis *J. Commun. Disord.* **44** 655–65

[24] Goodwin S J and Carpenter A F 2016 Successful treatment of paroxysmal ataxia and dysarthria in multiple sclerosis with levetiracetam *Mult. Scler. Relat. Disord.* **10** 79–81

[25] Codeluppi L, Bigliardi G, Chiari A and Meletti S 2013 Isolated paroxysmal dysarthria caused by a single demyelinating midbrain lesion *BMJ Case Rep.* **2013** bcr2013200777

[26] Iorio R, Capone F, Plantone D and Batocchi A 2014 Paroxysmal ataxia and dysarthria in multiple sclerosis *J. Clin. Neurosci.* **21** 174–5

[27] Li Y, Zeng C and Luo T 2011 Paroxysmal dysarthria and ataxia in multiple sclerosis and corresponding magnetic resonance imaging findings *J. Neurol.* **258** 273–6

[28] Marcel C *et al* 2010 Symptomatic paroxysmal dysarthria-ataxia in demyelinating diseases *J. Neurol* **257** 1369–72

[29] Friedrich G and Dejonckere P H 2005 The voice evaluation protocol of the European Laryngological Society (ELS)—first results of a multicenter study *Laryngorhinootologie* **84** 744–52

[30] Remacle M and Eckel H E 2010 *Surgery of Larynx and Trachea* (London: Springer)

[31] Fourcin A J and Abberton E 1971 First applications of a new laryngograph *Med. Biol. Illus.* **21** 172–82

[32] Fabre P 1957 Un procédé électrique percutané d'inscription de l'accolement glottique au cours de la phonation *Bull. Acad. Natl. Méd.* **141** 66–99

[33] Abberton E R M, Howard D M and Fourcin A J 1989 Laryngographic assessment of normal voice: A tutorial *Clin. Linguist. Phon.* **3** 281–96

[34] Fourcin A J 1981 Laryngographic assessment of phonatory function *ASHA Rep.* **11** 116–27

[35] Baken R J 1996 *Clinical Measurement of Speech and Voice* (San Diego, CA: Singular Publishing)

[36] Orlikoff R F 1995 Vocal stability and vocal tract configuration: an acoustic and electro-glottographic investigation *J. Voice* **9** 173–81

[37] Fant G 1960 *Acoustic Theory of Speech Production* (The Hague: Mouton)

[38] Kent R D and Read C 1992 *The Acoustic Analysis of Speech* (San Diego, CA: Singular Publishing)

[39] Fourcin A 2000 Voice quality and electrolaryngography *Voice Quality Measurement* ed R D Kent and M J Ball (San Diego, CA: Singular Publishing) ch 13

[40] Fourcin A and Abberton E 2008 Hearing and phonetic criteria in voice measurement: Clinical applications *Logop. Phoniatr. Vocol.* **33** 35–48

[41] Abberton E R M and Fourcin A J 1997 Electrolaryngography *Instrumental Clinical Phonetics* ed M J Ball and C Code (London: Whurr) 119–47

[42] Fourcin A J, Abberton E R M, Miller D and Howells D 1995 Laryngograph: Speech pattern element tools for therapy, training, and assessment *Eur. J. Disord. Commun.* **30** 101–15
[43] Hartelius L, Nord L and Buder E H 1995 Acoustic analysis of dysarthria associated with multiple sclerosis *Clin. Linguist. Phon.* **9** 95–120
[44] Beukelman D R, Kraft G H and Freal J 1985 Expressive communication disorders in persons with multiple sclerosis: a survey *Arch. Phys. Med. Rehabil.* **66** 675–7
[45] Stipancic K L, Tjaden K and Wilding G J 2016 Comparison of intelligibility measures for adults with Parkinson's disease, adults with multiple sclerosis, and healthy controls *J. Speech Lang. Hear. Res.* **59** 230–8
[46] Kuo C, Tjaden K and Sussman J E 2014 Acoustic and perceptual correlates of faster-than-habitual speech produced by speakers with Parkinsons disease and multiple sclerosis *J. Commun. Disord.* **52** 156–69
[47] Bauer V *et al* 2013 Subjective and perceptual analysis of voice quality and relationship with neurological disfunction in multiple sclerosis patients *Clin. Neurol. Neurosurg.* **115** 17–20
[48] Dogan M *et al* 2007 Objective and subjective evaluation of voice quality in multiple sclerosis *J. Voice* **21** 735–40
[49] Darley F L, Brown J R and Goldstein N P 1972 Dysarthria in multiple sclerosis *J. Speech Hear. Res.* **15** 229–45
[50] Hartelius L, Svensson P and Bubach A 1993 Clinical assessment of dysarthria: Performance on a dysarthria test by normal adult subjects, and by individuals with Parkinson's disease or with multiple sclerosis *Scand. J. Logop. Phoniatr.* **18** 131–41
[51] Tjaden K and Watling E 2003 Characteristics of diadochokinesis in Multiple Sclerosis and Parkinson's Disease *Folia Phoniatr. Logop.* **55** 241–59
[52] Yamout B *et al* 2013 Predictors of quality of life among multiple sclerosis patients: a comprehensive analysis *Eur. J. Neurol.* **20** 756–64
[53] Vavougios G, Doskas T and Konstantopoulos K 2018 An electroglottographical analysis-based discriminant function model differentiating multiple sclerosis patients from healthy controls *Neurol. Sci.* **39** 847–50
[54] Feijó A V *et al* 2004 Acoustic analysis of voice in multiple sclerosis patients *J. Voice* **18** 341–7
[55] Hartelius L, Buder E H and Strand E A 1997 Long-term phonatory instability in individuals with multiple sclerosis *J. Speech Lang. Hear. Res.* **40** 1056–72
[56] Kuo C and Tjaden K 2016 Acoustic variation during passage reading for speakers with dysarthria and healthy controls *J. Commun. Disord.* **62** 30–44
[57] Tjaden K, Lam J and Wilding G 2013 Vowel acoustics in Parkinson's disease and multiple sclerosis: comparison of clear, loud, and slow speaking conditions *J. Speech Lang. Hear. Res.* **56** 1485–502
[58] Tjaden K and Martel-Sauvageau V 2017 Consonant acoustics in Parkinsons disease and multiple sclerosis: comparison of clear and loud speaking conditions *Am. J. Speech-Lang. Pathol.* **26** 569
[59] Hartelius L, Runmarker B, Andersen O and Nord L 2000 Temporal speech characteristics of individuals with multiple sclerosis and ataxic dysarthria: 'scanning speech' revisited *Folia Phoniatr. Logop.* **52** 228–38
[60] Rosen K M, Goozée J V and Murdoch B E 2008 Examining the effects of multiple sclerosis on speech production: does phonetic structure matter? *J. Commun. Disord.* **41** 49–69

[61] Arnett P A, Smith M M, Barwick F H, Benedict R H and Ahlstrom B P 2008 Oral motor slowing in multiple sclerosis: relationship to neuropsychological tasks requiring an oral response *J. Int. Neuropsychol. Soc.* **14** 454–62

[62] Noffs G *et al* 2018 What speech can tell us: A systematic review of dysarthria characteristics in Multiple Sclerosis *Autoimmun. Rev.* **17** 1202–9

IOP Publishing

Neurological Disorders and Imaging Physics, Volume 2
Engineering and clinical perspectives of multiple sclerosis
Ayman El-Baz and Jasjit S Suri

Chapter 14

Novel approaches for segmenting cerebral vasculature

Heba Kandil, Ahmed Soliman, Ali Mahmoud, Ahmed Shalaby, Fatma Taher, Mohammed Ghazal, Adel Elmagraby and Ayman El-Baz

Multiple sclerosis (MS) is a disorder of the immune system disease that affects a human brain, spinal cord, and the eyes optic nerves. Patients of this long-lasting disease usually have problems with basic body functions such as muscle control, balance, and vision. An MS patient suffers from symptoms such as muscle weakness or spasms, troubles in walking and vision, depression, and problems in focusing and remembering. Causes of MS are not yet clear, however, there are some factors that make the disease occurrence more potential. People with certain genes, who smokes, who have some viral infections, or who have blood vessel disease are more vulnerable to this disease than others. Correlation between MS and changes in cerebral vascular tree structure or function has been suggested in literature before. Different vascular abnormalities have been correlated with MS including cerebral hypoperfusion, increased risk of ischemic disease, impaired venous drainage, and abnormalities of endothelial cells. It is hypothesized that tracking these vascular alterations and abnormalities would potentially help clinicians to avoid disease complications by initiating medical plans that are appropriate to mitigate any adverse events. Segmentation of the human brain's anatomical structures is an essential and inevitable step before the analysis, tracking, or diagnosis of vascular changes. The complex geometric nature of human brains have made it challenging to propose automatic and effective segmentation approaches. In this chapter, we propose two segmentation approaches that are able to segment cerebral vasculature automatically and accurately. This would potentially help experts in the early analysis and diagnosis of severe diseases, specifically, MS.

doi:10.1088/978-0-7503-1762-7ch14

14.1 Introduction

Cerebral changes in human brains' anatomical structures such as the alterations in cerebral blood vessels' diameters and tortuosity have been clinically linked to many vascular and non-vascular diseases. Cerebrovascular change is known to be a major factor in the development of severe diseases such as hypertension, Alzheimer, dementia, strokes, brain lesions, cognitive impairment, ischemic cerebral injury, and multiple sclerosis (MS). It is clinically hypothesized that the early detection and quantification of cerebrovascular changes would help physicians to the early diagnosis of patients with potential severe vascular or non-vascular diseases. This early diagnosis would help in initiating medical treatment plans to mitigate any adverse events and to control the development of such diseases. The first step in the process of detecting and quantifying these cerebral vascular changes is to segment the vascular tree of the human brain accurately. This segmentation is challenging due to the complex nature of human brains and the similar appearance of blood vessels and some of the brain's fat tissues. In this chapter, we will present two approaches that are able to segment cerebral vasculature efficiently.

MS is a disease known as a disorder of the immune system, which can affect a human brain, spinal cord, and the eyes optic nerves. Patients of this long-lasting disease usually have problems with basic body functions such as muscle control, balance, and vision. MS occurs when a human immune system attacks a material called myelin. Myelin is a fatty material that wraps around nerve fibers in the human body to protect them from damage. Loss of myelin may also lead to scar tissue formation. An MS patient suffers from symptoms such as muscle weakness or spasms, trouble with walking and vision, depression, and problems in focusing and remembering. These symptoms happen because the patient's brain cannot control sending signals through the body correctly and the nerves cannot accomplish their appropriate work in controlling feelings and movements. However, these symptoms differ from one patient to another. While some patients have trouble in doing their basic daily tasks and may have attacks when the illness condition gets worse, others may have mild symptoms that might not need medical intervention or treatment. Despite the fact that causes of MS are not yet clear, there are some factors that make the disease occurrence more potential. For example, people with certain genes, people who smoke, people who have some viral infections, or who have blood vessel disease are more vulnerable to this disease than others. A recent clinical hypothesis suggests that there is a correlation between MS and narrowed head and neck veins. Moreover, there are clinical hypotheses that MS might be caused by blood vessel changes. The hypothesis suggests that veins that are responsible for transferring blood from the brain and spine back to the heart might become too narrow and cause blood leakage into brain tissue. This blood leakage could potentially trigger inflammation which in turn could affect balance and muscle control associated with MS. In addition, this inflammation could result in microvascular damage. The relationship between MS and changes in cerebral vascular tree structure or function has been analyzed in literature in many studies [1–3]. Different vascular abnormalities have been correlated with MS including cerebral hypoperfusion, increased risk of ischemic disease, impaired venous drainage, and abnormalities of endothelial cells.

Segmentation of cerebral vasculature plays an important role in studying the correlation between MS and changes in cerebral blood vessels. It is an inevitable step before experts could be able to track the changes of cerebral vasculature. In the following section, we will present two different approaches to segment the brain's vasculature automatically and accurately.

14.2 Cerebral blood vessels segmentation

Image segmentation could be categorized into four approaches; pixel-based, boundary-based, region-based, and hybrid techniques. Pixel-based approaches make use of intensity information. They assume that pixels residing within a specific range are of the same class. These methods use thresholding based on pixel values. The accuracy of these methods is limited as they neglect all other spatial information. Boundary-based approaches rely on the fact that values of pixels change rapidly at boundaries between regions. These methods detect intensity rapid high-values change of pixels and consider these pixels candidates for boundary pixels. Then, these candidates are being further processed to find closed curves that represent separate regions. The conversion of disjoint pixels into closed curves is not an easy task, though. Local-similarity-analysis, Hough-transform-based global analysis, and global processing by graph-theoretic techniques are examples of algorithms used in this category. Region-based approaches can be classified into two categories; region growing methods and region splitting. Region growing methods which start with a seed-pixel and grow a region by appending spatially connected neighboring pixels that meet a specific homogeneity criterion. The basic challenge in these methods is to find the best homogeneity criterion. Several algorithms were developed that use statistical homogeneity criteria based on regional random fields, seed-controlled homogeneity competition, intensity information, texture, and surface measures.

Cerebral vasculature segmentation is a basic and essential operation in medical research that focuses on brains and is usually accomplished before any related diagnostic process. Different methods have been presented in literature to segment blood vessels and we can approximately classify these methods into six categories, namely: pattern recognition techniques, model-based techniques, tracking-based techniques, neural network-based techniques, artificial intelligence-based techniques. Many medical technologies have been introduced in literature to enhance the visualization and analysis of cerebral vasculature such as magnetic resonance angiography (MRA).

14.2.1 Magnetic resonance angiography

The value of MRA as an imaging modality is accepted for head and brain. It is usually used to visualize the intracranial circulation and extracranial carotid vessels, to depict the peripheral arterial occlusive disease, to evaluate the abnormalities of the central veins of the body and much more. MRAs are acquired using magnetic resonance imaging (MRI) scanners. MRA is useful in imaging vessels and blood flow. Despite the advancement in MRA techniques, vascular filtering and segmentation challenges have not been solved completely due to the complex nature of body vasculature, and the small diameters of blood vessels. A sample MRA image is shown in figure 14.1. In this chapter we introduce two presented approaches to segment cerebral vasculature from MRA data.

14.2.2 A three-dimensional (3D) CNN-based segmentation approach

Deep learning belongs to machine learning approaches whose task is to learn data representations in either a supervised, semi-supervised, or unsupervised way. The concept of deep learning is inspired by communication patterns and information processing in biological nervous systems. However, it has its own different structural and functional properties.

Deep machine learning approaches could be employed in medical systems for classification, detection, analysis, or segmentation of different human organs such as lung, liver, heart, or brain to help clinicians in disease diagnosis and in managing appropriate treatment plans. A deep learning technique known as a convolutional neural network (CNN) has been used recently to segment blood vessels in different human organs [4–11]. CNN is a deep feed-forward artificial neural network that has a connectivity pattern inspired by the human visual cortex. It consists of a fully-connected and convolutional set of layers. Each neuron in a fully connected layer is connected to every activation in the previous layer. It has been discouraged to use three-dimensional (3D) CNNs because of the expensive cost of the 3D computations. Nowadays however, there are many trials to solve this issue so that we can benefit from the 3D correlation and contextual information of the volumetric data.

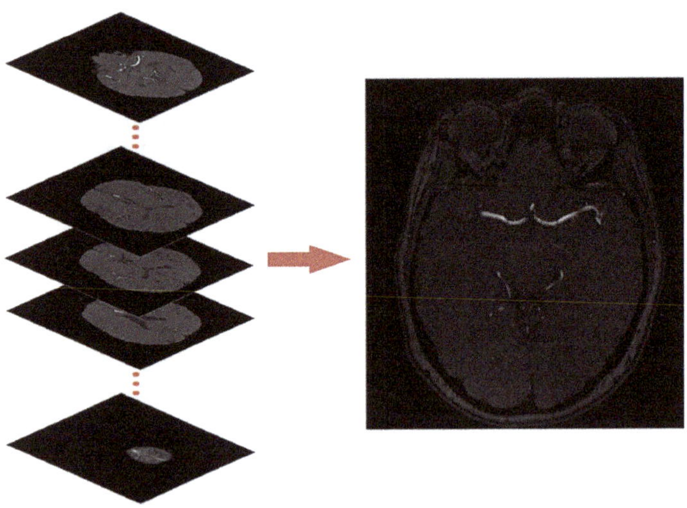

Figure 14.1. A sample of an MRA image.

In this context, we propose a deep learning approach to segment the vasculature of a human brain using a 3D CNN. The presented approach was inspired by the 3D CNN presented by Kamnitsas *et al* [12]. This approach does not impose any preprocessing of the input data and does not require any prior knowledge about existing tissue classes. However, to increase the accuracy of our segmentation and help the CNN to perform its job in an easier way, we applied a non-parametric bias field correction algorithm on the input to handle and correct any non-uniformities in the input MRA images.

14.2.2.1 An overview of the 3D deep CNN

A deep 3D CNN which is composed of eleven layers was used for the vasculature segmentation task to provide more discriminative power. In the baseline scheme of the presented 3D CNN, a feature extraction task was performed using layers of 5^3 kernels each. The receptive field (i.e. the input voxel neighborhood that influences the activation of the neuron) was of size 17^3. The classification layer has 1^3 kernels. Basically, this 3D CNN has two major components. The first component takes the MRA data volumes and extracts adjacent image patches from each volume and densely trains them into one pass of the network using an effective dense training scheme that also considers the adaptation to inherent class imbalance in data automatically. Moreover, input MRA images are being processed at multiple scales simultaneously using parallel convolutional pathways to incorporate as much local and contextual information as possible to enrich and enhance the segmentation process. The first component of the deep 3D CNN approach produces the soft segmentation maps which are then being post-processed using the second component, which is a 3D fully connected conditional random field (CRF) that removes any false positives and produces the final hard labels. Extra layers have been added to the baseline scheme to make the network deeper. To handle the expensive cost of computations and the need for additional trainable parameters associated with the nature of deep neural networks, smaller kernels have been used to reduce the number of convolutional operations and the number of training parameters by approximately a factor of 5. Each layer in the baseline scheme, which is composed of 5^3 kernels, has been replaced by two successive layers, each of which is composed of 3^3 kernels without altering the receptive field. This replacement resulted in the reduction of the number of weight parameters and the computational cost. Additionally, a second pathway operating on down-sampled volume is added to incorporate both local and larger contextual information in the 3D CNN. While the first pathway is responsible for capturing the detailed local appearance of the blood vessels, the second pathway could capture the higher-level features. Figure 14.2 shows a diagram of the basic components of this approach.

14.2.2.2 Incorporation of the local blood flow information to improve segmentation accuracy

We suggest that incorporating the information associated with the variability of the strength of blood flow signals (either increase or decrease) throughout the range of slices of an MRA volume would potentially enhance the accuracy of the vasculature

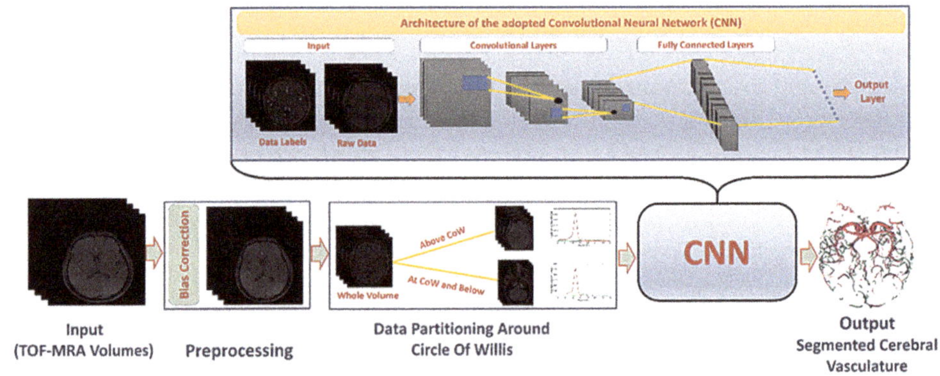

Figure 14.2. A block diagram representing the 3D CNN-based approach to segment cerebral vasculature.

segmentation results. To incorporate the local information of the blood flow, we suggested partitioning each volume into two compartments relative to a famous brain biological marker known as circle of Willis (coW) where each compartment tends to include blood vessels of similar appearance, and brightness. Also, the diameters' sizes of blood vessels in each compartment are supposed to have little difference between their values. The first compartment includes all MRA volume slices above coW and the second compartment includes all MRA volume slices starting at coW and what is below.

14.2.2.3 Evaluation data

Thirty MRA volumes have been used to test the presented segmentation approach. Each MRA volume consists of an average of 160 slices of a grid size of 696 × 768, a voxel spacing of 0.26 × 0.26, and a slice thickness of 0.5 mm. The gold standard ground truth segmentation was delineated manually by a medical imaging expert. The thirty datasets have been divided into twenty datasets used for training and ten datasets used for testing. We normalized the intensities of each MRA volume such that it has a zero-mean and a unit variance. This normalization improves CNN results and leads to a faster convergence.

14.2.2.4 Results and discussion

Two experiments have been conducted to test the efficacy of the presented approach and to validate the hypothesis that considering the variability of blood flow signals in the brain's blood vessels over time would potentially enhance the segmentation accuracy. In the first experiment, we fed the 3D CNN with the MRA volumes without partitioning them and we called this experiment the global experiment because the segmentation is performed globally over the entire MRA volume regardless of the variability of the blood flow strength over time in different slices. In the second experiment, the partitioned volumes were fed into the 3D CNN and we called this experiment the local experiment because it considers local blood flow strength variability between different sections of the brain. The final segmentation in the case of the second experiment is the combination of the output of each compartment. To evaluate the efficacy of using 3D CNNs in segmenting the brain's vasculature, common segmentation evaluation metrics have been used including dice similarity coefficient (DSC) which is evaluated as (DSC = 2TP/(2TP + FP + FN)) such that (TP) is true positive, (TN) is true negative, (FP) is false positive, and (FN) is false negative, specificity that is evaluated as (SPEC = TN/(TN + FP)), and sensitivity that is evaluated as (SENS = TP/(TP + FN)). The results proved the efficacy of the presented 3D CNN in segmenting cerebral vasculature. Also, the results showed that the local experiment outperformed the global one which validates the hypothesis that the incorporation of blood flow signal information into the presented approach would enhance the segmentation accuracy. The global experiment recorded a DSC of 83.20%, a SPEC of 99.00%, and a SENS of 83.79%, while the local experiment recorded a DSC of 84.37%, a SPEC of 99.00%, and a SENS of 86.14%. Also, we have conducted a comparison between the 3D CNN presented approach and the global statistical-based segmentation approach [13] and the results showed that the 3D CNN approach result outperformed in terms of DSC, SPEC, and SENS (table 14.1). Figure 14.3 presents the output probability for the background (class 0), the blood vessels (class 1), and the final hard labels. In addition, the qualitative results (figure 14.4) prove that applying the 3D CNN approach on the partitioned volumes produces more accurate segmented vasculature in terms of fewer gaps between the blood vessel segments and more detected vessels' voxels compared to the resulted vasculature of the global experiment.

Table 14.1. Evaluation of cerebral segmentation of the 3D CNN approach (local and global experiment) and the global statistical approach in terms of DSC, SPEC, and SENS.

Approach	DSC, %	SPEC, %	SENS, %
3D CNN (Local experiment)	84.37	99.00	86.14
3D CNN (Global experiment)	83.20	99.00	83.79
Global Statistical Approach [13]	80.12	97.50	85.28

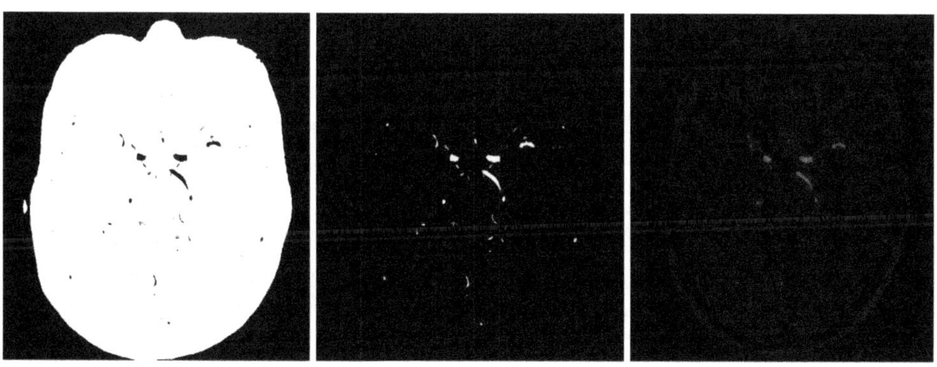

(a) (b) (c)

Figure 14.3. A sample of the output probability for the background (class 0) (a), and blood vessels (b), in addition to the final hard segmentation labels (c).

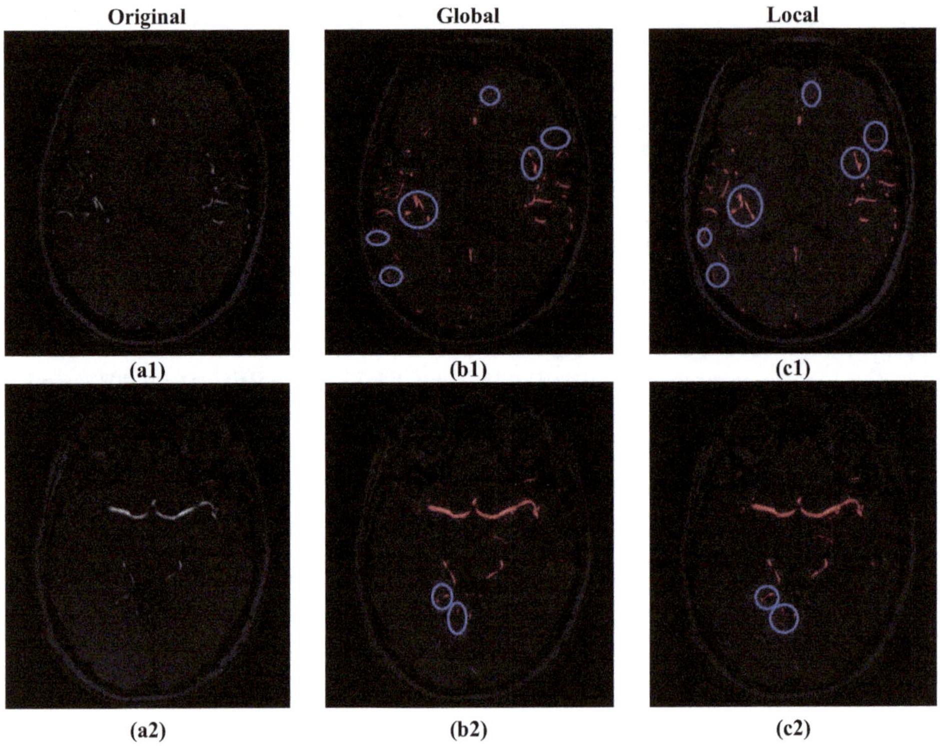

Figure 14.4. A sample of 2D segmentation results for two different cross sections (a1), (a2) using the entire MRA volume as an input (b1), (b2); and using the above circle of Willis volume (c1), and below circle of Willis volume (c2) as inputs to the 3D CNN. Segmented blood vessels are colored in red and enhanced segmentation in the local experiment (both above circle of Willis and below it) are contoured in blue.

To sum up, a novel 3D CNN based segmentation approach that takes into account the increase and decrease of blood flow signals in the brain's blood vessels over time was presented to segment cerebral vasculature from MRA data. Evaluation of the experimental results suggest that partitioning input MRA volumes into different compartments where each compartment has a homogenous range of intensities instead of processing the entire MRA volume without partitioning would potentially enhance the segmentation results. The accurate segmentation of cerebral vasculature resulting from this approach would have a very good impact on any further analysis of the brain or clinical diagnosis.

14.2.3 A 3D local adaptive segmentation approach

Experts in the field of blood vessels segmentation suggest that approaches that are based on statistical models are better than other approaches because they are less computationally intensive [14]. However, some statistical models require predefined probability models. Those probability models are not suitable for all applications due to the inevitable variability in the intensity distribution of blood vessels arising from patients, or the scanning conditions or parameters.

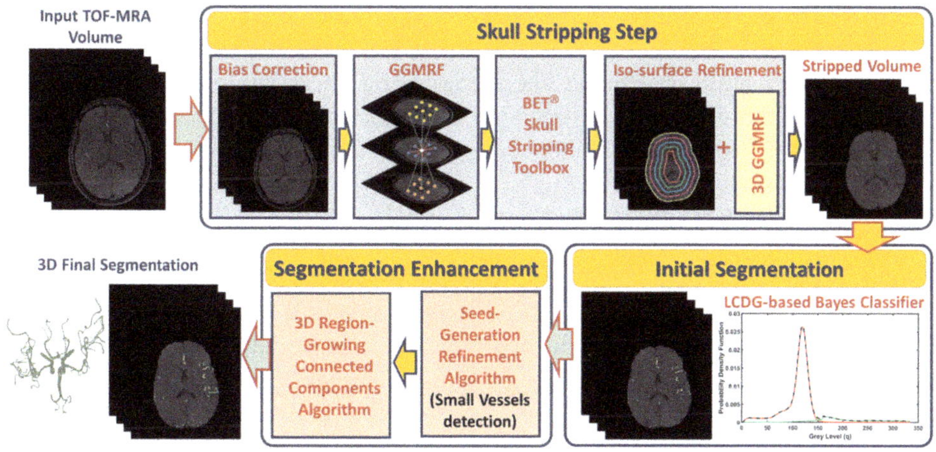

Figure 14.5. A block diagram of the 3D local adaptive segmentation approach.

It was a challenge to develop a blood vessel segmentation approach that is automatic and does not need the intervention of a human operator. Instead, there are manual segmentation approaches that are done by typical experts and semi-automatic approaches that require initialization of blood vessels seed points. Manual segmentation consumes much time and effort, is error-prone, and is subject to inter-observer variability. Semi-automatic segmentation approaches might require much more investigation, revision and evaluation by experts. In the next few paragraphs, we will present our novel fully automated approach to segment brain vasculature using a visual appearance model that is applied globally in the MRA volume and applied locally around the initial detected vascular tree using an adaptive window to increase the segmentation accuracy and to reduce the computational cost.

14.2.3.1 Main steps of the segmentation approach

This approach is composed of three main steps namely skull striping, initial segmentation using a linear combination of discrete Gaussians (LCDG), and the refinement of the initial segmentation (figure 14.5). These steps will be explained in more detail next.

14.2.3.1.1 Skull stripping algorithm

The human brain contains fat tissues whose visual appearance is similar to the appearance of the brain's blood vessels. To increase the efficiency of the segmentation process, we removed the skull from the MRA images and retained the brain tissue only before performing the segmentation task. To perform skull stripping, the MRA volumes were first processed by a nonparametric bias correction approach [15] to remove any bias in the MRA images that might occur due to magnetic field, to diminish noise effects, and to remove inconsistencies of the MRA images by taking into account the 3D spatially homogeneous pair-wise interactions between the grey levels of the MRA data. MRA data were then processed using a 3D generalized Gauss–Markov random field (GGMRF) model [16] to reduce or remove inhomogeneities in the MRA scans and to preserve the 3D edges between blood vessels and other brain structures. The 3D GGMRF model finds the best grey level that minimizes the difference between the centered voxel and its 26 neighborhood using the energy function that follows:

$$\hat{q}_s = \arg\min_{\tilde{q}_s}\left[|q_s - \tilde{q}_s| + \rho^{\alpha} \lambda^{\beta} \sum_{r \epsilon \upsilon_s} \eta_{s,r} \mid \tilde{q}_s - q_r \mid \right]$$

where q_s is the original gray-level; $\tilde{q}_s$ is the new estimated grey level; υ_s is the 26 neighborhood system; $\eta_{s,r}$ is the GGMRF potential; ρ and λ are scaling factors; $\alpha \in \{1,2\}$ is used to determine the prior distribution of the estimator ($\alpha = 1$ for Laplace or $\alpha = 2$ for Gaussian); and β was used to control the smoothing level such that $\beta \in [1.01, 2.0]$ ($\beta = 2$ for smoothing and $\beta = 1.01$ for relatively abrupt edges). The preprocessed MRA volume is then fed into a brain extraction tool (BET [17]) to obtain the initial skull. The Euclidian distance map inside the binary mask obtained from the previous step is calculated and a set of N iso-surfaces is created. After that, the marginal density of the brain voxels and non-brain voxels were estimated to obtain the initial map using the LCDG model. The Gibbs potentials for the pairwise Markov–Gibbs random field (MGRF) model of the initial map were then estimated to identify the MGRF probability. The following step is to classify the voxels inside each iso-surface using a Bayes classifier which is responsible for combining the visual appearance features (first and second order ones). If the iso-surface still contained non-brain tissues, the Bayes classifier was applied again until no non-brain tissue was found. Finally, the connected component analysis algorithm was used to extract only brain tissues and get rid of any non-brain tissues.

14.2.3.1.2 Initial blood vessels segmentation using LCDG

The initial cerebral vasculature was determined using a Bayesian framework which used the LCDG as a marginal density estimator for both blood vessels and brain tissues [13, 18]. The following equation represents the LCDG model used where C_p and C_n are the positive and negative components for blood vessels and other brain tissues.

$$P_{w,\Theta}(q) = \sum_{r=1}^{C_p} w_{p,r}\, \psi(q|\theta_{p,r}) - \sum_{l=1}^{C_n} w_{n,l}\, \psi(q|\theta_{n,l})$$

where $\Phi\theta(q)$ is the cumulative Gaussian function with $\theta = (\mu, \sigma2)$ for the mean, μ, and variance, σ^2 such that $\psi(q|\theta) = \Phi_\theta(q + 0.5) - \Phi_\theta(q - 0.5)$ for $q = 1, \ldots, Q - 2$, $\psi(0|\theta) = \Phi_\theta(0.5)$ and $\psi(Q - 1|\theta) = 1 - \Phi_\theta(Q - 1.5)$. The summation of all non-negative weights of the LCDG is equal to one. The parameters of prior probability, number of Gaussian components, mean, and variance of the model were estimated using a modified expectation–maximization algorithm (EM) [10]. To extract the cerebral blood vessels, the following Bayesian rule was used: $P(\upsilon)p(q|\upsilon) \geqslant P(O)p(q|O)$. $P(\upsilon)$, and $P(O)$ are the prior probabilities of the blood vessels and other brain tissues, respectively.

14.2.3.1.3 Blood vessels segmentation refinement using an automatic local adaptive segmentation algorithm

The initial cerebral vascular tree segmented using the LCDG was missing some important details, specifically smaller blood vessels. So, a following step to refine the segmentation results was required. We developed an automatic local adaptive segmentation algorithm that takes the initial vascular tree as an input and divides each segment of this tree into a set of connected components. Then, a search window of adaptive size was centered around each connected component to find a specific separation threshold for each region. The threshold value was estimated as $T = \frac{\mu_b + \mu_o}{2}$, where μ_b is the average intensity of blood vessels and μ_o is the average intensity of other cerebral tissues. An additional proposed seed-generation procedure was applied to find more blood vessel seeds that might have been missed by the segmentation algorithm. The general main steps for the segmentation approach are the following.

Main steps of the segmentation approach:

1. Preprocess each MRA volume by removing the skull and retaining only the brain tissue.
2. Remark the brain tissue as the region of interest for the segmentation algorithm.
3. Estimate the marginal density distribution for the blood vessels and other brain tissues using the LCDG model to obtain the initial vascular tree (see figure 14.6).
4. Apply a refinement segmentation algorithm on the initial vasculature (see figure 14.7):
    a. Using a proposed seed-generation algorithm which finds potential vessels seeds for regions of missing small vessels which were missed by the LCDG algorithm and accumulate them to the final segmented vascular tree.

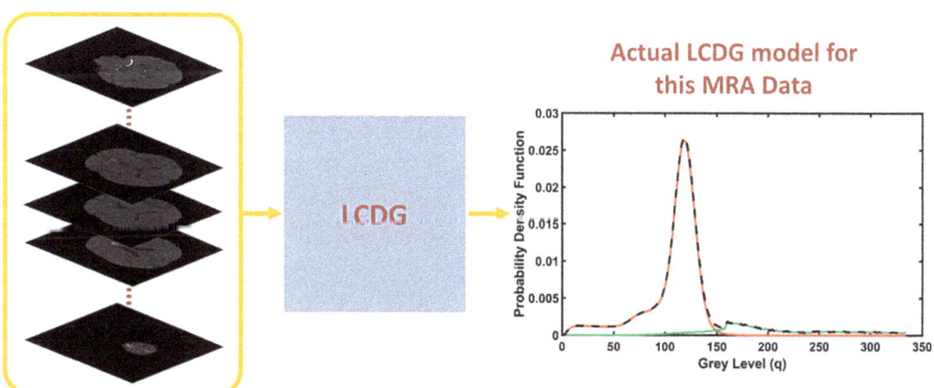

Figure 14.6. Normalized empirical density using the LCDG model.

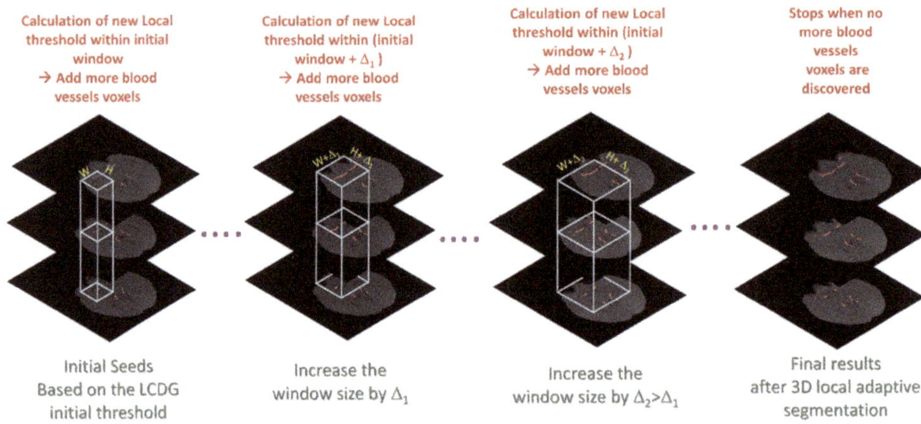

Figure 14.7. A diagram of the process of the local adaptive segmentation.

b. Determining an *N* odd number of seeds to be used for the extraction of *N* connected 3D vasculature using a 3D region-growing connected components.
c. Applying the majority voting approach to obtain the final segmented cerebral vascular tree.

14.2.3.1.4 Experimental results

The presented approach was tested using 200 MRA volumes. Each volume has an average of 160 slices of matrix size of 696 × 768. Qualitive and quantitative results of the presented segmentation algorithm were obtained and will be explained next. A sample output for the segmentation algorithm projected in a 2D axial plane and overlaid on the corresponding raw MRA slice is shown in figure 14.8. As shown in figure 14.8, it was noticed that in the initial segmented vasculature obtained from LCDG, the algorithm captured the center part of the blood vessels (area of maximal flow) that has voxels with a high certainty to be a blood vessel (pixels with pink color).

The improvement of segmentation obtained after applying the seed-generation algorithm in the same axial plane (pixels overlaid in red or green). Pixels colored in yellow and blue represent the results of the segmentation enhancement after applying the local adaptive algorithm which is processed in two consecutive stages, each used a different color (yellow and blue). The neighboring false negative voxels were correctly included as true positive voxels. Another sample output for the final result of the entire approach is shown in figure 14.9 where all segmented blood vessels are colored in white and the segmented vascular tree was overlaid on the corresponding MRA slice.

For the quantitative evaluation, the segmented cerebral vasculature was compared to ground truth and evaluated using common segmentation evaluation metrics. Ground truths were generated by an MRA expert. The used evaluation metrics were the DSC (has been defined in the first presented approach), and the absolute volume difference (AVD). AVD was estimated as the percentage volume

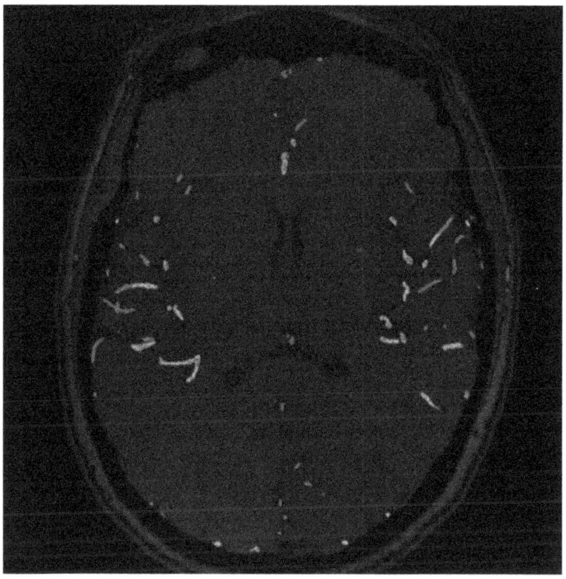

Figure 14.8. A sample output that shows different segmentation stages in different colors. Initial segmentation (using LCDG) is colored in pink. Results after applying the seed-generation procedures are colored in red and green. The application of the local adaptive search window resulted in yellow and blue colored pixels.

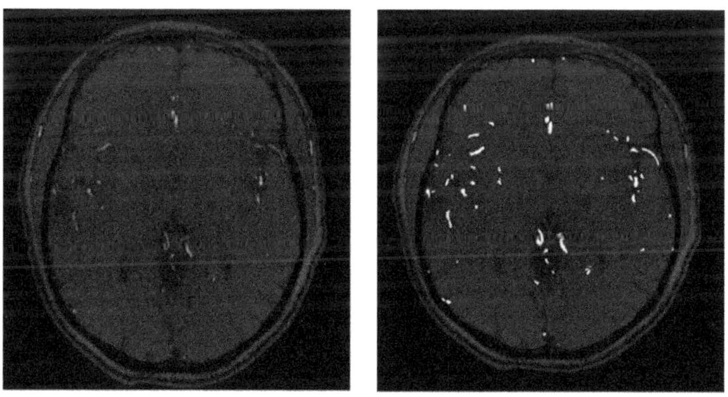

(a) **(b)**

Figure 14.9. A sample output of the 3D local adaptive segmentation approach. (a) Original image, and (b) the resulted segmentation where segmented blood vessels are overlaid in white.

difference between ground truth and segmentation results. A comparison has been conducted between the presented automatic segmentation approach and one of the famous state-of-the-art segmentation methods (global statistical method [13]), and the results are given in table 14.2. As shown in the table the presented approach had recorded higher accuracy in terms of DSC and AVD.

Table 14.2. DSC and AVD values for both the presented automatic local adaptive segmentation algorithm and the global statistical segmentation approach.

Segmentation approach	DSC (%)	AVD (%)
The 3D automatic local adaptive algorithm (presented)	~ 86.4	~ 10
Global statistical based approach [13]	~ 80	~ 23.6

14.2.3.1.5 Results and discussion

We presented an automated blood vessel segmentation approach that succeeded in segmenting both large and small cerebral blood vessels of diameter size larger than 1 mm accurately. The approach starts with removing the skull from the MRA images and retains only brain tissues using a novel appearance-geometric approach. Then an initial segmentation step is performed using the LCDG algorithm to produce the initial vascular tree. After that, a refinement step was performed on the initial vascular tree using the presented local adaptive segmentation approach. The segmentation approach was tested using clinical MRA data and proved to be accurate and effective in segmenting the brain's blood vessels. The presented approach was compared to traditional approaches and proved its outperformance and efficacy.

14.3 Summary

MS is a long-lasting severe disease that affects patients' lives in a severe way, making them unable to do their basic daily tasks. MS was found to be correlated to some cerebral changes. It is hypothesized that detecting these changes and tracking them over time would potentially help in controlling the progress of MS and might help in managing appropriate medical plans to reduce further medical complications. It is essential to segment cerebral structures accurately before tracking the alteration that could affect them. The segmentation task is very challenging due to reasons relative to the human brain's complex geometric nature and other scanner-related limitations. Only a few studies in literature targeted the task of automatic segmentation of cerebral structures due to the aforementioned problems. In this chapter, we have presented two different approaches to solve this segmentation challenge. The two approaches had higher accuracy rates in segmenting human cerebral vasculature automatically. This would potentially help clinicians in any further analysis or diagnosis of MS and hopefully could reduce further disease complications. A future plan is to develop a computer-aided diagnosis system that employs these efficient brain's vasculature segmentation approaches to help clinicians in detecting, quantifying, and tracking the progress of MS and potentially other vascular-related diseases. In addition to blood vessels [19–23], this work could also be applied to various other applications in medical imaging, such as the kidney, the heart, the prostate, the lung, and the retina. One application is renal transplant functional assessment. Chronic kidney disease (CKD) affects about 26 million people in the US with 17,000 transplants being performed each year. In renal transplant patients, acute rejection is the leading cause of renal dysfunction. Given the limited number of donors, routine clinical post-transplantation evaluation is of immense importance to help clinicians initiate timely interventions with appropriate treatment and thus prevent the graft loss. In recent years an increased area of research has been dedicated to developing noninvasive CAD systems for renal transplant function assessment, utilizing different image modalities (e.g. ultrasound, computed tomography (CT), MRI, etc). Accurate assessment of renal transplant function is critically important for graft survival. Although transplantation can improve patient well-being, there is a potential post-transplantation risk of kidney dysfunction that, if not treated in a timely manner, can lead to the loss of the entire graft, and even patient death. Thus, accurate assessment of renal transplant function is crucial for the identification of proper treatment. In recent years, an increased area of research has been dedicated to developing non-invasive image-based CAD systems for the assessment of renal transplant function. In particular, dynamic and diffusion MRI-based systems have been clinically used to assess transplanted kidneys with the advantage of providing information on each kidney separately. For more details about renal transplant functional assessment, please read [24–49]. The heart is also an important application to this work. The clinical assessment of myocardial perfusion plays a major role in the diagnosis, management, and prognosis of ischemic heart disease patients. Thus, there have been ongoing efforts to develop automated systems for accurate analysis of myocardial perfusion using first-pass images [50–66]. Another application for this work could be the detection of retinal abnormalities. The majority of ophthalmologists depend on visual interpretation for the identification of diseases types. However, inaccurate diagnosis will affect the treatment procedure which may lead to fatal results. Hence, there is a crucial need for computer automated diagnosis systems that yield highly accurate results. Optical coherence tomography (OCT) has become a powerful modality for the non-invasive diagnosis of various retinal abnormalities such as glaucoma, diabetic macular edema, and macular degeneration. The problem with diabetic retinopathy (DR) is that the patient is not aware of the disease until the changes in the retina have progressed to a level that treatment tends to be less effective. Therefore, automated early detection could limit the severity of the disease and assist ophthalmologists in investigating and treating it more efficiently [67, 68]. Abnormalities of the lung could also be another promising area of research and a related application to this work. Radiation-induced lung injury is the main side effect of radiation therapy for lung cancer patients. Although higher radiation doses increase the radiation therapy effectiveness for tumor control, this can lead to lung injury as a greater quantity of normal lung tissues is included in the treated area. Almost one third of patients who undergo radiation therapy develop lung injury following radiation treatment. The severity of radiation-induced lung injury ranges from ground-glass opacities and consolidation at the early phase to fibrosis and traction bronchiectasis in the late phase. Early detection of lung injury will thus help to improve management of the treatment [69–109]. This work can also be applied to other brain abnormalities, such as dyslexia and autism. Dyslexia is one of the most complicated developmental brain disorders that affect children's learning abilities. Dyslexia leads to the failure to develop age-appropriate reading skills in spite of the normal intelligence level and adequate reading instructions. Neuropathological studies have revealed an abnormal anatomy of some structures, such as the corpus callosum in dyslexic brains. There has been a lot of work in the literature that aims at developing CAD systems for diagnosing such a disorder, along with other brain disorders [110–132].

References

[1] Wuerfel J 2013 Multiple sclerosis, blood flow, and CSF circulation *J. Cereb. Blood Flow Metab.* **33** 1313

[2] Gaitán M I *et al* 2013 Multiple sclerosis shrinks intralesional, and enlarges extralesional, brain parenchymal veins *Neurology* **80** 145–51

[3] Caprio M G, Russo C, Giugliano A, Ragucci M and Mancini M 2016 Vascular disease in patients with multiple sclerosis: a review *J. Vasc. Med. Surg.* **4** 259

[4] Xue D-X, Zhang R, Feng H and Wang Y-L 2016 Cnn-svm for microvascular morphological type recognition with data augmentation *J. Med. Biol. Eng.* **36** 755764

[5] Wang S, Yin Y, Cao G, Wei B, Zheng Y and Yang G 2015 Hierarchical retinal blood vessel segmentation based on feature and ensemble learning *Neurocomputing* **149** 708717

[6] Ganin Y and Lempitsky V S 2014 N4-fields: Neural network nearest neighbor fields for image transforms *ACCV*

[7] Smistad E and Lvstakken L 2016 Vessel detection in ultrasound images using deep convolutional neural networks *Deep Learning and Data Labeling for Medical Applications* (Berlin: Springer) p 3038

[8] Liskowski P and Krawiec K 2016 Segmenting retinal blood vessels with deep neural networks *IEEE Trans. Med. Imaging* **35** 23692380

[9] Maninis K-K, Pont-Tuset J, Arbelaez P and Gool L V 2016 Deep retinal image understanding *Int. Conf. on Medical Image Computing and Computer Assisted Intervention* (Berlin: Springer) p 140148

[10] Fu H, Xu Y, Lin S, Wong D W K and Liu J 2016 Deepvessel: Retinal vessel segmentation via deep learning and conditional random field *Int. Conf. on Medical Image Computing and computer Assisted Intervention* (Berlin: Springer) p 132139

[11] Kandil H, Soliman A, Taher F, Mahmoud A, Elmaghraby A and El-Baz A 2018 Using 3-D CNNs and local blood flow information to segment cerebral vasculature *IEEE Int. Symp. on Signal Processing and Information Technology (ISSPIT).*

[12] Kamnitsas K, Ledig C, Newcombe V F J, Simpson J P, Kane A D, Menon D K, Rueckert D and Glocker B 2017 Efficient multi-scale 3d cnn with fully connected crf for accurate brain lesion segmentation *Med. Image Anal.* **36** 6178

[13] El-Baz A, Elnakib A, Khalifa F, AbouEl-Ghar M, McClure P, Soliman A and Gimelrfarb G 2012 Precise segmentation of 3-d magnetic resonance angiography *IEEE Trans. Biomed. Eng.* **59** 20192029

[14] Kandil H, Soliman A, Fraiwan L, Shalaby A, Mahmoud A, ElTanboly A, Elmaghraby A, Giridharan G and El-Baz A 2018 A novel MRA framework based on integrated global and local analysis for accurate segmentation of the cerebral vascular system *2018 IEEE 15th Int. Symp. on Biomedical Imaging (ISBI 2018)* (Piscataway, NJ: IEEE) pp 1365–8

[15] Tustison N J, Avants B B, Cook P A, Zheng Y, Egan A, Yushkevich P A and Gee J C 2010 N4itk: improved n3 bias correction *IEEE Trans. Med. Imaging* **29** 1310–20

[16] Bouman C and Sauer K 1993 A generalized gaussian image model for edge-preserving map estimation *IEEE Trans. Image Process.* **2** 296–310
[17] Smith S M 2002 Fast robust automated brain extraction *Hum. Brain Mapp.* **17** 143–55
[18] El-Baz and Gimel'farb G 2007 Em based approximation of empirical distributions with linear combinations of discrete gaussians *IEEE Int. Conf. on. Image Processing, 2007 (ICIP 2007)* vol 4 (Piscataway, NJ: IEEE) pp 300–73
[19] El-Baz A, Farag A A, Gimel'farb G L, El-Ghar M A and Eldiasty T 2006 Probabilistic modeling of blood vessels for segmenting mra images *ICPR (3)* 917–20
[20] El-Baz A, Farag A A, Gimelfarb G, El-Ghar M A and Eldiasty T 2006 A new adaptive probabilistic model of blood vessels for segmenting mra images *Medical Image Computing and Computer-Assisted Intervention–MICCAI 2006* vol 4191 (Berlin: Springer) pp 799–806
[21] Shalaby A, Taher F, El-Baz M, Ghazal V, Abou El-Ghar M, Takieldeen A and El-Baz A 2017 Probabilistic modeling of blood vessels for segmenting magnetic resonance angiography images *Medical Research Archive-MRA KEI* 34–42
[22] Chowdhury A S, Rudra A K, Sen M, Elnakib A and El-Baz A 2010 Cerebral white matter segmentation from MRI using probabilistic graph cuts and geometric shape priors *ICIP* 3649–52
[23] Mahmoud A, El-Barkouky A, Farag H, Graham J and Farag A 2013 A non-invasive method for measuring blood flow rate in superficial veins from a single thermal image *Proc. of the IEEE Conf. on Computer Vision and Pattern Recognition Workshops* pp 354–9
[24] Ali A M, Farag A A and El-Baz A 2007 Graph cuts framework for kidney segmentation with prior shape constraints *Proc. of Int. Conf. on Medical Image Computing and Computer-Assisted Intervention, (MICCAI'07) (Brisbane, Australia, October 29–November 2)* **vol 1** pp 384–92
[25] Chowdhury A S, Roy R, Bose S, Elnakib F K A and El-Baz A 2012 Non-rigid biomedical image registration using graph cuts with a novel data term *Proc. of IEEE Int. Symp. on Biomedical Imaging: From Nano to Macro, (ISBI'12) (Barcelona, Spain, May 2–5)* pp 446–9
[26] El-Baz A, Farag A A, Yuksel S E, El-Ghar M E A, Eldiasty T A and Ghoneim M A 2007 Application of deformable models for the detection of acute renal rejection *Deformable Models* vol 1 ed A A Farag and J S Suri (New York, NY: Springer) pp 293–333
[27] El-Baz A, Farag A, Fahmi R, Yuksel S, El-Ghar M A and Eldiasty T 2006 Image analysis of renal DCE MRI for the detection of acute renal rejection *Proc. of IAPR Int. Conf. on Pattern Recognition (ICPR'06) (Hong Kong, August 20–24)* pp 822–25
[28] El-Baz A, Farag A, Fahmi R, Yuksel S, Miller W, El-Ghar M A, El-Diasty T and Ghoneim M 2006 A new CAD system for the evaluation of kidney diseases using DCE-MRI *Proc. of Int. Conf. on Medical Image Computing and Computer-Assisted Intervention, (MICCAI'08) (Copenhagen, Denmark, October 1–6)* pp 446–53
[29] El-Baz A, Gimel'farb G and El-Ghar M A 2008 A novel image analysis approach for accurate identification of acute renal rejection *Proc. of IEEE Int. Conf. on Image Processing, (ICIP'08) (San Diego, California, USA, October 12–15)* pp 1812–5
[30] El-Baz A, Gimel'farb G and El-Ghar M A 2008 Image analysis approach for identification of renal transplant rejection *Proc. of IAPR Int. Conf. on Pattern Recognition, (ICPR'08) (Tampa, Florida, USA, December 8–11)* pp 1–4
[31] El-Baz A, Gimel'farb G and El-Ghar M A 2007 New motion correction models for automatic identification of renal transplant rejection *Proc. of Int. Conf. on Medical Image

Computing and Computer-Assisted Intervention, (MICCAI'07) (Brisbane, Australia, October 29–November 2) pp 235–43

[32] Farag A, El-Baz A, Yuksel S, El-Ghar M A and Eldiasty T 2006 A framework for the detection of acute rejection with Dynamic Contrast Enhanced Magnetic Resonance Imaging *Proc. of IEEE Int. Symp. on Biomedical Imaging: From Nano to Macro, (ISBI'06) (Arlington, Virginia, USA, April 6–9)* pp 418–21

[33] Khalifa F, Beache G M, El-Ghar M A, El-Diasty T, Gimel'farb G, Kong M and El-Baz A 2013 Dynamic contrast-enhanced MRI-based early detection of acute renal transplant rejection *IEEE Trans. Med. Imaging* **32** 1910–27 Prostate Cancer Diagnosis using SNCAE 23

[34] Khalifa F, El-Baz A, Gimel'farb G and El-Ghar M A 2010 Non-invasive image-based approach for early detection of acute renal rejection *Proc. of Int. Conf. Medical Image Computing and Computer-Assisted Intervention, (MICCAI'10) (Beijing, China, September 20–24)* pp 10–8

[35] Khalifa F, El-Baz A, Gimel'farb G, Ouseph R and El-Ghar M A 2010 Shapeappearance guided level-set deformable model for image segmentation *Proc. of IAPR Int. Conf. on Pattern Recognition, (ICPR'10) (Istanbul, Turkey, August 23–26)* pp 4581–4

[36] Khalifa F, El-Ghar M A, Abdollahi B, Frieboes H, El-Diasty T and El-Baz A 2013 A comprehensive non-invasive framework for automated evaluation of acute renal transplant rejection using DCE-MRI *NMR Biomed.* **26** 1460–70

[37] Khalifa F, El-Ghar M A, Abdollahi B, Frieboes H B, El-Diasty T and El-Baz A 2014 Dynamic contrast-enhanced MRI-based early detection of acute renal transplant rejection *2014 Annual Scientific Meeting and Educational Course Brochure of the Society of Abdominal Radiology, (SAR'14) (Boca Raton, FL, March 23–28)* CID: 1855912

[38] Khalifa F, Elnakib A, Beache G M, Gimel'farb G, El-Ghar M A, Sokhadze G, Manning S, McClure P and El-Baz A 2011 3D kidney segmentation from CT images using a level set approach guided by a novel stochastic speed function *Proc. of Int. Conf. Medical Image Computing and Computer-Assisted Intervention, (MICCAI'11) (Toronto, Canada, September 18–22)* pp 587–94

[39] Khalifa F, Gimel'farb G, El-Ghar M A, Sokhadze G, Manning S, McClure P, Ouseph R and El-Baz A 2011 A new deformable model-based segmentation approach for accurate extraction of the kidney from abdominal CT images *Proc. of IEEE Int. Conf. on Image Processing, (ICIP'11) (Brussels, Belgium, September 11–14)* pp 3393–6

[40] Mostapha M, Khalifa F, Alansary A, Soliman A, Suri J and El-Baz A 2014 Computer-aided diagnosis systems for acute renal transplant rejection: Challenges and methodologies *Abdomen and Thoracic Imaging* ed A El-Baz, J Saba and L Suri (Berlin: Springer) pp 1–35

[41] Shehata M *et al* 2016 A new non-invasive approach for early classification of renal rejection types using diffusion-weighted mri *IEEE Int. Conf. on Image Processing (ICIP), 2016* (Piscataway, NJ: IEEE) pp 136–40

[42] Khalifa F *et al* 2016 Kidney segmentation from CT images using a 3D NMF-guided active contour model *IEEE 13th Int. Symp. on Biomedical Imaging (ISBI), 2016* (Piscataway, NJ: IEEE) pp 432–5

[43] Shehata M, Khalifa F, Soliman A, Takieldeen A, El-Ghar M A, Shaffie A, Dwyer A C, Ouseph R, El-Baz A and Keynton R 2016 3d diffusion mri-based cad system for early diagnosis of acute renal rejection *2016 IEEE 13th Int. Symp. On Biomedical Imaging (ISBI)* (Piscataway, NJ: IEEE) pp 1177–80

[44] Shehata M *et al* 2015 A level set-based framework for 3d kidney segmentation from diffusion mr images *IEEE Int. Conf. on Image Processing (ICIP), 2015* (Piscataway, NJ: IEEE) 4441–5

[45] Shehata M, Khalifa F, Soliman A, El-Ghar M A, Dwyer A C, Gimelfarb G, Keynton R and El-Baz A 2016 A promising non-invasive cad system for kidney function assessment *Int. Conf. on Medical Image Computing and Computer-Assisted Intervention* (Berlin: Springer) pp 613–21

[46] Khalifa F, Soliman A, Elmaghraby A, Gimelfarb G and El-Baz A 2017 3d kidney segmentation from abdominal images using spatial-appearance models *Comput. Math. Methods Med.* **2017** 1–10

[47] Hollis E, Shehata M, Khalifa F, El-Ghar M A, El-Diasty T and El-Baz A 2016 Towards non-invasive diagnostic techniques for early detection of acute renal transplant rejection: A review *Egypt. J. Radiol. Nucl. Med.* **48** 257–69

[48] Shehata M, Khalifa F, Soliman A, El-Ghar M A, Dwyer A C and El-Baz A 2017 Assessment of renal transplant using image and clinical-based biomarkers *Proc. of 13th Annual Scientific Meeting of American Society for Diagnostics and Interventional Nephrology (ASDIN'17)* (*New Orleans, LA, USA* February 10–12, 2017)

[49] Shehata M, Khalifa F, Soliman A, El-Ghar M A, Dwyer A C and El-Baz A 2017 Early assessment of acute renal rejection *Proc. of 12th Annual Scientific Meeting of American Society for Diagnostics and Interventional Nephrology (ASDIN'16)* (*Pheonix, AZ, USA* February 19–21, 2016)

[50] Khalifa F, Beache G, El-Baz A and Gimel'farb G 2010 Deformable model guided by stochastic speed with application in cine images segmentation *Proc. of IEEE Int. Conf. on Image Processing, (ICIP'10) (Hong Kong, September 26–29)* pp 1725–8

[51] Khalifa F, Beache G M, Elnakib A, Sliman H, Gimel'farb G, Welch K C and El-Baz A 2013 A new shape-based framework for the left ventricle wall segmentation from cardiac first-pass perfusion MRI *Proc. of IEEE Int. Symp. on Biomedical Imaging: From Nano to Macro, (ISBI'13) (San Francisco, CA, April 7–11)* pp 41–4

[52] Khalifa F, Beache G M, Elnakib A, Sliman H, Gimel'farb G, Welch K C and El-Baz A 2012 A new nonrigid registration framework for improved visualization of transmural perfusion gradients on cardiac first–pass perfusion MRI *Proc. of IEEE Int. Symp. on Biomedical Imaging: From Nano to Macro, (ISBI'12) (Barcelona, Spain, May 2–5)* pp 828–31

[53] Khalifa F, Beache G M, Firjani A, Welch K C, Gimel'farb G and El-Baz A 2012 A new nonrigid registration approach for motion correction of cardiac first-pass perfusion MRI *Proc. of IEEE Int. Conf. on Image Processing, (ICIP'12) (Lake Buena Vista, Florida, September 30–October 3)* pp 1665–8

[54] Khalifa F, Beache G M, Gimel'farb G and El-Baz A 2012 A novel CAD system for analyzing cardiac first-pass MR images *Proc. of IAPR Int. Conf. on Pattern Recognition (ICPR'12) (Tsukuba Science City, Japan, November 11–15)* pp 77–80

[55] Khalifa F, Beache G M, Gimel'farb G and El Baz A 2011 A novel approach for accurate estimation of left ventricle global indexes from short-axis cine MRI *Proc. of IEEE Int. Conf. on Image Processing, (ICIP'11) (Brussels, Belgium, September 11–14)* pp 2645–9

[56] Khalifa F, Beache G M, Gimel'farb G, Giridharan G A and El-Baz A 2011 A new image-based framework for analyzing cine images *Handbook of Multi Modality State-ofProstate Cancer Diagnosis using SNCAE 25 the-Art Medical Image Segmentation and Registration*

Methodologies vol 2 ed A El-Baz, U R Acharya, M Mirmedhdi and J S Suri (New York: Springer) pp 69–98

[57] Khalifa F, Beache G M, Gimel'farb G, Giridharan G A and El-Baz A 2012 Accurate automatic analysis of cardiac cine images *IEEE Trans. Biomed. Eng.* **59** 445–55

[58] Khalifa F, Beache G M, Nitzken M, Gimel'farb G, Giridharan G A and El-Baz A 2011 Automatic analysis of left ventricle wall thickness using short-axis cine CMR images *Proc. of IEEE Int. Symp. on Biomedical Imaging: From Nano to Macro, (ISBI'11) (Chicago, Illinois, March 30–April 2)* pp 1306–9

[59] Nitzken M *et al* 2012 Accurate modeling of tagged cmr 3D image appearance characteristics to improve cardiac cycle strain estimation *2012 19th IEEE Int. Conf. on Image Processing (ICIP) (Orlando, FL, September 2012) (Piscataway, NJ: IEEE)* pp 521–4

[60] Nitzken M, Beache G, Elnakib A, Khalifa F, Gimel'farb G and El-Baz A 2012 Improving full-cardiac cycle strain estimation from tagged cmr by accurate modeling of 3D image appearance characteristics *2012 9th IEEE Int. Symp. on Biomedical Imaging (ISBI), (Barcelona, Spain)* (Piscataway, NJ: IEEE) pp 462–5 (Selected for oral presentation)

[61] Nitzken M J, El-Baz A S and Beache G M 2012 Markov-gibbs random field model for improved full-cardiac cycle strain estimation from tagged cmr *J. Cardiovasc. Magn. Reson.* **14** 1–2

[62] Sliman H, Elnakib A, Beache G, Elmaghraby A and El-Baz A 2014 Assessment of myocardial function from cine cardiac MRI using a novel 4D tracking approach *J. Comput. Sci. Syst. Biol.* **7** 169–73

[63] Sliman H, Elnakib A, Beache G M, Soliman A, Khalifa F, Gimel'farb G, Elmaghraby A and El-Baz A 2014 A novel 4D PDE-based approach for accurate assessment of myocardium function using cine cardiac magnetic resonance images *Proc. of IEEE Int. Conf. on Image Processing (ICIP'14) (Paris, France, October 27–30)* pp 3537–41

[64] Sliman H, Khalifa F, Elnakib A, Beache G M, Elmaghraby A and El-Baz A 2013 A new segmentation-based tracking framework for extracting the left ventricle cavity from cine cardiac MRI *Proc. of IEEE Int. Conf. on Image Processing, (ICIP'13) (Melbourne, Australia, September 15–18)* pp 685–9

[65] Sliman H, Khalifa F, Elnakib A, Soliman A, Beache G M, Elmaghraby A, Gimel'farb G and El-Baz A 2013 Myocardial borders segmentation from cine MR images using bi-directional coupled parametric deformable models *Med. Phys.* **40** 1–13

[66] Sliman H, Khalifa F, Elnakib A, Soliman A, Beache G M, Gimel'farb G, Emam A, Elmaghraby A and El-Baz A 2013 Accurate segmentation framework for the left ventricle wall from cardiac cine MRI *Proc. of Int. Symp. on Computational Models for Life Science, (CMLS'13) (Sydney, Australia, November 27–29)* **vol 1559,** pp 287–96

[67] Eladawi N, Elmogy M M, Ghazal M, Helmy O, Aboelfetouh A, Riad A, Schaal S and El-Baz A 2018 Classification of retinal diseases based on OCT Images *Front. Biosci.* **23** 247–64

[68] ElTanboly A, Ismail M, Shalaby A, Switala A, El-Baz A, Schaal S, Gimel'farb G and El-Azab M 2017 A computer-aided diagnostic system for detecting diabetic retinopathy in optical coherence tomography images *Med. Phys.* **44** 914–23

[69] Abdollahi B, Civelek A C, Li X F, Suri J and El-Baz A 2014 PET/CT nodule segmentation and diagnosis: A survey *Multi Detector CT Imaging* ed L Saba and J S Suri (London: Taylor and Francis) pp 639–51

[70] Abdollahi B, El-Baz A and Amini A A 2011 A multi-scale non-linear vessel enhancement technique *Annual Int. Conf. of the IEEE Engineering in Medicine and Biology Society, EMBC, 2011* (Piscataway, NJ: IEEE) pp 3925–9
[71] Abdollahi B, Soliman A, Civelek A, Li X F, Gimel'farb G and El-Baz A 2012 A novel gaussian scale space-based joint MGRF framework for precise lung segmentation *Proc. of IEEE Int. Conf. on Image Processing, (ICIP'12)* (Piscataway, NJ: IEEE) pp 2029–32
[72] Abdollahi B, Soliman A, Civelek A, Li X F, Gimelfarb G and El-Baz A 2012 A novel 3D joint MGRF framework for precise lung segmentation *Machine Learning in Medical Imaging* (Berlin: Springer) pp 86–93
[73] Ali A M, El-Baz A S and Farag A A 2007 A novel framework for accurate lung segmentation using graph cuts *Proc. of IEEE Int. Symp. on Biomedical Imaging: From Nano to Macro, (ISBI'07)* (Piscataway, NJ: IEEE) pp 908–11
[74] El-Baz A, Beache G M, Gimel'farb G, Suzuki K and Okada K 2013 Lung imaging data analysis *Int. J. Biomed. Imaging* **2013** 1–2
[75] El-Baz A, Beache G M, Gimel'farb G, Suzuki K, Okada K, Elnakib A, Soliman A and Abdollahi B 2013 Computer-aided diagnosis systems for lung cancer: Challenges and methodologies *Int. J. Biomed. Imaging* **2013** 1–46
[76] El-Baz A, Elnakib A, Abou El-Ghar M, Gimel'farb G, Falk R and Farag A 2013 Automatic detection of 2D and 3D lung nodules in chest spiral CT scans *Int. J. Biomed. Imaging* **2013** 1–11
[77] El-Baz A, Farag A A, Falk R and La Rocca R 2003 A unified approach for detection, visualization, and identification of lung abnormalities in chest spiral CT scans *Int. Congress Ser.* **1256** 998–1004
[78] El-Baz A, Farag A A, Falk R and La Rocca R 2002 Detection, visualization and identification of lung abnormalities in chest spiral CT scan: Phase-I *Proc. of Int. conf. on Biomedical Engineering (Cairo, Egypt,* ***vol 12***
[79] El-Baz A, Farag A, Gimel'farb G, Falk R, El-Ghar M A and Eldiasty T 2006 A framework for automatic segmentation of lung nodules from low dose chest CT scans *Proc. of Int. Conf. on Pattern Recognition, (ICPR'06)* vol 3 (Piscataway, NJ: IEEE) pp 611–4
[80] El-Baz A, Farag A, Gimelfarb G, Falk R and El-Ghar M A 2011 A novel level setbased computer-aided detection system for automatic detection of lung nodules in low dose chest computed tomography scans *Lung Imaging and Computer Aided Diagnosis* **10** 221–38
[81] El-Baz A, Gimel'farb G, Abou El-Ghar M and Falk R 2012 Appearance-based diagnostic system for early assessment of malignant lung nodules *Proc. of IEEE Int. Conf. on Image Processing, (ICIP'12)* (Piscataway, NJ: IEEE) pp 533–6
[82] El-Baz A, Gimel'farb G and Falk R 2011 A novel 3D framework for automatic lung segmentation from low dose CT images *Lung Imaging and Computer Aided Diagnosis* ed A El-Baz and J S Suri (London: Taylor and Francis) pp 1–16
[83] El-Baz A, Gimel'farb G, Falk R and El-Ghar M 2010 Appearance analysis for diagnosing malignant lung nodules *Proc. of IEEE Int. Symp. on Biomedical Imaging: From Nano to Macro (ISBI'10)* (Piscataway, NJ: IEEE) pp 193–6 Prostate Cancer Diagnosis using SNCAE 27
[84] El-Baz A, Gimel'farb G, Falk R and El-Ghar M A 2011 A novel level set-based CAD system for automatic detection of lung nodules in low dose chest CT scans *Lung Imaging and Computer Aided Diagnosis* vol 1 ed A El-Baz and J S Suri (London: Taylor and Francis) pp 221–38

[85] El-Baz A, Gimel'farb G, Falk R and El-Ghar M A 2008 A new approach for automatic analysis of 3D low dose CT images for accurate monitoring the detected lung nodules *Proc. of Int. Conf. on Pattern Recognition, (ICPR'08)* (Piscataway, NJ: IEEE) pp 1–4

[86] El-Baz A, Gimel'farb G, Falk R and El-Ghar M A 2007 A novel approach for automatic follow-up of detected lung nodules *Proc. of IEEE Int. Conf. on Image Processing, (ICIP'07)* vol 5 (Piscataway, NJ: IEEE) p V-501

[87] El-Baz A, Gimel'farb G, Falk R and El-Ghar M A 2007 A new CAD system for early diagnosis of detected lung nodules *IEEE Int. Conf. on Image Processing, 2007. ICIP 2007* vol 2 (Piscataway, NJ: IEEE) p II-461

[88] El-Baz A, Gimel'farb G, Falk R, El-Ghar M A and Refaie H 2008 Promising results for early diagnosis of lung cancer *Proc. of IEEE Int. Symp. on Biomedical Imaging: From Nano to Macro, (ISBI'08)* (Piscataway, NJ: IEEE) pp 1151–4

[89] El-Baz A, Gimel'farb G L, Falk R, Abou El-Ghar M, Holland T and Shaffer T 2008 A new stochastic framework for accurate lung segmentation *Proc. of Medical Image Computing and Computer-Assisted Intervention, (MICCAI'08)* pp 322–30

[90] El-Baz A, Gimel'farb G L, Falk R, Heredis D and Abou El-Ghar M 2008 A novel approach for accurate estimation of the growth rate of the detected lung nodules *Proc. of Int. Workshop on Pulmonary Image Analysis* pp 33–42

[91] El-Baz A, Gimel'farb G L, Falk R, Holland T and Shaffer T 2008 A framework for unsupervised segmentation of lung tissues from low dose computed tomography images *Proc. of British Machine Vision, (BMVC'08)* pp 1–10

[92] El-Baz A, Gimelfarb G, Falk R and El-Ghar M A 2011 3D MGRF-based appearance modeling for robust segmentation of pulmonary nodules in 3D LDCT chest images *Lung Imaging and Computer Aided Diagnosis* 51–63

[93] El-Baz A, Gimelfarb G, Falk R and El-Ghar M A 2009 Automatic analysis of 3D low dose CT images for early diagnosis of lung cancer *Pattern Recognit.* **42** 1041–51

[94] El-Baz A, Gimelfarb G, Falk R, El-Ghar M A, Rainey S, Heredia D and Shaffer T 2009 Toward early diagnosis of lung cancer *Proc. of Medical Image Computing and Computer-Assisted Intervention, (MICCAI'09)* (Berlin: Springer) pp 682–9

[95] El-Baz A, Gimelfarb G, Falk R, El-Ghar M A and Suri J 2011 Appearance analysis for the early assessment of detected lung nodules *Lung Imaging and Computer Aided Diagnosis* 395–404

[96] El-Baz A, Khalifa F, Elnakib A, Nitkzen M, Soliman A, McClure P, Gimel'farb G and El-Ghar M A 2012 A novel approach for global lung registration using 3D Markov Gibbs appearance model *Proc. of Int. Conf. Medical Image Computing and Computer-Assisted Intervention, (MICCAI' 12) (Nice, France, October 1–5)* pp 114–21

[97] El-Baz A, Nitzken M, Elnakib A, Khalifa F, Gimel'farb G, Falk R and El-Ghar M A 2011 3D shape analysis for early diagnosis of malignant lung nodules *Proc. of Int. Conf. Medical Image Computing and 28 Authors Suppressed Due to Excessive Length Computer-Assisted Intervention, (MICCAI'11) (Toronto, Canada, September 18–22)* pp 175–82

[98] El-Baz A, Nitzken M, Gimelfarb G, Van Bogaert E, Falk R, El-Ghar M A and Suri J 2011 Three-dimensional shape analysis using spherical harmonics for early assessment of detected lung nodules *Lung Imaging and Computer Aided Diagnosis* 421–38

[99] El-Baz A, Nitzken M, Khalifa F, Elnakib A, Gimel'farb G, Falk R and El-Ghar M A 2011 3D shape analysis for early diagnosis of malignant lung nodules *Proc. of Int. Conf. on*

Information Processing in Medical Imaging, (IPMI'11) (Monastery Irsee, Germany (Bavaria), July 3–8) pp 772–83
[100] El-Baz A, Nitzken M, Vanbogaert E, Gimel'Farb G, Falk R and Abo El-Ghar M 2011 A novel shape-based diagnostic approach for early diagnosis of lung nodules *2011 IEEE Int. Symp. on Biomedical Imaging: From Nano to Macro* (Piscataway, NJ: IEEE) pp 137–40
[101] El-Baz A, Sethu P, Gimel'farb G, Khalifa F, Elnakib A, Falk R and El-Ghar M A 2011 Elastic phantoms generated by microfluidics technology: Validation of an imaged-based approach for accurate measurement of the growth rate of lung nodules *Biotechnol. J.* **6** 195–203
[102] El-Baz A, Sethu P, Gimel'farb G, Khalifa F, Elnakib A, Falk R and El-Ghar M A 2010 A new validation approach for the growth rate measurement using elastic phantoms generated by state-of-the-art microfluidics technology *Proc. of IEEE Int. Conf. on Image Processing, (ICIP'10) (Hong Kong, September 26–29)* pp 4381–3
[103] El-Baz A, Sethu P, Gimel'farb G, Khalifa F, Elnakib A, Falk R and Suri M A E G J 2011 Validation of a new imaged-based approach for the accurate estimating of the growth rate of detected lung nodules using real CT images and elastic phantoms generated by state-of-the-art microfluidics technology *Handbook of Lung Imaging and Computer Aided Diagnosis* ed A El-Baz and J S Suri vol 1 (New York: Taylor & Francis) pp 405–20
[104] El-Baz A, Soliman A, McClure P, Gimel'farb G, El-Ghar M A and Falk R 2012 Early assessment of malignant lung nodules based on the spatial analysis of detected lung nodules *Proc. of IEEE Int. Symp. on Biomedical Imaging: From Nano to Macro, (ISBI'12)* (Piscataway, NJ: IEEE) pp 1463–6
[105] El-Baz A, Yuksel S E, Elshazly S and Farag A A 2005 Non-rigid registration techniques for automatic follow-up of lung nodules *Proc. of Computer Assisted Radiology and Surgery, (CARS'05)* vol 1281 (Amsterdam: Elsevier) pp 1115–20
[106] El-Baz A S and Suri J S 2011 *Lung Imaging and Computer Aided Diagnosis* (Boca Raton, FL: CRC Press)
[107] Soliman A, Khalifa F, Shaffie A, Liu N, Dunlap N, Wang B, Elmaghraby A, Gimelfarb G and El-Baz A 2016 Image-based cad system for accurate identification of lung injury *Proc. of IEEE Int. Conf. on Image Processing, (ICIP'16)* (Piscataway, NJ: IEEE) pp 121–5
[108] Soliman A, Khalifa F, Dunlap N, Wang B, El-Ghar M and El-Baz A 2016 An isosurfaces based local deformation handling framework of lung tissues *2016 IEEE 13th Int. Symp. on Biomedical Imaging (ISBI)* (Piscataway, NJ: IEEE) pp 1253–9
[109] Soliman A, Khalifa F, Shaffie A, Dunlap N, Wang B, Elmaghraby A and El-Baz A 2016 Detection of lung injury using 4d-ct chest images *2016 IEEE 13th International Symposium on Biomedical Imaging (ISBI)* (Piscataway, NJ: IEEE) pp 1274–7 Prostate Cancer Diagnosis using SNCAE 29
[110] Dombroski B, Nitzken M, Elnakib A, Khalifa F, El-Baz A and Casanova M F 2014 Cortical surface complexity in a population-based normative sample *Transl. Neurosci.* **5** 17–24
[111] El-Baz A, Casanova M, Gimel'farb G, Mott M and Switala A 2008 An MRI-based diagnostic framework for early diagnosis of dyslexia *Int. J. Comput. Assist. Radiol. Surg.* **3** 181–9
[112] El-Baz A *et al* 2008 A new CAD system for early diagnosis of dyslexic brains *Proc. Int. Conf. on Image Processing (ICIP'2008)* (Piscataway, NJ: IEEE) pp 1820–3

[113] El-Baz A, Casanova M F, Gimel'farb G, Mott M and Switwala A E 2007 A new image analysis approach for automatic classification of autistic brains *Proc. IEEE Int. Symp. on Biomedical Imaging: From Nano to Macro (ISBI'2007)* (Piscataway, NJ: IEEE) pp 352–5

[114] El-Baz A, Elnakib A, Khalifa F, El-Ghar M A, McClure P, Soliman A and Gimel'farb G 2012 Precise segmentation of 3-D magnetic resonance angiography *IEEE Trans. Biomed. Eng.* **59** 2019–29

[115] El-Baz A, Farag A A, Gimel'farb G L, El-Ghar M A and Eldiasty T 2006 Probabilistic modeling of blood vessels for segmenting MRA images *Int. Conf. on Pattern Recognition (ICPR) (3)* 917–20

[116] El-Baz A, Farag A A, Gimelfarb G, El-Ghar M A and Eldiasty T 2006 A new adaptive probabilistic model of blood vessels for segmenting mra images *Medical Image Computing and Computer-Assisted Intervention–MICCAI 2006* vol 4191 (Berlin: Springer) pp 799–806

[117] El-Baz A, Farag A A, Gimelfarb G and Hushek S G 2005 Automatic cerebrovascular segmentation by accurate probabilistic modeling of tof-mra images *Medical Image Computing and Computer-Assisted Intervention–MICCAI 2005* (Berlin: Springer) pp 34–42

[118] El-Baz A, Farag A, Elnakib A, Casanova M F, Gimel'farb G, Switala A E, Jordan D and Rainey S 2011 Accurate automated detection of autism related corpus callosum abnormalities *J. Med. Syst.* **35** 929–39

[119] El-Baz A, Farag A and Gimelfarb G 2005 Cerebrovascular segmentation by accurate probabilistic modeling of tof-mra images *Image Analysis* vol 3540 (Berlin: Springer) pp 1128–37

[120] El-Baz A, Gimelfarb G, Falk R, El-Ghar M A, Kumar V and Heredia D 2009 A novel 3D joint Markov-gibbs model for extracting blood vessels from PC–mra images *Medical Image Computing and Computer-Assisted Intervention–MICCAI 2009* vol 5762 (Berlin: Springer) pp 943–50

[121] Elnakib A, El-Baz A, Casanova M F, Gimel'farb G and Switala A E 2010 Imagebased detection of corpus callosum variability for more accurate discrimination between dyslexic and normal brains *Proc. IEEE Int. Symp. on Biomedical Imaging: From Nano to Macro (ISBI'2010)* (Piscataway, NJ: IEEE) pp 109–12

[122] Elnakib A, Casanova M F, Gimel'farb G, Switala A E and El-Baz A 2011 Autism diagnostics by centerline-based shape analysis of the corpus callosum *Proc. IEEE Int. Symp. on Biomedical Imaging: From Nano to Macro (ISBI'2011)* (Piscataway, NJ: IEEE) pp 1843–6

[123] Elnakib A, Nitzken M, Casanova M, Park H, Gimel'farb G and El-Baz A 2012 Quantification of age-related brain cortex change using 3D shape analysis *2012 21st Int. Conf. on, IEEE Pattern Recognition (ICPR)* pp 41–4

[124] Mostapha M *et al* 2014 A statistical framework for the classification of infant DT images *2014 IEEE Int. Conf. on Image Processing (ICIP)* (Piscataway, NJ: IEEE) pp 2222–6

[125] Nitzken M *et al* 2011 3D shape analysis of the brain cortex with application to dyslexia *2011 18th IEEE Int. Conf. on Image Processing (ICIP) (Brussels, Belgium)* (Piscataway, NJ: IEEE) pp 2657–60 (Selected for oral presentation. Oral acceptance rate is 10 percent and the overall acceptance rate is 35 percent)

[126] El-Gamal F E, Elmogy M M, Ghazal M, Atwan A, Barnes G N, Casanova M F, Keynton R and El-Baz A S 2017 A novel CAD system for local and global early diagnosis of Alzheimer's disease based on PIB-PET scans *2017 IEEE Int. Conf. on Image Processing (ICIP)* pp 3270–74

[127] Ismail M, Soliman A, Ghazal M, Switala A E, Gimel'farb G, Barnes G N, Khalil A and El-Baz A 2017 A fast stochastic framework for automatic MR brain images segmentation *PLoS One* **12** e0187391

[128] Ismail M M, Keynton R S, Mostapha M M, ElTanboly A H, Casanova M F, Gimel'farb G L and El-Baz A 2016 Studying autism spectrum disorder with structural and diffusion magnetic resonance imaging: a survey *Front. Hum. Neurosci.* **10** 211

[129] Alansary A, Ismail M, Soliman A, Khalifa F, Nitzken M, Elnakib A, Mostapha M, Black A, Stinebruner K and Casanova M F *et al* 2016 Infant brain extraction in t1-weighted mr images using bet and refinement using lcdg and mgrf models *IEEE J. Biomed. Health Inform.* **20** 925–35

[130] Ismail M *et al* 2017 A new deep-learning approach for early detection of shape variations in autism using structural mri *2017 IEEE International Conference on Image Processing (ICIP)* (Piscataway, NJ: IEEE) pp 1057–61

[131] Ismail M, Soliman A, ElTanboly A, Switala A, Mahmoud M, Khalifa F, Gimel'farb G, Casanova M F, Keynton R and El-Baz A 2016 Detection of white matter abnormalities in MR brain images for diagnosis of autism in children *2016 IEEE 13th Int. Symp. on Biomedical Imaging (ISBI)* (Piscataway, NJ: IEEE) pp 6–9

[132] Ismail M, Mostapha M, Soliman A, Nitzken M, Khalifa F, Elnakib A, Gimel'farb G, Casanova M F and El-Baz A 2015 Segmentation of infant brain MR images based on adaptive shape prior and higher-order MGRF *2015 IEEE Int. Conf. on Image Processing (ICIP)* (Piscataway, NJ: IEEE) pp 4327–31

Lightning Source UK Ltd.
Milton Keynes UK
UKHW051327190220
358970UK00003B/99

9 780750 317603